Sport, Physical Activity and Public Health

Edited by
Louise Mansfield and Joe Piggin

Routledge
Taylor & Francis Group
LONDON AND NEW YORK

First published 2018
by Routledge
2 Park Square, Milton Park, Abingdon, Oxon, OX14 4RN, UK

and by Routledge
711 Third Avenue, New York, NY 10017, USA

Routledge is an imprint of the Taylor & Francis Group, an informa business

British Library Cataloguing in Publication Data
A catalogue record for this book is available from the British Library

ISBN 13: 978-1-138-08368-4

Typeset in Myriad Pro
by RefineCatch Limited, Bungay, Suffolk

Publisher's Note
The publisher accepts responsibility for any inconsistencies that may have arisen during the conversion of this book from journal articles to book chapters, namely the possible inclusion of journal terminology.

Contents

Citation Information vii
Notes on Contributors xi

Introduction: Sport, physical activity and public health 1
Louise Mansfield and Joe Piggin

1. Bodies of knowledge: connecting the evidence bases on physical activity and health inequalities 7
Tess Kay

2. Should we privilege sport for health? The comparative effectiveness of UK Government investment in sport as a public health intervention 27
Mike Weed

3. The State and management of partnership arrangements in France: an analysis of the implementation of the 'Sport, Health and Well-being' plan 45
Marina Honta

4. A political spectator sport or policy priority? A review of sport, physical activity and public mental health policy 61
Andy Smith, Jon Jones, Laura Houghton and Tom Duffell

5. Olympic sport and physical activity promotion: the rise and fall of the London 2012 pre-event mass participation 'legacy' 77
Paul Bretherton, Joe Piggin and Guillaume Bodet

6. Group fitness instructors as local level health promoters: a Foucauldian analysis of the politics of health/fitness dynamic 93
Pirkko Markula and Jocelyn Chikinda

7. Health, physical activity and the body: an inquiry into the lives of female migrant cleaners in Denmark 115
Verena Lenneis and Gertrud Pfister

8. Are they 'worth their weight in gold'? Sport for older adults: benefits and barriers of their participation for sporting organisations 131
Claire R. Jenkin, Rochelle M. Eime, Hans Westerbeek, Grant O'Sullivan and Jannique G. Z. van Uffelen

9. What difference does dance make? Critical conversations across dance, physical activity and public health 149
Beccy Watson, Brett Lashua and Pip Trevorrow

10. Examining the integration of sport and health promotion: partnership or paradox? 163
Laura Misener and Katie E. Misener

11. Resourcefulness, reciprocity and reflexivity: the three Rs of partnership in sport for public health research 181
Louise Mansfield

Research Notes

12. Exercise on referral: evidence and complexity at the nexus of public health and sport policy 199
E. J. Oliver, C. L. Hanson, I. A. Lindsey and C. J. Dodd-Reynolds

13. The world turned upside down: sport, policy and ageing 205
Michael Gard and Rylee A. Dionigi

14. The sociopolitics of sport, physical education, and school health in the United States 213
James D. Ressler, K. Andrew R. Richards and Paul M. Wright

Index 217

Citation Information

The chapters in this book were originally published in the *International Journal of Sport Policy and Politics*, volume 8, issue 4 (November 2016). When citing this material, please use the original page numbering for each article, as follows:

Editorial

Sport, physical activity and public health
Louise Mansfield and Joe Piggin
International Journal of Sport Policy and Politics, volume 8, issue 4 (November 2016), pp. 533–537

Chapter 1

Bodies of knowledge: connecting the evidence bases on physical activity and health inequalities
Tess Kay
International Journal of Sport Policy and Politics, volume 8, issue 4 (November 2016), pp. 539–557

Chapter 2

Should we privilege sport for health? The comparative effectiveness of UK Government investment in sport as a public health intervention
Mike Weed
International Journal of Sport Policy and Politics, volume 8, issue 4 (November 2016), pp. 559–576

Chapter 3

The State and management of partnership arrangements in France: an analysis of the implementation of the 'Sport, Health and Well-being' plan
Marina Honta
International Journal of Sport Policy and Politics, volume 8, issue 4 (November 2016), pp. 577–591

Chapter 4

A political spectator sport or policy priority? A review of sport, physical activity and public mental health policy
Andy Smith, Jon Jones, Laura Houghton and Tom Duffell
International Journal of Sport Policy and Politics, volume 8, issue 4 (November 2016), pp. 593–607

Chapter 5

Olympic sport and physical activity promotion: the rise and fall of the London 2012 pre-event mass participation 'legacy'
Paul Bretherton, Joe Piggin and Guillaume Bodet
International Journal of Sport Policy and Politics, volume 8, issue 4 (November 2016), pp. 609–624

Chapter 6

Group fitness instructors as local level health promoters: a Foucauldian analysis of the politics of health/fitness dynamic
Pirkko Markula and Jocelyn Chikinda
International Journal of Sport Policy and Politics, volume 8, issue 4 (November 2016), pp. 625–646

Chapter 7

Health, physical activity and the body: an inquiry into the lives of female migrant cleaners in Denmark
Verena Lenneis and Gertrud Pfister
International Journal of Sport Policy and Politics, volume 8, issue 4 (November 2016), pp. 647–662

Chapter 8

Are they 'worth their weight in gold'? Sport for older adults: benefits and barriers of their participation for sporting organisations
Claire R. Jenkin, Rochelle M. Eime, Hans Westerbeek, Grant O'Sullivan and Jannique G. Z. van Uffelen
International Journal of Sport Policy and Politics, volume 8, issue 4 (November 2016), pp. 663–680

Chapter 9

What difference does dance make? Critical conversations across dance, physical activity and public health
Beccy Watson, Brett Lashua and Pip Trevorrow
International Journal of Sport Policy and Politics, volume 8, issue 4 (November 2016), pp. 681–693

Chapter 10

Examining the integration of sport and health promotion: partnership or paradox?
Laura Misener and Katie E. Misener
International Journal of Sport Policy and Politics, volume 8, issue 4 (November 2016), pp. 695–712

Chapter 11

Resourcefulness, reciprocity and reflexivity: the three Rs of partnership in sport for public health research
Louise Mansfield
International Journal of Sport Policy and Politics, volume 8, issue 4 (November 2016), pp. 713–729

Chapter 12

Exercise on referral: evidence and complexity at the nexus of public health and sport policy
E. J. Oliver, C. L. Hanson, I. A. Lindsey and C. J. Dodd-Reynolds
International Journal of Sport Policy and Politics, volume 8, issue 4 (November 2016), pp. 731–736

Chapter 13

The world turned upside down: sport, policy and ageing
Michael Gard and Rylee A. Dionigi
International Journal of Sport Policy and Politics, volume 8, issue 4 (November 2016), pp. 737–743

Chapter 14

The sociopolitics of sport, physical education, and school health in the United States
James D. Ressler, K. Andrew R. Richards and Paul M. Wright
International Journal of Sport Policy and Politics, volume 8, issue 4 (November 2016), pp. 745–748

Notes on Contributors

Guillaume Bodet is Senior Lecturer at the School of Sport, Exercise and Health Sciences, Loughborough University, UK.

Paul Bretherton is Senior Lecturer in Sport Management and Policy at the School of Sport, Exercise and Health Sciences, Loughborough University, UK.

Jocelyn Chikinda is Professor at the Faculty of Physical Education and Recreation, University of Alberta, Canada.

Rylee A. Dionigi is Associate Professor at the School of Exercise Science, Sport and Health, Charles Sturt University, Australia.

C. J. Dodd-Reynolds is Lecturer in Sport at the School of Applied Social Sciences, Durham University, UK.

Tom Duffell is based at the Department of Sport and Physical Activity, Edge Hill University, UK.

Rochelle M. Eime is Associate Professor at the Institute of Sport, Exercise and Active Living (ISEAL), Victoria University, Australia.

Michael Gard is based at the School of Human Movement and Nutrition Sciences, The University of Queensland, Australia.

C. L. Hanson is based at the School of Applied Social Sciences, Durham University, UK.

Marina Honta is a Professor at Centre Emile Durkheim (UMR CNRS 5116), University of Bordeaux, France.

Laura Houghton is based at the Department of Sport and Physical Activity, Edge Hill University, UK.

Claire R. Jenkin is based at the Institute of Sport, Exercise and Active Living (ISEAL), Victoria University, Australia.

Jon Jones is based at the Department of Sport and Physical Activity, Edge Hill University, UK.

Tess Kay is Professor in Sport and Social Sciences at the Division of Sport, Health and Exercise Sciences, Brunel University London, UK.

Brett Lashua is Senior Lecturer at the Carnegie School of Sport, Leeds Beckett University, UK.

Verena Lenneis is a Research Assistant at the Copenhagen Centre for Team Sport and Health, Department of Nutrition, Exercise and Sports, University of Copenhagen, Denmark.

I. A. Lindsey is Lecturer in Sport at the School of Applied Social Sciences, Durham University, UK.

Louise Mansfield, PhD, is Senior Lecturer in Sport, Health and Social Sciences at Brunel University London, UK.

Pirkko Markula is Professor at the Faculty of Physical Education and Recreation, University of Alberta, Canada.

Katie E. Misener is Assistant Professor at the University of Waterloo, Canada.

Laura Misener is Associate Professor at the School of Kinesiology, Western University, Canada.

E. J. Oliver is Senior Lecturer and Programme Director in the School of Applied Social Sciences, Durham University, UK.

Grant O'Sullivan is based at the Institute of Sport, Exercise and Active Living (ISEAL), Victoria University, Australia.

Gertrud Pfister is based at the Copenhagen Centre for Team Sport and Health, Department of Nutrition, Exercise and Sports, University of Copenhagen, Denmark.

Joe Piggin, PhD, is a Senior Lecturer at Loughborough University's School of Sport, Exercise and Health Sciences in the UK.

James D. Ressler is Associate Professor at the Department of Kinesiology and Physical Education, Northern Illinois University, USA.

K. Andrew R. Richards is a Faculty Member at the Department of Kinesiology, University of Alabama, USA.

Andy Smith is Associate Head of Sport Studies and Sport Development, Edge Hill University, UK.

Pip Trevorrow is a Research Fellow at the Carnegie School of Sport, Leeds Beckett University, UK.

Jannique G. Z. van Uffelen is a Senior Research Fellow in Active Aging at the Institute of Sport, Exercise and Active Living (ISEAL), Victoria University, Australia.

Beccy Watson is a Reader at the Carnegie School of Sport, Leeds Beckett University, UK.

Mike Weed is Professor of Applied Policy Sciences and Head of the School of Human and Life Sciences at Canterbury Christ Church University, UK.

Hans Westerbeek is Dean of the College of Sport and Exercise Science at the Institute of Sport, Exercise and Active Living (ISEAL), Victoria University, Australia.

Paul M. Wright is EC Lane and MN Zimmerman Endowed Professor at the Department of Kinesiology and Physical Education, Northern Illinois University, USA.

INTRODUCTION

Sport, physical activity and public health

The aim of this special issue is to encourage critical discussions about the political issues connected to the contemporary role of sport and physical activity in public health. There is evidence of a late twentieth-century resurgence in the importance of physical activity in public health policy. For example, increasingly explicit recommendations on physical activity levels in global health strategies and national physical activity policies and continued and updated position statements from specialist medicine and exercise working groups are available. In addition, local promotion, delivery, governance and monitoring of individual and community-based sport and physical activity programmes are intensifying. While there is an established corpus of policy-orientated research articles on public health and lifestyle factors including physical activity, sport is remarkably absent from the public health research agenda. This omission is evident despite the sport sector currently being a priority area for increasing population rates of physical activity. Very little is known about the contribution of sport to physical activity and health. Whilst there has been extensive and recent investment in policy and practice aspects of physical activity, both in the UK and worldwide, population-level responses have had limited success in arresting the upward trend in inactivity and reducing inequalities in activity levels. The requirements for successful individual, community and national promotion of sport and physical activity programmes are not well understood and there is scope to bring critical work to the fore on the impact and consequences (both intended and unintended) of such programmes for diverse groups of people. The relationships between sport, physical activity and health are not neutral but reflect complex temporal and spatial struggles over political positions, social ideologies, policymaking and policy enactment. It is, thus, timely and significant for this special issue to raise questions and present critical analyses about the politics and policy of the sport/physical activity/health dynamic.

Public health is an established and powerful policymaking sector in the UK and worldwide. Public health policymaking involves several approaches connected to research and evidence-building, commissioning and managing, service delivery and public participation in programmes intended to prevent disease, promote health and prolong life at a population level (WHO 2007). This is of course a complicated policy arena. Public health involves various methods of monitoring and evaluation, a range of interventions and many health professionals working with diverse people in varying contexts (Douglas *et al.* 2007). There is a growing awareness and intensifying morality surrounding the potential public health threats posed by a lack of physical activity as well as the benefits of sustained engagement in physical activity. Much of this narrative is driven by medical and behavioural science. However, some critical research has identified the complex relationships between sport, physical activity and health (Waddington 2000). Other research has addressed the policy dimensions of physical activity, commercialisation and marketing (Piggin 2014, Piggin and Bairner 2014). Some work has explored the complex political arena of sports medicine and health (Malcolm and Scott 2011) and another focus has been on critical understandings of the structures, processes, experiences and health consequences of fitness-based physical activity (Markula 1995, Maguire 2008, Mansfield 2011). Questions about ageing, disability, socio-economic status, ethnicity and gender have also come to the fore in discussions about the policies and politics of sport and physical activity for health (see, for example, Wilkinson and Marmot 2003, Howe 2004, Wray 2007, Phoenix and Grant 2009, Kay and Spaaij 2012). Despite such critiques, stemming from disciplines as varied as social gerontology, the sociology of sport, social psychology, gender studies, international development, policy studies and policy science, there is space for more overt discussions of the increasing relevance and complexities of the politics and policy implications of sport, physical activity and public health.

In this special issue, we include articles from a variety of disciplinary foundations that engage in critical examinations of sport and physical activity allied to public health policy. The papers selected cover both the analysis *of* policy and analysis *for* policy (Houlihan *et al.* 2009), ensuring that a critical focus on the politics of each is at the centre of discussions. Our contributors discuss issues connected to the politics and policy of sport, physical activity and public health by focusing on a range of theoretical themes including evidence and knowledge production, national policies and the political promotion of sport and physical activity for health, sports mega-events and public health, social diversity in community sport for health programming, education and training in physical education and fitness sectors, and critical perspectives on partnership working in sport and public health. Overall, the papers reflect debate about the motivations of national and local government intervention in policymaking on public health that includes the role of sport and/or physical activity, and the polemic about the impact that such policy decisions have on people and their communities.

This special issue reflects a current expansion in academic, policy and practice interest in sport and physical activity for public health. There are 11 research articles representing high-quality empirical approaches to advancing knowledge about sport or physical activity and public health. We also include three research notes; shorter discussion pieces drawing attention to particular ideas; and critical perspectives on the promotion of sport for public health improvement. *Tess Kay* leads the collection by identifying the absence of social science theories and evidence in physical activity policy guidance. More specifically, she argues that there is a perceptible failure in such guidance to recognise and include well-established debates about health inequalities and the social determinants of health despite levels of physical activity being the lowest amongst those in the lower social gradient. Expanding the scope of the knowledge base on physical activity for health, perhaps by bringing together communities of experts in health behaviour research and those working on social science perspectives on the social determinants of health, is proposed as a key step in ensuring a better understanding of the relationship between health inequalities and physical activity. It is also perhaps a route towards better-informed and more relevant physical activity guidance. Taking up a discussion of the relationship between evidence-based policy and the promotion of sport for public health, *Mike Weed* interrogates evidence for the effectiveness of sport for raising population levels of physical activity and delivering public health outcomes amongst the least active. Analysing UK national survey data, Weed argues that sport participation has stagnated or fallen since 1990 despite continued Government investment and that from 1997, any increases in population levels of physical activity are not associated with sport. Coupled with what Weed identifies as a limited evidence-base for the effectiveness of sport interventions in raising activity levels amongst inactive people, he concludes that national agendas for increasing physical activity for public health should privilege choice of opportunities for a range of physical activities rather than prioritise sport.

Marina Honta presents a discussion of the role of the state in the implementation of the 'Sport, Health and Wellbeing Plan' in France. She identifies inter-ministerial governance as an acclaimed approach to effective enactment of the national plan. However, by Honta's view, the complex and fractured nature of French state departments curtails the possibility of effective implementation of national programming at the local level. Honta argues that inter-ministerial partnerships, and the power struggles that prevail in such cross-government working, have meant that the regional and local implementation of the 'Sport, Health and Wellbeing Plan' is limited. The challenges of raising population levels of physical activity through national programming are also considered in the first of our research notes by *Oliver, Hanson, Lindsey and Dodd-Reynolds* in a critical commentary about the recent extension of the UK Exercise on Referral programmes to include sport; an approach the authors identify as Sport-based Exercise on Referral. Two important issues are raised: (1) the weak evidence base for supporting exercise on referral means that there is questionable potential to scale up a national programme to include sport; and (2) including sport in exercise on referral schemes may exacerbate existing challenges associated with providing appropriately targeted activities for those with complex barriers to exercising.

Recognition of the complex relationship between sport, physical activity and public health is the subject of *Smith, Jones, Houghton and Duffell's* paper, which turns the attention of the special issue to mental health. The authors offer an overview of sport, physical activity and mental health policy in England, UK. In it they identify that whilst the use of exercise and other modes of physical activity are an explicit part of health policy goals to prevent and treat mental illness and promote mental health, a focus on mental health is largely absent from national and local sport and physical activity policy. Coupled with a lack of clear practice guidelines, little reference to monitoring and evaluating sport and physical activity for mental health and complex political and funding contexts for commissioning physical activity for mental health programmes, the authors conclude there are significant challenges in designing, implementing and evaluating sport and physical activity projects for mental health outcomes. They offer a rallying call to sport and mental health organisations, researchers, programme deliverers and policymakers to address these challenges through community sport policy development, enactment and evaluation.

Presenting a policy content analysis of London 2012's Olympic pre-event documentation on participation legacy, *Bretherton, Piggin and Bodet* examine the destruction, construction and reconstruction of competing discourses presented by different organisations responsible for legacy delivery. Employing a governmentality framework, the authors identify inconsistencies in the representation of participation legacy which contribute to failings in delivering legacy outcomes. The authors conclude that host governments cannot rely on elusory concepts like 'inspiration' for positive legacy effects of mega-events like the Olympic Games. Strategic approaches that recognise the wider social and political impact on legacy efforts are required for legacy policy to be effectively enacted. In our second research note, *Gard and Diongi* illustrate how sport, more broadly seen as a social policy instrument, appears to be endlessly flexible and is used to support a range of political and health-based ideologies across the life course. Using examples connected to the political imperative of public health, their discussion illustrates the rhetoric of sport's public health utility. In the context of the so-called crises of obesity, ageing and lifestyle diseases, the authors conclude that sport promotion provides a plethora of opportunities for over-stating the benefits of physical activity and representing dominant public health discourses of self-serving institutions.

The contribution by *Markula and Chikinda* and the third and final of our research notes by *Ressler, Richards and Wright* focus on the promotion of public health in education and training. Markula and Chikinda's small-scale qualitative study identifies traditional fitness instructors as potential new local public health promoters but highlights incongruity between fitness instructor training and qualifications, and public health priorities. Fitness instructor training, dominated as it is by narrow, exacting and overbearing approaches to fit bodies, and reinforcing medical discourses and models of health based solely on the absence of disease, leave little room for instructors to teach and learn about health inequalities, health and social diversity, and more holistic strategies for public health promotion. Offering a discussion of the socio-politics of physical education, sport, schools and health in the USA, Ressler et al. argue that physical education programmes are also failing to make an impact in enhancing public health as they are currently making little impact in increasing physical activity or encouraging active lifestyles. Physical education, it is argued, is marginalised in the curriculum in the USA, dominated by competitive athletic programming and dogged by conflicts over teaching and coaching. The result is the continued exclusion of those not interested in traditional sports and ongoing challenges for physical education as a public health intervention. Ressler et al. do, however, propose a more fruitful dialogue between physical education and public health through knowledge exchange between the sectors and higher expectations and more rigorous accountability of PE as a mechanism for public health.

Our next two contributions shift the emphasis of debate to the complexities of participant experience in selected sport and physical activity opportunities. For *Lenneis and Pfister*, gender and ethnicity intersect to foreground conceptions of healthy bodies and physical activity in female migrant cleaners in Denmark. The authors emphasise that minority ethnic groups in Denmark are more at risk of ill health than native populations but that little is known about their lifestyle behaviours, including their attitudes to and practices and of physical activity. Exploring the views of female migrant cleaners through in-depth interviews, Lenneis and Pfister identify that weight loss and management are motivating factors for becoming and being physically active but that work and unpaid domestic constraints serve to create often insurmountable barriers to participation. For these authors, policy needs to recognise the constraining features of organised work and the gendered character of unpaid domestic labour in shaping opportunities for and barriers to physical activity for ethnic minority women. *Jenkin, Eime, Westerbeck, O'Sullivan* and *van Uffelen* examine the role of sports organisations in promoting and delivering sports for older adults. Focus group research with representatives of the Australian National Sports Organisations (ANSOs) and older people revealed personal and organisational barriers to the engagement of older people in sport but Jenkin et al. argue that these can be countered by a series of identified participation benefits for those in older age groups. The authors conclude that there are emerging opportunities for sports clubs to engage older people and the possibility that this demographic can experience health benefits from taking part in sport.

Our final three contributions address issues associated with evidence-building and knowledge production in sport, physical activity and public health partnership work. *Watson, Lashua and Trevorrow* introduce some of the challenges of developing research-practice partnerships in youth community dance projects where practitioners experience an intensifying requirement for evaluation to demonstrate 'what works' in public health terms. Presenting collective, critical conversations between dance practitioners, academic researchers and local authority commissioners, the authors highlight different disciplinary, dance practice, management, research and public health views that need to be considered in developing relevant and effective approaches to monitoring and evaluating community dance programmes. Ongoing dialogue focused on positioning dance as a meaningful sociocultural activity and a sporting leisure pursuit with innumerable possibilities for health and well-being benefits. Such critical conversations served to navigate a path in a direction away from dominant discourses of 'measuring' the public health impact of dance and towards evaluation strategies that captured the creative, artistic and altogether more innovative possibilities for impact from engagement in practices of dance.

Our final two contributions examine in detail the complexities of partnership working in the current climate of monitoring, evaluation and evidence-building in the sport and public health sectors. *Misener and Misener* examine the role of sport organisations in public health promotion in Canada using observational and interview methods. They provide a case study of a local cross-sector partnership between sport and public health agencies for increasing physical activity for health through a strategic marketing project. Despite the national imperative for sport–public health promotion partnerships, the authors highlight a misalignment in local collaborations as a result of different and competing values, discourses and objectives. For these authors, higher-order priorities emphasising partnerships as a means to achieving public health outcomes underestimate local constraints in capacity in achieving health policy goals. *Mansfield* focuses on the complexities of collaborative working in knowledge production about sport for public health benefits. Drawing on her experiences of working in evidence-building projects involving multiple and diverse stakeholder groups, she explores the competing and converging interests in the roles, responsibilities and values that shape such work. Mansfield identifies resourcefulness, reciprocity and reflexivity as central characteristics of partnership working. She presents them in a conceptualisation of the three Rs of research-policy-practice (RPP) partnerships; a way of understanding and addressing the sociodynamics of partnership work. Mansfield argues her conceptual approach as a way of demythologising the role of sport in achieving public health outcomes via an interrogation of resource allocation, ownership and use in partnerships, and through a thorough analysis of the relationships that characterise them.

We do not wish to suggest that the contributions in this special issue bring the politics and policy issues associated with sport, physical and public health to a close. Rather, we present this collection as a starting point for debate and for the development of research, policy and practice based on the diversity of the arguments proposed. We invite scholars in both sport and public health, alongside stakeholders from policy and practice, to engage with the issues our contributors have raised in advancing knowledge and developing future directions for understanding the politics of sport, physical activity and public health. For us, the current agenda for research on sport, physical activity and public health might best be focused on five areas of work; rigorous empirical studies on sport for public health, critical analyses of knowledge production methods and strategies for evidence-building, assessments of partnership working in the design, delivery and evaluation of sport for health programmes, critical policy analysis where sport is prioritised for public health objectives, and examinations of the place and status of sport and physical activity in wider political agendas for public health, particularly in relation to current concerns about mental health and well-being.

Disclosure statement

No potential conflict of interest was reported by the author.

References

Douglas, J., *et al.*, 2007. *A reader in promoting public health*. London: Sage.

Houlihan, B., Bloyce, D., and Smith, A., 2009. Developing the research agenda in sport policy. *International journal of sport policy and politics*, 1, 1–12. doi:10.1080/19406940802681186

Howe, P.D., 2004. *Sport, professionalism, and pain: ethnographies of injury and risk*. Psychology Press. New York, NY: Routledge.

Kay, T. and Spaaij, R., 2012. The mediating effects of family on sport in international development contexts. *International review for the sociology of sport*, 47 (1), 77–94. doi:10.1177/1012690210389250

Maguire, J.S., 2008. *Fit for consumption: sociology and the business of fitness*. London: Routledge.

Malcolm, D. and Scott, A., 2011. Professional relations in sport healthcare: workplace responses to organisational change. *Social science & medicine*, 72, 513–520. doi:10.1016/j.socscimed.2010.11.016

Mansfield, L., 2011. 'Sexercise': working out heterosexuality in Jane Fonda's fitness books. *Leisure studies*, 30 (2), 237–255. doi:10.1080/02614367.2010.523837

Markula, P., 1995. Firm but shapely, fit but sexy, strong but thin. The postmodern aerobicizing female bodies. *Sociology of Sport Journal*, 12, 424–453.

Phoenix, C. and Grant, B.C., 2009. *Expanding the agenda for research on the physically active aging body. Journal of Ageing and Physical Activity*. 17 (3), 362–379.

Piggin, J., 2014. Designed to move? Physical activity lobbying and the politics of productivity. *Health education journal*, 74, 16–27.

Piggin, J. and Bairner, A., 2014. The global physical inactivity pandemic: An analysis of knowledge production. *Sport education and society*, 21, 131–147.

Waddington, I., 2000. Sport, health and drugs: A critical sociological perspective. Oxford: Taylor & Francis.

Wilkinson, R.G. and Marmot, M.G., eds., 2003. *Social determinants of health: the solid facts*. Geneva: World Health Organization.

World Health Organisation (WHO), 2007. *Working for health: an introduction to the World Health Organization*. Geneva: WHO Switzerland.

Wray, S., 2007. Health, exercise, and well-being: the experiences of midlife women from diverse ethnic backgrounds. *Social theory & health*, 5 (2), 126–144. doi:10.1057/palgrave.sth.8700100

Louise Mansfield
Joe Piggin

Bodies of knowledge: connecting the evidence bases on physical activity and health inequalities

Tess Kay

ABSTRACT

This paper addresses the absence of social science perspectives in physical activity policy guidance. Physical activity is a universal health focus, a priority for global, regional and national agencies acting on public health (e.g. the World Health Organisation; WHO Regional Office for Europe; Public Health England). Current UK guidance about being physically active was published in 2011, during a period of intense economic downturn and 'austerity' welfare. Physical activity is known to be lowest among sectors of the population at the lower end of the social gradient, making marginalised and disadvantaged groups priorities for initiatives to raise activity levels. Although much emphasis was given to the robust scientific underpinning of the 2011 guidance, it failed to engage with either the national or global debate around health inequalities, and gave no consideration to the social processes affecting health. This paper considers this omission. It first overviews patterns of health inequalities and explains the potential contribution of physical activity to addressing them. It then reviews the content of UK physical activity guidance, examines the role of health behaviour research in informing them, and suggests a number of ways in which social science knowledge could have enhanced its analysis. The paper then considers the process of knowledge production which informed the guidance, and considers the value of incorporating research into the social determinants of health (SDH) into the evidence base that informs physical activity guidance. It concludes with suggestions about how this might be done.

Introduction

Physical activity is a universal health focus, a priority for global, world regional and national action on public health (e.g. WHO 2010, Public Health England 2014, WHO Regional Office for Europe 2016). In the UK, it has featured more than a dozen times in guidance issued by the National Institute for Health and Care Excellence (NICE) addressing a wide range of health conditions and contexts including workplace health, child and youth health, cardiovascular disease, obesity, brief advice and exercise referral schemes (NICE 2008, 2009, 2010, 2013a, 2013b, 2014). For Public Health England, physical activity is a key contributor to its priorities of *Helping people to live longer and more healthy lives* and *Reducing the burden of disease and disability in life* (e.g. Public Health England 2013). With national sport strategies such as Sport England's *Towards an active nation* (Sport England 2016) signifying an increasing focus on health outcomes, the position of PA in public health policy is an important context for policy, practice and knowledge production in sport.

It is in this context that this paper reflects on the potential contribution of social science perspectives in informing the promotion of physical activity for health benefits. Current guidance was published in 2011 in the *Start Active, Stay Active* (SASA) report (Department of Health 2011) and provides the scientific underpinning for more recent statements (e.g. Public Health England 2014).SASA was a joint endeavour by the UK's four home countries (England, Scotland, Wales and Northern Ireland) to update and synthesise the available evidence and develop guidance from it. On its launch, much emphasis was given to its scope and scientific quality. Intended as the first link in a communication chain that would extend through practitioners to the general public, its review of scientific evidence was leavened with accounts of how people might incorporate physical activity in everyday life.

The inclusion of these descriptions is illuminating in providing insight into how 'scientists' view, and present, their social world. The SASA report was commissioned in the shadow of the global economic crisis of 2008; by 2009, when its contributors began their deliberations, UK unemployment was rising, and two years later reached its highest level for 17 years. Yet the SASA report made no reference to poverty, deprivation or material hardship; on the contrary, it suggested the challenge was to help people to fit activity into 'busy lives' (Department of Health 2011, p. 8), not barren and impoverished ones. A brief reference was made to differences in physical activity levels between age groups and by gender, but the wider issue of inequalities in health, connected to social and economic stratification, went unexamined. Like much UK public health policy, the report focused only on individually-focused strategies promoting health behaviour change, and ignored the material and structural factors that are known to inhibit this (Bambra *et al.* 2011, p. 403).

Yet the existence of health inequalities is not a niche phenomenon and the debate surrounding it is not confined to specialists: when the SASA experts first convened in 2009 the UK discussion on health inequalities was already three decades old and strongly established in the public and policy domains. It had been launched 30 years previously by the Black Report (Black 1980) and reinvigorated in 1998 by the first of three 'New Labour' governments through the Acheson Inquiry into Health Inequalities (Acheson 1998). It was the third of these governments, then headed by Prime Minister Gordon Brown, that had commissioned SASA. More significantly, the health inequalities debate was very current – the work of the SASA expert groups (2009–2011) was contemporaneous with the *Strategic Review of Health Inequalities in England* led by Sir Michael Marmot (2008–2010). Marmot had recently led the World Health Organisation's global analysis of the social determinants of health (SDH) (WHO 2008a, 2008b); his report on the UK situation, *Fair society, healthy lives* (Marmot 2010a) was published to wide public exposure in 2010 – being featured, for example, on nationally broadcast television news programmes – when writing on SASA had yet to begin (Department of Health, Annex A, pp. 50–52). There is, however, no mention of Marmot's UK work in SASA, nor of the WHO's earlier work on inequalities – despite members of the SASA expert groups having worked on WHO PA policy (Department of Health, Annex D, pp. 55–56). The UK's guidance to increase levels of physical activity, known to be lowest among poorer sectors of the population, therefore failed to engage with either the national or global debate around health inequalities. In short, it gave no consideration to the social processes affecting health.

This paper considers this omission. It first overviews patterns of health inequalities and explains the potential contribution of physical activity to addressing them. It then examines the content of the SASA report, and suggests a number of ways in which attention to social structural factors could have enhanced its analysis. The paper then considers the process of knowledge production which informed the guidance, and considers the value of incorporating social science into the evidence base that informs physical activity guidance. The paper concludes with suggestions about how this should be done.

Health and inequality

The central premise of this paper is that responses to physical inactivity by policymakers, practitioners and research communities have all been weakened by the collective failure to draw on expert analyses of the dynamics of health inequalities. The purpose of this section is therefore to establish why consideration of health inequalities is relevant to approaches to address physical activity, and should underpin them. Later sections of the paper then consider the implications this shift in focus would have for the range of evidence that PA experts draw on.

Health inequalities are easily demonstrated, most commonly through comparisons of life expectancy: in 2008, 29 countries of the world had a life expectancy over 80 years, while 12 had life expectancy under 50 (WHO 2008a). Such discrepancies are not explained by biology, but by multiple factors including access to healthcare and health education, to a safe living environment and to the basic resources for living including food security and sanitation (WHO 2008a). But more striking than comparisons between countries of very different economic status, where large discrepancies might be expected, are the inequalities between population groups *within* single nations. In England in 2009–2011, the average life expectancy for men and women in the most affluent 10% of neighbourhoods was 83 and 86 years, respectively, while for men and women in the poorest 10%, it was 73 and 79 years. The gap doubled when comparisons took into account health quality: men and women in the top 10% averaged 71 and 72 years of healthy life, while those in the bottom 10% averaged only 52 and 53 years (ONS 2013).

The forms of ill health that produce these patterns are mostly non-communicable diseases (NCDs) – non-infectious and non-transmissible conditions that include physical ailments (such as heart disease, asthma, cancer and diabetes) and mental, neurological and substance use disorders (e.g. depression, dementia and alcoholism). Exposure to NCDs is strongly influenced by individuals' health behaviours, including their diet and levels of physical activity, leading to extensive investment in strategies to promote healthy lifestyles. NCDs are not, however, only associated with individual behaviours, but also show a strong social gradient, and have higher prevalence among poorer groups in all nations. The distribution of NCDs therefore indicates significant structural influences on health that are not addressed by strategies that focus only on individual behaviour. Initially mainly a concern in high income countries, NCDs are now also the main causes of the disease burden in low and middle income countries (LMICs), fuelled by three global trends – population ageing; rapid unplanned urbanisation and globalisation (WHO 2008a). Regardless of a country's overall economic status, however, health inequalities within nations persist: in every country in the world, lower socio-economic position correlates with worse health. For individuals, health inequality stems not so much from the distribution of power and wealth between nations, but from their distribution within them.

While physical activity policy has not addressed the connection between health and structural inequality, this has been extensively examined in wider analyses that frame public health. The landmark study in this field is the work of the WHO's Commission on the social determinants of health, established to synthesise scientific evidence of health inequalities and foster a global movement to address them. Its comprehensive report, *Closing the gap in a generation* (WHO 2008a) argued that health inequities were inextricably bound to wide processes of inequality and could not be addressed within health policy alone; rather, they required action to address inequities in the way in which power and resources are distributed in society, led by national governments but involving a plurality of actors (WHO 2008a, p. 44). The Commission identified required areas: policy coherence (ensuring health equity was addressed in all relevant government policies); action for equity; financial policy to improve equity (including the taxation system and public sector funding) and measurement, evaluation and training, to monitor progress towards health equity and raise awareness of it (WHO 2008a, pp. 44–45). This cross-cutting approach was evident in the treatment of physical activity, which was identified as important for alleviating NCDs. The report emphasised that physical activity could be constrained by 'the conditions of daily living' and recognised the need to address this through policies shaping the distribution of economic resources, such as welfare support, and those affecting the physical environment, including housing and transport provision. In similar vein, the European Commission's 2013 review of health inequalities (European Commission 2013) drew attention to the wide spectrum of policies that could affect the context within which physical activity might occur. The review depicted health behaviours as 'proximate causes' of health and ill health, that is, factors which exerted influence on health but were themselves only the manifestations of underlying health inequalities, rather than their root causes. It advocated attention to the 'causes of the causes' – that is, the need to look beyond healthy behaviours to address the social and economic factors that influenced and constrained them. This perspective gives greater consideration to contextual factors which influence how and why people become physically active, rather than focusing narrowly on individuals' immediate motivations and 'choices'.

Despite the advocacy of transnational organisations such as WHO and the European Commission, there has been limited progress in establishing integrated policy approaches to address health inequalities. The neglect of inequalities in the SASA physical activity guidance is not, therefore, unusual in comparison to other areas of health policy. There are nonetheless a number of reasons why it is fruitful to examine how this omission has arisen and how it might therefore be overcome in future. For one thing, the capacity of physical activity to reduce risk of NCDs makes it central to strategies to reduce health inequalities – so there is a strong policy rationale. For another, the UK is especially prominent in scholarship and policy guidance on health inequalities, and was engaged in such an exercise contemporaneously to the development of the SASA report; this makes it all the more incongruous that this expertise has not informed its PA policy, and more important to know why. Finally, physical activity expertise is often informed by the sport and exercise sciences, and this offers an opportunity for social scientists of sport to contribute their expertise on inequality and exclusion to this multidisciplinary academic community. It is from this perspective that the next section therefore subjects the UK physical activity guidance provided by the SASA report to a critical reading. This has two purposes: to consider the substantive knowledge that the report offers, and the process through which this knowledge was produced.

Representing health: the portrayal of active lifestyles in physical activity guidance

The SASA report on which the following analysis focuses was published in 2011. Previous guidance to promote physical activity had limited success: across the four UK countries, only 33–43% of men were meeting the recommended levels of activity in 2010, and even fewer women (23–32%) (Department of Health 2011). The most acute problems were however in the lowest income neighbourhoods, where the proportion of the population achieving recommended levels of activity was only half that of the highest (Public Health England 2014). As Marmot (2010a) has noted, improving the health outcomes of the least healthy groups is not a marginal concern for public health – it is a core strategy, because it leads to the greatest aggregate health gains at population level. The SASA report might therefore have been expected to address the situations of those in adverse circumstances, given the significance of physical activity as a risk factor for NCDs that are most prevalent among lower socio-economic groups. Yet what the following account shows is that far from being a prominent focus, low-income and marginalised groups were wholly invisible in SASA – an incongruous omission at any time, but all the more remarkable in a period of global economic downturn and 'austerity' welfare.

The SASA report took the form of a new 60-page publication on 'physical activity for health' endorsed by the UK's four Chief Medical Officers. The report drew on a wide evidence base on physical activity to establish 'a UK-wide consensus on the amount of physical activity we should all aim to do at each stage of our lives' (Department of Health 2011, p. 6). Adopting a life course approach, it for the first time, provided age-appropriate guidance. It also highlighted the risk of sedentary behaviour, and emphasised the importance of being active on a daily basis. Its seven chapters define physical activity and explain its contribution to health (Chapter 1); outline the approach taken to developing the guidance (Chapter 2); present evidence and guidance about physical activity for four phases in the life course (Chapters 3–6) and offer conclusions about how the guidelines can be applied, including suggestions for 'new opportunities' for action by different organisational actors (Chapter 7). The report also contains appendices which detail the methodology adopted to produce the guidelines, including the evidence base used and the work undertaken by the five expert groups that contributed – one for each of the four SASA age groups, and a fifth focused on sedentary behaviour. Membership overlapped between groups.

The critique below focuses on the four age group chapters, Chapters 3–6, which cover 'early years' (under 5 s), 'children and young people' (5–18 years), 'adults' (19–64 years) and 'older adults' (65+ years). Each chapter sets out the developmental and health characteristics of the age group, presents the guidelines for recommended levels and types of PA, and provides a summary of the scientific evidence on which they are based. Each also contains a section on 'Understanding the guidelines', which discusses how they may translate into practice. This includes two or three 'boxed' examples to illustrate how activity may be incorporated in daily life for the relevant age group. The examples are ~200 words descriptions of individuals/families in everyday life, including their household and employment arrangements and the forms of physical activity in which they engage.

The inclusion of the examples recognises the importance of contextualising individuals' behaviour. This is consistent with the increased use of social ecological models (SEMs) of health (discussed in detail below) to underpin analyses of health behaviour; although underpinned by cognitivism, these models so aim to locate individuals within their wider social context. The descriptions are also potentially helpful to the 'chain of communication' through which the SASA guidance aims to be accessible for practitioners, who can in turn transmit it to the public (Department of Health 2011, p. 3). Although the examples are not factually based, they are intended to have practical utility – to be relevant and realistic in their representations of how individuals at different points in the life course can incorporate physical activity into their lifestyles, especially those who are in the less active groups of the population. It is instructive to examine how well they do this.

The content of the SASA examples

The 10 SASA examples are populated by 15 adults and 8 children. The content and detail in each example varies – for example, some descriptions mention employment details while others do not – which limits the analysis that can be offered here. The commentary below considers how population diversity and 'everyday life' are portrayed in SASA, and considers what additional content it would have been useful to include from health inequalities perspective:

- *Early years (0–4 years): two children, each living with their two parents. All four parents employed, with one mother on maternity leave.* The families portrayed in the 'early years' category facilitate their children's physical activity in the context of full employment and financial security, living in neighbourhoods that give them excellent access to facilities for being active.

  In contrast, a health inequalities focus would direct attention to vulnerable households for this age group – lone parents, single-income households and households with one or more unemployed parents. The situation of low income families offers multiple challenges to healthy lifestyles for children and adults. In 2009, even government statistics recognised that more than 3 million of the nation's children were living in poverty (Brewer *et al.* 2009, 2011). Maternal employment is an especially strong differentiator across social-economic classifications: mothers with lower educational qualifications who have children below school age have low employment rates.
- *Child/youth (5–18 years): 3 young people, aged 7 (male) 14 and 14 (females), attending school; 2 live with both parents and one with a lone parent; one has a disability; other siblings mentioned.* The SASA child/youth examples for the 5–18 age group all consist of reconfined to focus on

young people attending school and living in their parental home, in financially secure households. There are multiple examples of access to high quality, easily accessible provision for physical activity, much of it within walking distance of home.

In the UK, young people's lives diverge when compulsory schooling ends at age 16: those leaving school then have low qualifications which is associated with a lifetime trajectory of low and insecure income. Such issues are missing from the SASA report, as are any of the negative behaviours associated with youth – illicit and illegal behaviour, teen pregnancy, high unemployment, rising alcohol consumption (Wright *et al.* 2012). The SASA examples overlook these, and also omit the well-documented declines in PA levels associated with education transitions, especially among females.

The child/youth category contains the report's single representation of a lone parent family, headed by a father in full-time employment. This is an atypical representation of lone parenthood in the UK in 2010, where mothers headed >90% of these households (ONS 2015) and were the most economically insecure of the working-age population, especially constrained by the absence of affordable childcare. In the UK, lone parents are at risk of low income and time shortage; for children, living in a lone parent household doubles the risk of living in poverty (ONS 2015). These circumstances can constrain healthy behaviour.

- *Adult (18–64 years): two men and one woman, aged 27, 37 and 22, respectively; two in employment and one due to start employment. The younger male is a wheelchair user. All are childless and single.* Two of the adults in these examples are in employment and the third is waiting to begin a job she has secured. The two able-bodied adults make use of multiple small opportunities to be active. The examples show more insight into the situation of the wheelchair user, detailing a number of practical and psychological barriers that he has overcome.

  The examples of adults are notable for their narrow representation of ages and family situations; despite the importance attached to family life as a context for PA, each case study focuses on a single, childless person, and adults in their 40 s, 50 s and 60 s are completely omitted. The impact of parenthood on men and women's activity patterns is not addressed, despite policy recognition of the challenges of achieving work-life balance; the sizeable literature on gendered patterns of activity within families, including constraints on mothers, is also omitted. There are no references to material deprivation.
- *Older adults (65+ years): one married man age 70 and one widow age 81, both retired from previous paid employment and living in their own home*: The two older adults are both retirees, who worked until 51 (man) and 76. They live in their own homes and lead active, sociable, unconstrained lives – the man is a basketball referee and leads walking tours, while the woman has set up a local walking group where she has 'progressed to the fast group'. They have secure living conditions, good access to services, strong social networks, high levels of confidence and uncompromised physical and mental ability.

  The older adults included in the SASA report are notable for being wholly unaffected by any negative factors associated with ageing. These are nonetheless national and global policy concerns, and include low income, social isolation and dependency on care services. It is particularly striking that no mention is made to constraints or reductions in physical and mental capacities associated with biological ageing including chronic illness (Banks *et al.* 2012).

Overall it would appear that the examples in the SASA report are designed to emphasise the capacity of individuals to take opportunities to be active. It is notable that those in the lower reaches of the social gradient are not in evidence, despite being the population sectors that are least active and stand most to gain from changing this behaviour. These are also the groups with poor aggregate health status, with whom health professionals are most likely to work, for whom the SASA report is supposed to be a link in the communication chain for PA guidance. It therefore appears that while a health inequalities focus would address issues of structural disadvantage, current dominant expertise in physical activity does not. The next section explores how this arises.

Informing PA policy: from individual behaviour change to the social determinants of health

The above analysis of the SASA 'examples' has highlighted how physical activity guidance fails to address issues of health inequalities. To the critical social scientific eye the descriptions in the report appear uninformed even at the descriptive level, failing to identify those at the bottom of the social gradient, let alone examine the structural factors that may affect them. This section discusses how this arises from the theoretical underpinning of such guidance in cognitivism, and suggests how an alternative approach could overcome this.

There is of course a well-established social science critique of the failure of health related research to recognise individuals as social actors, to understand their interaction with social context and to recognise the constraints that may arise from the unfavourable circumstances in which unhealthy behaviour occurs. Yet much of the theorisations that underpin physical activity guidance *do* purport to recognise the existence of multiple, multilevel influences on individuals, and do advocate that health interventions should address them. These principles are central to 'Social Ecological Models' (SEMs), first expounded in McLeroy *et al.*'s Ecological Model of Health Behaviours (1988), and increasingly used in analyses of physical activity behaviour, including several sources on which the SASA report drew. The fact that the SASA report nonetheless produced such limited social analysis suggests that further scrutiny is merited of the capacity of SEMs to provide this.

The SEM proposed by McLeroy *et al.* (1988) was not the first approach to address social context – a similar idea underpins social cognitive theory (e.g. Bandura 2004); rather, its originality lay in bringing together two concepts: health behaviour was affected by *multiple levels of influence*, and that it was shaped through *reciprocal causation* between individuals and these layers of context.

McLeroy *et al.*'s initial SEM specified five levels at which influence occurred – intrapersonal, interpersonal, organisational, community and public policy, and subsequent versions have produced multiple variants of this. They include Stokols (1992, 1996, six levels); the U.S. National Heart, Lung and Blood Institute (2004, six levels); Glanz *et al.* 2005; four); Story *et al.* (2008; four) and Sallis (2009; six). While they vary in detail, all recognise multiple factors and spheres of influence beyond the individual, including family, community and neighbourhood; multiple policy environments and various depictions of 'social', including social environment, social factors, social cultural environment and macro-level environment. And while Mcleroy *et al.*'s original SEM omitted key social structural variables (Winch 2012, n.p. commented 'it is not clear where culture, social class, racism, gender, economics/employment are supposed to fit, or if they fit anywhere'), in later versions these too appear, including gender, age, race/ethnicity and SES.

Where then do SEM approaches fall short? At the intervention level, Golden and Earp (2012) found fewer than 10% of interventions were based on SEMs, and among those, most only focused on individual factors and rarely addressed all levels of influence. They suggested that targeting upper levels of SEM 'is likely more challenging than adapting intrapersonal- and interpersonal-level programmes', and that there are particular difficulties in translating theories about 'higher level social and behavioural change' into practical action at intervention level (Golden and Earp 2012, p. 370). Burke *et al.* suggest however that the failure is not simply a failure of application, but reflects a more fundamental theoretical feature: that for all their emphasis on context and multilevel social influences, SEMs remain rooted in individual theories, and focus[ed] on changing individual motivations to stimulate behaviour change. Golden and Earp (2012, p. 370) similarly concluded that 'the predominant theories in the literature we reviewed continue to have an individual orientation'. Thus, while the promise of SE models lies in their concern with multiple levels of social and physical environments, this is undermined by their continued reliance on health behaviour theories rooted in cognitivism (Burke *et al.* 2009).

This becomes more apparent when the representation of social factors in SEMs is scrutinised. This reveals considerable difference between the social science view of 'social' influences and that which dominates policy guidance on health behaviour change. The commentary below considers three aspects of this: (i) which social structural factors (e.g. gender, age, race) are included and how they are (appear to be) defined/conceptualised; (ii) what is included in the levels of models specifically labelled as 'social', and (iii) what factors are contained in the 'highest' (structural) levels of SEMs (Table 1).

The incorporation of social structural factors in SEMs

SEMs incorporate a range of 'social' factors, including gender, age, ethnicity, and in some cases, social class and/or socio-economic position. All however appear only as individual characteristics; they are not conceptualised as structuring social processes. Confined to the 'individual' level in virtually all models and categorised as 'demographic' – or in some cases, 'biological' – characteristics, they are shorn of any 'social' dimensions. This narrow conceptualisation is evident in the treatment of 'gender' which is omitted by McLeroy *et al.* (1988 – 16 years after Title IX was enacted), labelled 'sex' in NHLBI (2004), and is classed as 'biological' (with 'age' and 'genes', and distinct from the 'demographic' factors, race/ethnicity and income) in Story *et al.* (2008). The disregard of the social nature of gender is an unexpected omission for a global north academic community, where gender equity legislation is formally embedded across all major social institutions including the welfare state, the labour market, the legal system and the institutions of government. Other examples include the conceptualisation of ageing as only a biological process (although even that was omitted from the SASA examples!), and references to culture which only allude to overt and conscious actions and practices (e.g. requirements for single-sex provision for some faith groups).

The constitution of the 'social' category in SEMs

'Social' factors are essential elements of SEMs. They are considered to be 'higher' level influences, which individuals interact. All the example models therefore address 'social' factors, albeit defined in varied ways and placed at different levels within the model. Three overarching trends emerge. First, the term 'social' is primarily applied to forms of direct social interaction and/or immediate social context: references are made to social networks, social settings (community, school, etc) and social environments. Second, several of the 'social' factors in SEMs are psychological concepts – for example, social support, role modelling and social climate. Finally, social factors commonly occur mid-model – in Level 3 ('social/cultural') of six in NHLBI; in Level 2 ('social environment') of four in Story *et al.* (2008) and in Level 4 ('Behaviour Settings') of six in Sallis (2009).

Structural factors: the highest level of SEMs

Social scientists would expect social structural influences on health to appear in the 'highest' level of SEMs. Instead these levels focus on institutional structures, not on social ones. Public policy is the focus of the highest level for McLeroy *et al.*, NHLBI and Glan *et al.*, and prominent in Story *et al.*'s 'macro-level environment', alongside other economic sectors. In Sallis's 2009 variant, policy features at Level 5, while the highest (Level 6) offers an eclectic mix of factors, including the natural and information environments; clubs, teams and programmes, and advocacy and social capital. Across all five SEMs, social structural phenomena are absent: the variables recognised at individual level (gender, race) do not reappear, and wider social trends (e.g. globalisation, urbanisation, population ageing) are not introduced.

Table 1. Multilevel approaches of selected social ecological models (SEMs) of health behaviour.

	McLeroy *et al.* (1988)	NHLBI (2004)	Glanz *et al.* (2005)	Story *et al.* (2008)	Sallis (2009)
Levels specified in SEM → Social variables ↓	L1 Intrapersonal L2 Interpersonal L3 Organisational L4 Community L5 Public policy	L1 Biological and demographic L2 Psychological L3 Social/cultural L4 Organisational L5 Physical environment L6 Policies/incentives	L1 Behaviour L2 Individual – socio-demographics L3 Environmental L4 Policy	L1 Individual – demographic, biological L2 Social environment (networks) L3 Physical environment (settings) L4 Macro-level environment (sectors)	L1 Intrapersonal – demographics, biological, psychological, family L2 Perceived environment qualities L3 Behaviour: active living domains L4 Behaviour settings L5 Policy environment L6 Overarching
Gender	–	L1 Biological/demographic	L2 Individual – socio-demographics	L1 Individual – biological	L1 Intrapersonal
Age	–	L1 Biological/demographic	L2 Individual – socio-demographics	L1 Individual – biological	L1 Intrapersonal
Race/ethnicity	–	L1 Biological/demographic	L2 Individual – socio-demographics	L1 Individual – demographic	L1 Intrapersonal
Culture	–	L3 Cultural beliefs, social norms	–	–	L6 Overarching – includes norms, culture, social cultural environment
Socio-econ status/ employment	–	L1 Biological/demographic	–	–	–
Income	–	–	–	L1 Individual – demographic	–
Notes	McLeroy *et al.* (1988)	*L1 Intrapersonal*: this covers individual characteristics that influence behaviour: knowledge, skills, self-efficacy; there is no mention of personal socio-demographic characteristics *L2 Interpersonal*: Family, friends, peers, interpersonal processes and groups providing identity and support			
	NHLBI (2004)	*L1 Individual*: includes 'sex'; no reference to gender			
	Glanz *et al.* (2005)	*L2 Individual – socio-demographics*: no indicators of social class or income			
	Story *et al.* (2008)	*L2 Social environment* – psychological terms (social support, role modelling, social norms); refers to social networks/interactions rather social structures			
	Sallis (2009)	*L6 Overarching*: very diverse category, includes information environment, natural environment; perceived crime; partners for activities; clubs, teams, programmes; advocacy; social capital			

Source: McLeroy *et al.* (1988), Glanz *et al.* (2005), NHLBI (2004), Story *et al.* (2008), Sallis (2009).

It is apparent that there are significant discrepancies between social science and health behaviourist approaches to conceptualising social influences on health behaviour. Within health psychology, Golden and Earp (2012) warn that approaches that claim to address social influences are in fact underpinned by theories that depict individuals as self-determining, unaffected by external influences. Burke *et al.* further highlight that this approach promotes a normative view of the individual, through which specific characteristics become universalised:

> One key assumption informing health behavior theories is the standard or 'norm' on which they are based..... The persistence of this assumed norm is linked to the social, cultural, and historical context of the practice of health behavior research and theory production.... (Burke *et al.* 2009, p. 59S)

Burke *et al.* draw attention to the significance that the *process* of knowledge production has for the evidence it yields. The next section now addresses this. It first examines the potential of the 'SDH' framework for improving understanding of health behaviour, then considers how this body of knowledge might be incorporated into the evidence base for PA.

The *social determinants of health* as a potential framework for conceptualising structural influences on physical activity

There are alternatives to SEMs for theorising how health behaviour is influenced by factors beyond the individual. They include variants of SEMs originating from critical health psychologists, such as Golden *et al.*'s (2015) proposal to 'upend' the SEM and place social policy at its centre. For physical activity specialists, there may be particular value in approaches that encourage a focus on health inequalities, ensuring that the adverse social circumstances of the least active sectors of the population will be addressed. It is with this in mind that this section examines the SDH framework which potentially might enable approaches to PA to be refocused to take greater account of the social gradient of health.

Theories about the SDH draw on a lengthy tradition. As Irwin and Scali (2007) note, 'Analysts have long observed that social and environmental factors decisively influence people's health' (Irwin and Scali 2007, p. 236). This thinking underpinned the health movements of the nineteenth century, which sought to alleviate the impacts of industrialisation on the working and living conditions of the poor. In the modern era, the focus on social determinants traces back to the emergence of community health approaches in the 1960s and 1970s. Although the highly regarded Black report (1980) on UK health inequalities was discarded by the incoming Thatcher government, the agenda re-emerged with new momentum in the 1990s and 2000s. More recently, the SDH framework has provided the theoretical underpinning for the World Health Organisation's Commission on the Social Determinants of Health (CSDH; cf. *Closing the gap in a generation*; WHO 2008a), the UK Marmot Review (*Fair society, healthy lives* 2010a), and the European Commission's *Commission* on *Health inequalities in the EU* (2013).

The core premise of the SDH framework is that individuals' health outcomes are influenced by a range of social structural factors which reflect the wider organisation of power and resources in society. The resulting inequalities underpin more immediate health 'determinants', which are the range of interacting factors that shape health and well-being. These include material circumstances, the social environment, psychosocial factors and biological factors, which are 'in turn... influenced by social position, itself shaped by education, occupation, income, gender, ethnicity and race' (Marmot 2010b, p. 11). These diverse social factors are more influential on individuals than those more obviously and directly associated with health, including health behaviour, genetic makeup and access to healthcare services. Serious health inequalities do not, therefore, arise by chance, or as a result of individual behaviour or characteristics; rather, 'Social and economic differences in health status reflect, and are caused by, social and economic inequalities in society'. (Marmot 2010b, p. 12). To address health inequalities, it is therefore *necessary* to address social

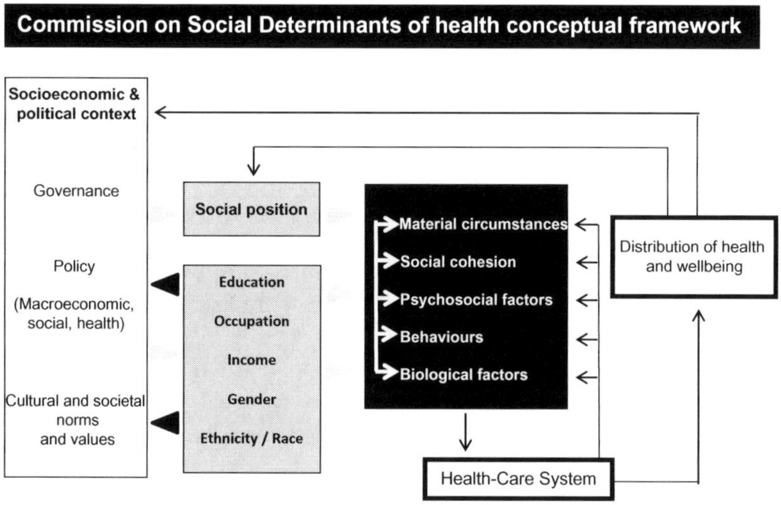

Figure 1. Conceptualising the social determinants of health. Reproduced from WHO, Closing the gap in a generation, Commission on Social Determinants of Health Report, Fig. 4.1, page 43. Copyright 2008.

structural factors, making it important that these are incorporated in health policy, guidance and interventions.

The conceptualisation of SDH presented below stems from the work of the WHO CSDH in 2007 and is underpinned by theories of the social production of health from three fields – psychosocial approaches; social production of disease/political economy of health, and eco-social frameworks. Each of these strongly emphasise the concept of 'social position' as playing a central role in the SDH inequalities (Solar and Irwin 2010, pp. 4–5), and this is a core focus reflected in the framework.

The resulting SDH framework recognises three forms of 'mechanism' which interact with each other to influence exposure to health risk (Figure 1). This is broadly equivalent to the 'multilevel' approach used in SEMs, although with fewer components than the 4–6 levels those use. The SDH framework also differs from SEMs by beginning its analysis at what would be their highest/most distant level mechanisms. In contrast to SEMs, which centre the individual and work up/outward to wider influences, this SDH framework starts with two categories of structural determinants ('socio-economic and political context' and 'social position'), before moving to the third category ('intermediary determinants') which are those directly experienced by individuals.

The CSDH conceptual framework

The three mechanisms of the SDH framework consist of two categories of 'structural determinants' (*context* and *social positioning)* which produce structural health inequalities, which give rise to a third category (*intermediary determinants*) which influence individuals' specific health outcomes.

(1) The 'highest' level of social influence emanates from the *socioe-conomic and political context*. 'Context' is the first of the two categories of 'structural determinants' which give rise to mechanisms which stratify populations as a whole. The socio-economic and political context consists of four domains of representation and policymaking (governance, macroeconomic policies, social policies and public policies), with the more open-ended 'culture and societal values' as the fifth. In the SDH framework, 'context' therefore includes 'all social and political mechanisms that generate, configure and maintain social hierarchies' (Solar and Irwin 2010, p. 5), including the labour market, the educational system and the welfare state.

(2) The second category of structural determinants is those that determine *social position*. These are closely interconnected with *context* as they emerge from socio-economic and political institutions to produce stratification and social class divisions which define individual socio-economic position within hierarchies of power, prestige and access to resources. Solar and Irwin identify the most important structural stratifiers and their proxy indicators as including income, education, occupation, social class, gender, race/ethnicity. In identifying these, the framework therefore demonstrates the connection between high-level contextual factors, and the resources and characteristics that position an individual in society.

(3) The final category consists of *intermediary determinants of health*. While the first two categories, were concerned with the overall structuring of society, including health inequalities, the 'intermediary' determinants are reflective of people's place within social hierarchies, and influence their material circumstances. The main intermediary determinants are material circumstances, psychosocial circumstances and behavioural and/or biological factors. Based on their social position, individuals experience differences in exposure and vulnerability to health-compromising conditions. The health system itself is recognised as a social determinant at this level, allowing many of the provision factors addressed in SEMs – such as availability of programmes and facilities – to be included.

It should be evident that the SDH framework has considerable common ground with the SEMs discussed previously. The two approaches address similar factors at individual, household, community and policy levels; in fact there are few factors named in one approach that are not included in the other – or could be. There are differences of degree, such as the compression of lower levels factors from SMEs into the single category of 'intermediary determinants' in the SDH framework. The SDH framework is, however, distinguished by the coherence across its three categories: any factor referred to in one domain can be linked to corresponding elements in the other two. This contrasts with SMEs where, for example, gender appears only as an individual factor and its structural properties are not addressed.

The SDH framework offers a number of potential benefits to PA policy, practice and analysis. At the aggregate level, it directs attention to those in hardship, including groups linked by their shared experiences (e.g. of low income). The SDH framework is not, however, an approach only concerned with those on the margins; the gradient of health affects the entire social spectrum. The Marmot review introduced the concept of 'proportionate universalism' to respond to this – the notion that interventions should be both universal and targeted to where there is more needs (Graham and Kelly 2004, in Bambra *et al.* 2011, p. 401). More significantly, by foregrounding constraining influences and barriers which are not of an individual's own making, it offers an alternative to a policy focus on 'weak' individuals who behave badly.

The SDH framework has two contributions to make to PA policy. First, by highlighting structural variation in social position, it can inform work with priority groups for PA. Second, by highlighting how structural influences shape individual circumstances, it provides a valuable counterbalance to the SEM focus on individual agency. Both of these have potential to contribute to the evidence base for PA, and the final section examines how this might occur.

Addressing the social in physical activity guidance: incorporating the social determinants of health perspective

Physical activity guidance has been limited by a failure to utilise informed analyses of the social world. The resulting policy has placed too much emphasis on the individual as an active agent, and ignored evidence of the constraints and barriers that can affect them. By omitting a body of knowledge on structural influences and the inequalities that result from them, the situation of the least healthy and least active has remained invisible.

This final section considers how the evidence base can be widened to address this gap. It proposes addressing four aspects of the process of knowledge production: (i) what additional evidence is necessary to inform PA policy and guidance; (ii) what additional evidence is available and accessible; (iii) what changes to the knowledge community are required and (iv) how knowledge might be translated.

Redefining the evidence base: connecting physical activity to health inequalities

The SASA report was 'evidence based' and contained authoritative statements to this effect. The evidence on which it drew consisted primarily of biomedical research into the benefits to people's bodies of being active. The approach was underpinned by a broad psychosocial theorisation of health behaviour that stresses the capacity of individuals to make themselves active. There is however little evidence to indicate that trying to improve people's psychosocial experiences without introducing accompanying interventions to address the material and structural determinants with which they are associated will succeed (Bambra *et al.* 2011, p. 403). This is why it is important for PA policy to also be informed by the evidence on the SDH and their effect on people's capacities to behave in healthy ways.

The increasing use of SEMs, which purport to address the wider social influences affecting individuals, has not introduced such analysis. SEMs do nonetheless recognise external contextual influences, and this opens the door to introducing relevant evidence. It would therefore seem beneficial for future PA guidance to be directly informed by the very substantial, long-standing literature that examines how social disadvantage maps on to poor health, and how individuals are affected by material (and other) deprivation. To date, the expert analysts who inform PA guidance have not accessed this body of knowledge.

Once individuals are conceptualised as being connected to and located within social structural influences the focus moves from interventions focusing on behaviour modification, to alternative approaches which address the structural influences affecting them. Connecting PA to health inequalities would lead to the use of evidence on the characteristics, situations and experiences of different population groups, and produce more informed guidance for interventions to increase physical activity levels. Such analyses are more likely to have relevance to those with whom health workers engage than the portrayals given in the SASA reports, in which no-one is deprived, disadvantaged or constrained.

Accessing evidence

The dynamics of health inequalities are complex and need to be understood through appropriate analysis. There is plentiful evidence available to reduce PA experts' ignorance about the people for whom PA is most relevant, important and difficult to achieve, including:

Social statistical data, including published analyses of it

This data is plentiful and accessible and would allow the made-up world of the SASA exemplars to be replaced by a factually based one. These data provide a detailed descriptive profile of population characteristics, socio-economic variables, characteristics and dynamics of poverty and disadvantage and patterns of health including the association of PA with health outcomes. Useful sources include the UK census, health survey, 'living in Britain', etc. They include focused analyses of some of the key variables that appear in SEMs – for example, families, detailing patterns of family structure, size, household composition, revealing how these vary with the social gradient (e.g. higher incidence of lone parent households, low-income households and larger families in low-income groups) At the time of writing, the UK office for National statistics holds over 1600 data sets categorised as 'health', 2000 on 'society' and 4000 on the environment. They provide substantial data on the geographic distribution of the population and the factors driving population change (increases/decreases in births, deaths and migration); and on topics such as families and older people, and other subgroups of specific relevance to the PA agenda. Policymakers and researchers make wide use of such data, making it something of an anomaly that academics providing guidance on physical activity do not. When they do, they will reveal an uncompromising picture of health inequalities, correlated to the social gradient. This recasts the health agenda:

> This link between social conditions and health is not a footnote to the 'real' concerns with health – health care and unhealthy behaviours – it should become the main focus. (Marmot 2010b, p. 4)

Research that examines how people are affected by adverse circumstances

Exposure to stressors in the social and physical environment is associated with both short-term changes in physiology, perceptions and behaviour; and longer-term risk of adverse outcomes including cardiovascular disease, diabetes and anxiety disorders (Thompson *et al.* 2015, p. 18). Between 2009 and 2011, the period during which the SASA report was produced, 2.5 million children were classed as living in poverty, along with 5.6 m working-age adults (Brewer *et al.* 2011). This equates to 1-in-5 children (19.7%), and nearly 1-in-6 working-age adults (16%); a further ~23% of pensioners (2.6 m people) were also in poverty. Evidence on the effects of material deprivation in the UK and internationally has a long tradition (e.g. Haan *et al.* 1987, Wilson *et al.* 2004, Weaver *et al.* 2014, in Thompson *et al.* 2015, p. 18), especially in periods of economic downturn or policy priority (the interwar depression; mass unemployment in the 1980s; child poverty in the 1990s; post-2008 austerity), and includes research into income poverty, food insecurity, low-quality housing and poor living environments. Among this work are also bodies of research addressing the complex and interrelated effects of deprivation on particular population groups, including, for example, women; lone parents; minority ethnic communities and of course older age adults.

> There is a strong strand of psychosocial work which holds particular interest for PA behaviourists: it consistently shows that material hardship induces high levels of stress that are disabling and are associated with increases in depressive illnesses, suicide and para suicide. As a result, coping mechanisms and capacity for agency are reduced – not through inadequacy, but as a rational, and involuntary, response to hardship. (Tomlinson and Walker 2009)

Evidence such as this may give us pause about policy approaches that focus on 'motivating' people to be active. As Bambra warns, policies are unlikely to succeed when they 'attempt to tackle health inequalities by trying to "empower" people or encouraging them to feel happier, more confident or more responsible, without necessarily addressing the key, underlying issues' (Bambra *et al.* 2011, p. 403).

Research which examines people's experiences of being active in everyday life, including the constraints they encounter

There has been a growth in UK-specific analyses of this type, stimulated by the award of the 2012 Olympic and Paralympic Games to London in 2005, with its claims of a legacy of increased sport participation that would benefit national health. As well as increasing funding to researchers, the 'legacy' agenda fostered public investment in initiatives to increase sports participation, some especially targeted at inactive people. In the period since the games, major programmes led by national lead agency Sport England have also had a remit to improve the evidence base, through rigorous evaluations; two programmes (Get healthy, get into sport (2013–2016) and its successor, Get healthy, get active (from 2016) have channelled more than £12 million into community-focussed initiatives accompanied by rigorous evaluations from which evidence is beginning to emerge. Other detailed analyses include Hills, Bradford and Johnston's (2013) study of national charity StreetGames' legacy-building programmes in disadvantaged areas; Edwards *et al.* (2015) analysis poverty and access to young people; and Mansfield *et al.* (2015) evaluation of a complex community intervention to encourage inactive people to be active.

Implicit in the above is the need for recognition of qualitative methodology. The area of physical activity exposes qualitative researchers very directly to resistance rooted in deep paradigmatic differences. This is epitomised by the oft-cited 'hierarchy of evidence' for health and medical research, which in its simplest form classes randomised controlled trials as the 'gold standard' of research and does not explicitly recognise qualitative research at all. Lester and O'Reilly (2015) suggest this leaves qualitative research arguing 'from the bottom of the pyramid' for its value, but this may understate its growing use in cognate areas. Qualitative methods are now well-established within research method training in university first and postgraduate degree programmes in public health (e.g. Tod and Hurst 2014), and increasingly feature in guidance for practitioners – e.g. *How to use qualitative research evidence when making decisions about interventions* (Department of Health, State Government of Victoria 2010) and *Using qualitative research to assess your impact* (New Philanthropy Capital/CLINKS 2014). If qualitative researchers in health are currently in an 'interesting position, somewhere between acceptance and promotion' (Lester and O'Reilly 2015, p. 628), this initial level of entry might be leveraged to achieve fuller participation within the PA expert community.

Diversifying the knowledge community

We have seen above that there is plentiful relevant additional evidence available to improve understanding of the factors affecting people's physical activity. A strong argument can be made for incorporating this knowledge into the evidence base to inform PA policy. Whether this argument is persuasive enough to convince the PA expert community as currently composed is less certain. In 2011 the SASA report dealt with the topic of 'health inequalities' in 111 words, in a brief section concerned only with 'inequalities' in levels of physical activity – between girls and boys, women and men, majority and minority ethnic groups and households of different income levels. Descriptions were brief – the statement about household income in its entirety was 'Physical activity is lower in low-income households'. There was no acknowledgement of structural inequalities in the UK population, or their influence on health.

This limited treatment is indicative of the lack of social science sensibility in much PA policy. It raises questions about whether the current knowledge community is equipped to identify, evaluate and make best use of the wider evidence available. As noted, the work of the SASA expert working groups was contemporaneous with the Marmot review, yet made no reference the Marmot report itself, or to the health inequalities agenda it addressed. The 2016 investigation into 'The Science of Using Science' on the use of research by decision makers (Langer *et al.* 2016) found that while decision makers were responsive to active, structured interventions, passive approaches – for example, making evidence 'available' without supporting strategies to motivate and guide users – had no effect on uptake. This suggests that simply making more diverse evidence available to the existing expert community on PA is unlikely to effect change; instead, action is needed to disrupt current structures and processes that shape the use of evidence in this area. Three dimensions to consider are:

- *Diversifying the disciplinary base*: participation of social scientists in the knowledge community that informs PA policy, to ensure knowledge pertaining to the social processes underpinning health inequalities is included in the evidence base, including the emerging literature on engaging inactive groups through sport; with this comes use of associated methodologies, especially the use of qualitative approaches advocated above.
- *Including expert knowledge from outside the academic community*: reliance on an academic evidence base may be insufficient to inform a complex, multilevel policy area. The Marmot review offered an extended model, also incorporating extensive consultation (including meetings, seminars and workshops) with public, private and third sector organisations, across a broad welfare agenda (including health, community, housing, youth and education). An online consultation was also conducted.

- *Obtaining lay knowledge*: individuals are considered to be unreliable informants about some aspects of their own health (e.g. Nisbett and Wilson 1977) – self-report measures of activity are notoriously inaccurate (Warren *et al.* 2010). They are however expert commentators on their own complex individual lifestyles and biographies within which their activity occurs or is constrained. Physical activity guidance would benefit from fuller knowledge about the explanations underlying activity patterns, including the practical, emotional and experiential factors that affect people, especially those who are inactive.

Translating and mobilising knowledge on the social determinants of health

The availability of evidence on the SDH would not automatically lead to its use in policy and practice. The WHO recognised this, noting that addressing health inequity through attention to social determinants would require investment in formal training of policymakers and health practitioners (WHO 2008a, p. 44). Golden and Earp (2012) view social science grand theory as highly relevant to healthcare but warn that although the 'appropriation of sociological perspectives.... makes sense, practitioners may be unfamiliar with these perspectives unless they are regularly included in public health training programs'. They further caution that 'even if taught.. ..these grand theories do not usually include the types of operationalized constructs that characterize psychological theories' (Golden and Earp 2012, p. 370). This suggests that if physical activity guidance is to benefit from the evidence about the SDH outlined in this paper, attention will need to be paid to how such knowledge is translated for potential users.

This issue of research 'use' is prominent in public health and has considerable wider currency – Breckon and Dodson (2016) refer to 'a whole industry' arising 'to help find more ways to link research to practice' (2016, p. 4). Their practice-focused discussion of *'Using Evidence – What Works?'* distils the key guidance from the 'science of using science' project on translating research for users. It identifies six mechanisms that can be effective: building awareness of evidence; building agreement on relevant policy questions and the evidence required to answer them; providing access to evidence; facilitating interaction between researchers and research users; developing users' skills to access and make sense of evidence and influencing decision-making structures and processes to include research use. In each of these the emphasis is on 'active' approaches that increase users' capability, motivation and opportunity (CMO) to use research evidence. At the practice level, Smith *et al.* (2015) provide a particularly valuable example of the forms in which physical activity knowledge might be made accessible to health professionals, through their exploration of narratives as a vehicle for knowledge translation for health professionals. A narrative approach exploits the capacity of qualitative data for capturing and conveying the 'everyday' manifestation of the SDH, and furthermore mirrors the use of 'examples' in the SASA report. The latter point may offer a potential entry point for persuading the current expert community to recognise the value of such methodologies; more fundamentally, it signifies the need for specific action to ensure such shifts occur.

Conclusion

Academic expert communities are significant gatekeepers to knowledge in policy-related fields that impact people's lives. The processes through this influence is exerted require continuous scrutiny to reflect on the voices and interests that are represented (Shortall 2013).

In the UK PA policy, there is little question that guidance for promoting physically activity to the population are scientifically informed. The concern of many social scientists is not about the quality of evidence, but its scope. At present PA is not drawing on expert analysis of SDH, despite a lengthy and continuing international literature documenting the impact of material and social deprivation on health. PA policy that is informed by such research will be better equipped to address the complexities of people's situations and the factors that constrain them from being active. This involves bringing together two complementary bodies of knowledge – health behaviourist accounts of physical activity, and socials science accounts of the SDH. This paper has also suggested, however, that PA policy will also benefit from an evidence base that is expanded in other ways too, and looks beyond academic expertise to other forms of expert knowledge.

Social scientists within the academic sport science community can help bridge this chasm, by contributing social scientific theories, methodologies and knowledge to this area. Such offers must be constructive: to dismiss health behaviourists as not addressing 'context' is not adequate, when their theoretical frameworks do; to argue that they do not address it 'properly' is not sufficient without elucidation and to elucidate by only offering grand theory is not only unhelpful but actively counterproductive, reinforcing the notion that 'social influences' exist only as some abstraction that is beyond translation into practice. Tangible specifics are required to demonstrate how social science knowledge can enhance understanding of health behaviour and efforts to enhance it.

The use evidence on health inequalities will not automatically guarantee a shift in PA policy focus. Bambra *et al.* (2011) warn against policies 'which attempt to tackle health inequalities by trying to "empower" people or encouraging them to feel happier, more confident or more responsible, without necessarily addressing the key, underlying issue' (Bambra *et al.* 2011, p. 403). Expanding the body of knowledge underpinning PA guidance is however a crucial step. It will rebalance the content of the underpinning evidence, in quite transformative ways.

Closing the health gap is a long-term project (WHO 2008a, 2008b). Closing the knowledge gap could occur in the blink of an eye – if the research communities involved could just make eye contact in the first place.

Disclosure Statement

No potential conflict of interest was reported by the author(s).

References

Acheson, D. (Chairman), 1998. *Independent enquiry into inequalities in health*. London: The Stationery Office.

Bambra, C., *et al.*, 2011. A labour of Sisyphus? Public policy and health inequalities research from the black and Acheson reports to the Marmot review. *Journal of Epidemiology & Community Health*, 65, 399–406. doi:10.1136/jech.2010.111195

Bandura, A., 2004. Health promotion by social cognitive means. *Health Education & Behavior*, 31 (2), 143–164. doi:10.1177/1090198104263660

Banks, J., Nazroo, J., and Steptoe, A., 2012. *The dynamics of ageing: evidence from the English longitudinal study of ageing 2002–10*. London: Institute of Fiscal Studies.

Black, D. (Chair), 1980. *Inequalities in health*. London: DHSS.

Breckon, J. and Dodson, J., 2016. *Using evidence: what works? A discussion paper*. London: Alliance for Useful Evidence.

Brewer, M., Browne, J., and Joyce, R., 2011. *Child and working-age poverty from 2010 to 2020, commentary 121*. London: Institute for Fiscal Studies.

Brewer, M., *et al.*, 2009. *Poverty and inequality in the UK: 2009, commentary 109*. London: Institute for Fiscal Studies.

Burke, N., *et al.*, 2009. Theorizing social context: rethinking behavioral theory. *Health Education & Behavior*, 36 (Suppl. 1), 55S–70S. doi:10.1177/1090198109335338

Department of Health, 2011. *Start active, stay active: a report on physical activity from the four home countries' chief medical officers*. London: HMSO.

Department of Health, State Government of Victoria, 2010. *How to use qualitative research evidence when making decisions about interventions*. Melbourne: State Government of Victoria. Available from: http://www.health.vic.gov.au/health promotion/evidence_evaluation/cdp_tools.htm [Accessed 24 January 2016].

Edwards, G., *et al.*, 2015. *Moving the goal posts: poverty and access to sport for young people. CASE report 95*. London: London School of Economics.

European Commission, 2013. *Health inequalities in the EU — final report of a consortium. Consortium lead: Sir Michael Marmot*. Available from: http://ec.europa.eu/health/social_determinants/docs/healthinequalitiesineu_2013_en.pdf [Accessed 14 December 2015].

Glanz, K., Saelens, B.E., and Frank, L.D., 2005. Healthy nutrition environments: concepts and measures. *American Journal of Health Promotion*, 19 (5), 330–333. doi:10.4278/0890-1171-19.5.330

Golden, S.D. and Earp, J.A.L., 2012. Social ecological approaches to individuals and their contexts: twenty years of health education & behavior health promotion interventions. *Health Education & Behavior*, 39 (3), 364–372. doi:10.1177/1090198111418634

Golden, S.D., *et al.*, 2015. Upending the social ecological model to guide health promotion efforts toward policy and environmental change. *Health Education & Behavior*, 42 (1S), 8S–14S. doi:10.1177/1090198115575098

Graham, H. and Kelly, M.P., 2004. *Health inequalities: concepts, frameworks and policy*. London: HAD.

Haan, N., Kaplan, G.A., and Camacho, T., 1987. Poverty and health: prospective evidence from the Alameda county study. *American Journal of Epidemiology*, 125, 989–998.

Hills, L., Bradford, S., and Johnston, C., 2013. *Building a participation legacy from the London 2012 Olympic and Paralympic games in disadvantage areas. Report for StreetGames*. London: Brunel University London.

Irwin, A. and Scali, E., 2007. Action on the social determinants of health: a historical perspective. *Global Public Health*, 2 (3), 235–256. doi:10.1080/17441690601106304

Langer, L., Tripney, J., and Gough, D., 2016. *The science of using science: researching the use of research evidence in decision-making*. London: EPPI-Centre, Social Science Research Unit, UCL Institute of Education, University College London.

Lester, J. and O'Reilly, M., 2015. Is evidence-based practice a threat to the progress of the qualitative community? Arguments from the bottom of the pyramid. *Qualitative Inquiry*, 21 (7), 628–632. doi:10.1177/1077800414563808

Mansfield, L., *et al.*, 2015. The health and sport engagement (HASE) intervention and evaluation project: protocol for the design, outcome, process and economic evaluation of a complex community sport intervention to increase levels of physical activity. *BMJ Open*, 5 (10), e009276–e009276. doi:10.1136/bmjopen-2015-009276

Marmot, M., 2010a. *The Marmot review: fair society, healthy lives strategic review of health inequalities in England post 2010*. Marmot Review Final Report. London: University College London.

Marmot, M., 2010b. *The Marmot review: fair society, healthy lives strategic review of health inequalities in England post 2010*. Marmot Review Executive Summary. London: University College London.

McLeroy, K.R., *et al.*, 1988. An ecological perspective on health promotion programs. *Health Education & Behavior*, 15 (4), 351–377. doi:10.1177/109019818801500401

New Philanthropy Capital/CLINKS, 2014. *Improving evidence: Using qualitative research to assess your impact*. Available from: http://www.clinks.org/sites/default/files/QualGuidanceFinal.pdf [Accessed 22 January 2016].

NHLBI, 2004. *Ecological model of diet, physical activity, and obesity*. US Department of Health and Human Services, National Heart, Blood and Lung Institute. Available from: http://www.nhlbi.nih.gov/research/reports/2004-obesity/abstracts-fig1 [Accessed 14 December 2015].

NICE, 2008. *Promoting physical activity in the workplace*. NICE public health guidance 13. Manchester: National Institute for Health and Clinical Excellence.

NICE, 2009. *Promoting physical activity for children and young people*. NICE public health guidance 17. Manchester: National Institute for Health and Clinical Excellence.

NICE, 2010. *Prevention of cardiovascular disease*. NICE public health guidance 25. Manchester: National Institute for Health and Clinical Excellence.

NICE, 2013a. *Obesity*. NICE clinical guideline 43. Manchester: National Institute for Health and Clinical Excellence.

NICE, 2013b. *Physical activity: brief advice for adults in primary care*. NICE public health guidance 44. Manchester: National Institute for Health and Clinical Excellence.

NICE, 2014. *Exercise referral schemes to promote physical activity*. NICE public health guidance 54. Manchester: National Institute for Health and Clinical Excellence.

Nisbett, R. and Wilson, T., 1977. Telling more than we can know: verbal reports on mental processes. *Psychological Review*, 84, 231–259. doi:10.1037/0033-295X.84.3.231

ONS, 2013. *Life expectancy at birth and at age 65 for local areas in England and Wales: 2009–11*. London: HMSO.

ONS, 2015. *Families and households, 2015*. London: HMSO.

Public Health England, 2013. *Our strategic priorities 2013–2014*. London: Public Health England.

Public Health England, 2014. *Everybody active, every day. An evidence-based approach to physical activity*. London: Public Health England.

Sallis, J.F., 9 Apr 2009. *Using research to create a less obesogenic world*. Presentation to the Texas Obesity Research Center. Available from: http://sallis.ucsd.edu/Documents/Pubs_documents/Slides_HoustonObesity_040909.pdf [Accessed 9 December 2015].

Shortall, S., 2013. The role of subjectivity and knowledge power struggles in the formation of public policy. *Sociology*, 47 (6), 1088–1103. doi:10.1177/0038038512454950

Smith, B., *et al.*, 2015. Narrative as a knowledge translation tool for facilitating impact: translating physical activity knowledge to disabled people and health professionals. *Health Psychology*, 34 (4), 303–313. doi:10.1037/hea0000113

Solar, O. and Irwin, A., 2010. *A conceptual framework for action on the social determinants of health*. Geneva: WHO.

Sport England, 2016. *Towards and active nation. Strategy 2016–2021*. London: Sport England.

Stokols, D., 1992. Establishing and maintaining healthy environments: toward a social ecology of health promotion. *American Psychologist*, 47 (1), 6–22. doi:10.1037/0003-066X.47.1.6

Stokols, D., 1996. Translating social ecological theory into guidelines for community health promotion. *American Journal of Health Promotion*, 10, 282–298. doi:10.4278/0890-1171-10.4.282

Story, M., *et al.*, 2008. Creating healthy food and eating environments: policy and environmental approaches. *Annual Review of Public Health*, 29, 253–272. doi:10.1146/annurev.publhealth.29.020907.090926

Thompson, C., *et al.*, 2015. "Everyone was looking at you smiling": East London residents' experiences of the 2012 Olympics and its legacy on the social determinants of health. *Health & Place*, 36, 18–24. doi:10.1016/j.healthplace.2015.08.008

Tod, A.M. and Hurst, J., 2014. *Health and inequality: applying public health research to policy and practice*. London: Routledge.

Tomlinson, M. and Walker, R., 2009. *Coping with complexity: child and adult poverty*. London: Child Poverty Action Group.

Warren, J.M., et al.; for the Experts Panel, 2010. Assessment of physical activity – a review of methodologies with reference to epidemiological research: a report of the exercise physiology section of the European association of cardiovascular prevention and rehabilitation. *European Journal of Cardiovascular Prevention & Rehabilitation*, 17, 127–139. doi:10.1097/HJR.0b013e32832ed875

Weaver, R.R., *et al.*, 2014. Health capabilities and diabetes self-management: the impact of economic, social, and cultural resources. *Social Science & Medicine*, 102, 58–68. doi:10.1016/j.socscimed.2013.11.033

WHO, 2008a. *Closing the gap in a generation: health equity through action on the social determinants of health* Commission on Social Determinants of Health Report Geneva: WHO.

WHO, 2008b. *Closing the gap in a generation: health equity through action on the social determinants of health* Commission on Social Determinants of Health Executive Summary. Geneva: WHO.

WHO, 2010. *Global recommendations on physical activity for health*. Geneva: WHO.

WHO Regional Office for Europe, 2016. *Physical activity strategy for the WHO European region 2016–2025*. Copenhagen: WHO.

Wilson, K., *et al.*, 2004. Linking perceptions of neighbourhood to health in Hamilton, Canada. *Journal of Epidemiology & Community Health*, 58, 192–198. doi:10.1136/jech.2003.014308

Winch, P., 2012. *Ecological models and multilevel interventions: health behavior change at the individual, household and community levels*. John Hopkins University. Available from: http://ocw.jhsph.edu/courses/healthbehaviorchange/PDFs/C14_2011.pdf [Accessed 9 November 2015].

Wright, C., Lodge, H., and Jacobson, B., 2012. *Childs play? The ante natal to adolescent health legacy in the Olympic boroughs*. London: London Health Observatory.

Should we privilege sport for health? The comparative effectiveness of UK Government investment in sport as a public health intervention

Mike Weed

ABSTRACT
Claimed links between sport and health are pervasive. This paper interrogates evidence for the UK Government's theory of change that sport can be used as a public health intervention to increase physical activity among the less and least active to deliver improvements in the physical health of the population. Regardless of efficacy evidence linking sport participation to improvements in physical health, effectiveness evidence to support the processes by which it is assumed that sport participation can be increased among the less and least active is unclear.

This paper reviews evidence from controlled designs and conducts two primary time-series analyses of current and historical national survey data explore evidence for the effectiveness of sport as a public health intervention for physical health.

Results show that there is no top-tier evidence from controlled designs to support, and some second-tier evidence from time-series analyses to undermine, the effectiveness of sport as a public health intervention to increase physical activity among the less and least active. Despite sustained UK Government investment, sport participation has stagnated or fallen from 1990, while since 1997 an additional 10% of the population have become physically active in ways that do not include sport.

Consequently, there is no evidence that sport is effective as a public health intervention to improve physical health. In comparison to the opportunity cost of not implementing potentially effective alternatives that promote wider physical activity choices that do not privilege sport, investment in sport as a public health intervention may cause net harm to the physical health of the UK population.

Introduction

The claimed link between sport and health is pervasive. The United Nations believes 'Sport's unique and universal power to attract, motivate and inspire makes it a highly effective tool for engaging and empowering individuals, communities and even countries to take action to improve their health' (SDPIWG 2008, p. 27). Similarly, the World Health Organisation claims 'the sports movement has a great influence on the level of health-enhancing physical activity in the general population' (WHOROE 2011, p. 15). In the UK, government justification for sport participation targets linked to the London 2012 Olympic and Paralympic Games made explicit claims about the impact of sport on health, particularly obesity (e.g., DCMS 2010). Furthermore, regardless of the contemporary government policy for sport, the implied justificatory link to health is never far away (e.g., DCMS 2002).

Now, however, the UK Government sport strategy, 'Sporting Future: A New Strategy for an Active Nation' (Cabinet Office 2015), puts the link to health front and centre. The Prime Minister at the time of publication claimed that sport 'encourages us all to lead healthier and more active lives' (Cameron 2015, p. 6), and the Minister for Sport that 'The impact sport has on physical and mental health… shows the power to transform people's wellbeing and create a fitter, healthier and happier nation' (Crouch 2015, p. 9). Furthermore, the Minister explicitly links this impact to major public health concerns: 'This has never been more important, when we are battling with growing levels of obesity and diabetes, mental health problems and other conditions associated with inactivity that cost the nation £7.4 bn each year' (p. 9).

The somewhat hyperbolic Ministerial claims are, however, underpinned by an explicit and fundamental change in the way that government supports, funds, and provides for sport. Specifically, sport will no longer be the sought outcome from government sport policy, rather:

> funding decisions will be made on the basis of the social good that sport and physical activity can deliver, not simply on the number of participants. We are redefining what success looks like in sport by concentrating on five key outcomes: physical wellbeing, mental wellbeing, individual development, social and community development and economic development. (Cabinet Office 2015, p. 10)

This approach comes with specific and measurable success indicators which, for physical wellbeing, are stated as being an increase in the percentage of the population in England meeting the Chief Medical Officer's (CMO) guidelines for physical activity and a decrease in the percentage of the population in England that are physically inactive (Cabinet Office 2015, p. 74). These success indicators clearly show that government is seeking to use sport as a public health intervention to improve the physical health of the less and least active. The most recent Health Survey for England data (2012) shows that 39% of the population in England are *less active*, in that they do not meet CMO guidelines that 150 min of moderate to vigorous physical activity each week is necessary to achieve health benefits. In addition, there is a subgroup within this *less active* group that comprise the *least active* 23% of the population, who do less than 30 min activity each week. It is this least active group that government considers to be 'physically inactive'. Thus, the UK Government's theory of change is that sport can be used as a public health intervention to increase the physical activity levels of less and least active members of the population (the 39% that do not meet CMO guidelines) to deliver improvements in the physical health of the population. The purpose of this paper is to interrogate the evidence for this theory of change, and in doing so assess the effectiveness of sport as a public health intervention to improve physical health,[1] including the possibility that, in comparison to the opportunity cost of not implementing alternatives that do not privilege sport, the UK Government investment in sport may cause net harm to population health.

But what are the alternatives? Broadly speaking, sport may be contrasted to wider activity choices including formal exercise and informal physical activity. While some approaches to defining sport have attempted to do so according to its features (e.g., being rule bound, or involving organised participation), others provide lists of activities (e.g., football, tennis). When the concern is with using sport as a public health intervention, the most appropriate definition is one that focuses on population perceptions, and these will be shaped by culture, history, school curricula, and media coverage in the population concerned. Therefore, while not precise and definitive, the definition of sport used for this paper is the set of activities that have come to be regarded as such by the UK population. These activities can be contrasted with wider activity choices, including formal exercise activities, such as aerobics or visiting the gym, that are undertaken for the purpose of exercising, and informal physical activity, such as gardening or walking a dog, in which the activity is largely incidental. Obviously the definitional boundaries between sport, exercise, and physical activity are fluid, but this reflects the fluidity of perceptions among the UK population. The advantage of this approach is that it recognises that if an individual perceives something to be sport, then their response will be determined by their attitudes towards sport, and this is the key to understanding the potential of sport as a public health intervention.

In considering distinctions between sport and physical activity, Sporting Future (Cabinet Office 2015, p. 27) notes that, 'Overwhelmingly, those who responded to the consultation told us that these distinctions are unhelpful, outdated and irrelevant'. Of course, those who responded to the strategy consultation are sport stakeholders, not the populations that are the targets of sport as a public health intervention. As such, a key question will be whether such populations, and specifically the less and least active that the strategy is seeking to target, also see such distinctions as unhelpful, outdated, and irrelevant? Or whether continuing to privilege sport by delivering physical activity under the auspices of sport as proposed by the strategy will come to be seen by the less and least active as branding those activities as sport, with their responses then being determined by their attitudes towards sport? This is a question to which the paper will return in its conclusion.

The first section of the paper provides its context, exploring the logic models that underpin the UK Government's theory of change that sport can be used as a public health intervention to increase physical activity among the less and least active to deliver improvements in the physical health of the population. It also explores how far top-tier evidence from studies with controlled designs supports the efficacy and effectiveness logic models, and identifies a lack of evidence for the latter. Given the lack of effectiveness evidence from controlled designs, the second section outlines two time-series analyses of current and historical national survey data presented in this paper. The results section notes that these time-series analyses provide no evidence to support, and some evidence to undermine, the effectiveness logic model that underpins the theory of change. The discussion section then explores provider acceptance, noting that sport stakeholders either do not appreciate or do not accept, that the effectiveness of sport as a public health intervention is not proven. The concepts of opportunity cost and comparative effectiveness are also discussed, and an extended theory of change and logic model that includes alternative ways of becoming active other than sport is suggested. Finally, and in conclusion, the paper notes that sport may not be the most effective public health intervention to improve physical health, and that, in comparison to the opportunity cost of not implementing potentially effective alternatives that promote wider activity choices that do not privilege sport, current UK Government investment in sport may result in net harm to population health.

Context

Public policy projects are increasingly expected to be underpinned by a 'theory of change' structure detailing how project objectives and inputs are assumed to lead through particular activities to project outputs and then to sought outcomes (PricewaterhouseCoopers 2009, p. 17). This theory of change structure is derived from basic programme theory (Rogers 2008) in which logic models are developed to detail and underpin theories of change (PricewaterhouseCoopers 2009), and the UK Government recommends that this approach should underpin any social policy intervention (HM Treasury 2013). A programme theory identifies which outcomes are sought but, importantly, the underpinning logic models also identify the processes by which such outcomes are assumed to be achievable. It is a way of ensuring that the effectiveness of public policy interventions can be measured, and that they are not speculative experiments on the public (House of Commons Health Committee 2009).

There are two logic models that underpin the government's theory of change for sport as a public health intervention. First, an efficacy logic model, which details the processes by which participation in sport is assumed to improve physical health; second, an effectiveness logic model, which details the processes by which it is assumed that sport participation can be increased among the less and least active. This section now details these logic models and explores existing evidence to underpin them, focusing on what has come to be accepted to be 'top-tier' evidence for interventions (Canadian Task Force on the Periodic Health Examination 1979, Sackett 1989, Barton 2000, Burns *et al.* 2011, Haynes *et al.* 2012), that from controlled designs (including randomised controlled trials, other controlled trials and case-controlled longitudinal cohort studies).

The efficacy logic model for sport as a public health intervention

Efficacy evidence relates to the performance of an intervention under ideal and controlled conditions (Singal *et al.* 2014), which in this case is that members of the public are compliant with the intervention and participate in sport. Consequently, efficacy evidence is concerned with the health benefits sport participation can confer, and the efficacy logic model is straightforward (Figure 1). The efficacy logic model is that sport participation results in increased physical activity which results in improved physical health, and the robustness of the evidence underpinning this logic model is uncontested. A recent systematic review for the UK Government's Culture and Sport Evidence programme[2] (Taylor *et al.* 2015) found 101 sources published between 1996 and 2012 that provided 'strong evidence' from controlled designs that participation in sport has a significant impact on primary and secondary prevention of non-communicable conditions via biological mechanisms that increase fitness and reduce obesity (Taylor *et al.* 2015). These conclusions assume the first step in the efficacy logic model, that sport increases physical activity, and focus on the second step, that physical activity improves health. If this first step is assumed, then a long-standing body of evidence from controlled designs shows physical activity improves physical health, which was summarised in the UK for the CMOs to underpin physical activity recommendations (DoH 2011), and more recently in Australia (Brown *et al.* 2012). These sources each provide evidence that can be summarised in an all-cause mortality curve that shows an inverse curvilinear relationship between physical activity participation and all-cause mortality risk reduction (see Figure 2). This curve shows that the greatest health benefits are gained from moving those that do less than 30 min physical activity per week to doing 60–90 min per week, where the all-cause mortality risk reduction is 15–20%. The curve also shows that at the CMO's recommended level of 150 min per week the all-cause mortality risk reduction is 25%. While there is a further risk reduction above 150 min – for example, the next 180 min of activity adds a further circa 10% risk reduction – the greatest public health benefits are clearly those gained by targeting the less and least active. Consequently, there is good top-tier evidence from controlled designs for the efficacy logic model underpinning the government's theory of change for sport as a public health intervention.

The effectiveness logic model for sport as a public health intervention

While there is good evidence for the efficacy logic model underpinning the government's theory of change for sport as a public health intervention, it is limited to the impact of sport as a public

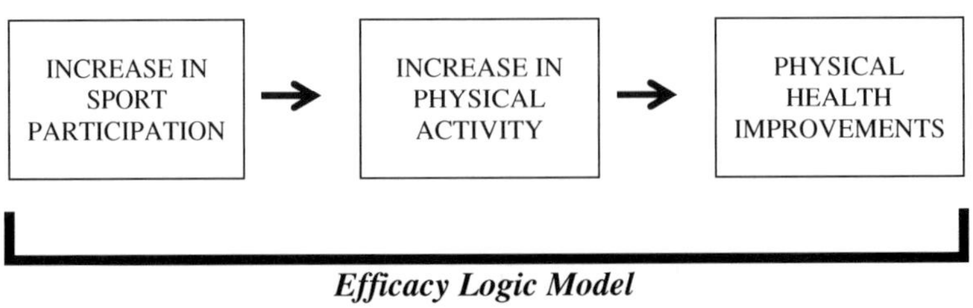

Figure 1. Efficacy logic model for sport as a public health intervention to improve physical health.

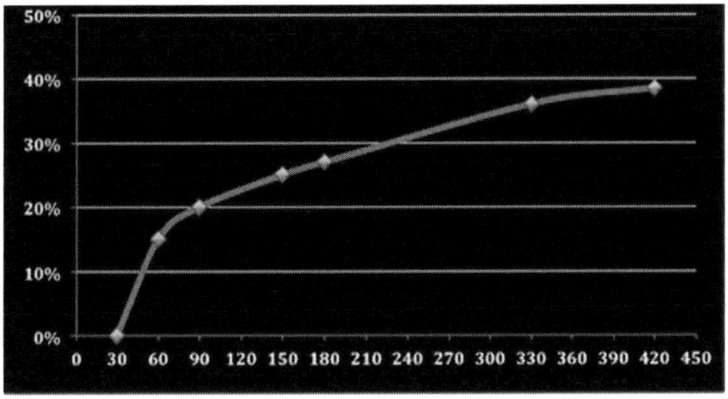

Figure 2. All cause mortality risk reduction by weekly minutes of moderate-to-vigorous physical activity. Source: derived from Brown *et al.* (2012).

health intervention only in the ideal circumstance in which people participate in sport. To understand the performance of sport as a public health intervention under 'real world' conditions, an effectiveness logic model must be developed (Singal *et al.* 2014), which details the processes by which it is assumed that sport participation can be increased among the UK Government's target audiences, the less and least active. Given it is dealing with processes leading to changes in attitudes and behaviours, the effectiveness logic model is more complex (Figure 3) than the efficacy logic model.

The effectiveness logic model starts with people's awareness of sport, from which the assumptions are that they then become interested in participating, they face no barriers to participation, or they overcome barriers, thus creating effective demand, supply is available to match demand, and participation results (Marsh *et al.* 2010). At the point of participation, the effectiveness logic model connects with the efficacy logic model described in Figure 1, with sport participation raising physical activity levels resulting in improved health. The effectiveness logic model can be used to highlight where intervention strategies are required, from which evidence to underpin the logic model can be derived. For example, it might be assumed that there is effective demand for sport participation, but that there are shortfalls in available supply. This is a convenient assumption to make, as a shortfall in supply is easy to address given sufficient investment. This assumption underpinned the UK Government's £135 million investment in supply infrastructure to raise sport participation through the London 2012 Olympic and Paralympic Games (Sport England 2010). Unfortunately, Weed *et al.*'s (2015) analysis of the sport participation legacy from London 2012 suggests this was a flawed assumption as there was little meaningful sustained increase in participation arising from hosting the games. A less convenient assumption is that there is interest in sport participation, but that structural and psychological barriers, such as lack of time or money, or fear of embarrassment, prevent this from becoming effective demand. There is a long history of initiatives that have sought to address structural barriers (Collins 2014), while Sport England's recent 'This Girl Can' campaign[3] sought to help women and girls overcome psychological barriers. The least convenient assumption is that awareness of sport does not translate into interest. This assumption is least convenient for two reasons: first, because it suggests people are simply not interested in sport and, second, because it is the first step of the logic model, so even if interest is stimulated, there remain a number of further steps before interest becomes participation.

Unfortunately, however, top-tier evidence to underpin the assumptions of the effectiveness logic model for sport as a public health intervention is limited. For example, two Cochrane systematic reviews exploring the effect of interventions through sport organisations on increasing participation in sport (Priest *et al.* 2008a) and on healthy behaviour change (Priest *et al.* 2008b)

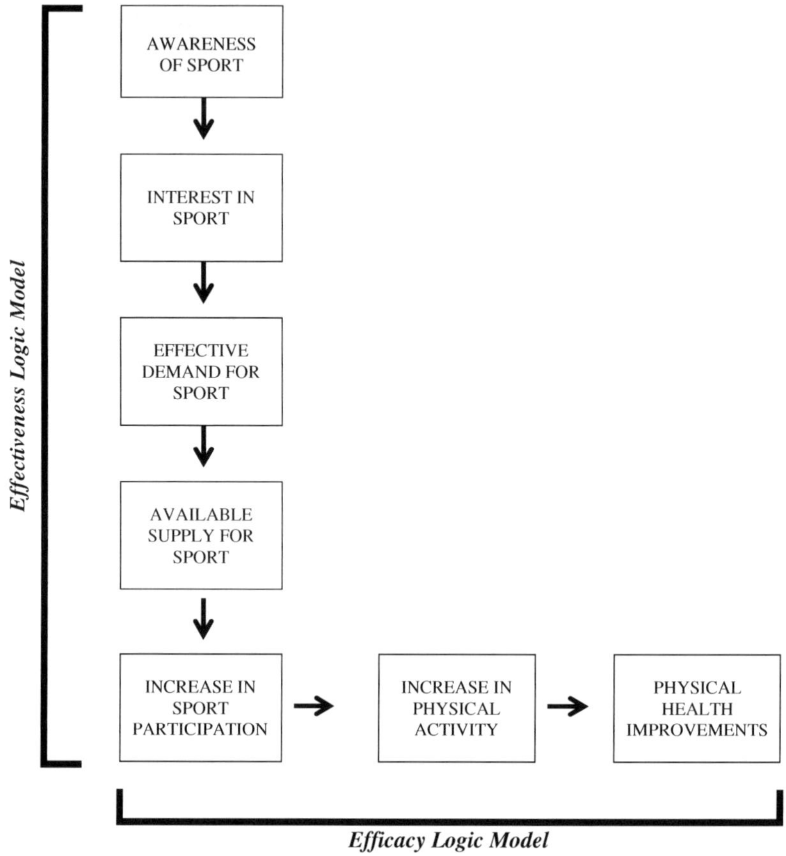

Figure 3. Effectiveness and efficacy logic models for sport as a public health intervention to improve physical health.

could, respectively, locate 'no rigorous studies evaluating the effects of interventions organised through sporting organisations to increase participation in sport' (Priest *et al.* 2008a, p. 2) and 'no rigorous studies evaluating the effectiveness of policy interventions organised through sporting organisations to increase healthy behaviours, attitudes, knowledge or the inclusion of health-oriented policies within the organisations' (Priest *et al.* 2008b, p. 2). Cavill *et al.* (2012), in a report commissioned by Sport England, suggest that this may be because there is no tradition of using controlled designs in sport. Consequently, their report examined evidence from controlled designs that focused on physical activity, but that Cavill *et al.* (2012) assessed as reporting sport specific results. A total of 11 studies were included, 10 of which focused on adults, from which Cavill *et al.* (2012) concluded: '[w]hile the body of evidence is not extensive, … there are a number of well-designed studies that provide evidence for the effectiveness of sporting interventions'. They identified 'group exercise sessions; use of running/jogging and static bikes and optional additional sessions at home' as well as 'counselling; fitness assessment; recording of activity levels; goal setting; and detailed follow-up' (p. 47) as effective aspects of the interventions. While this suggests that there may be evidence to underpin the assumptions of the effectiveness logic model, unfortunately a more detailed exploration of the included studies suggests otherwise.

Six of the studies considered by Cavill *et al.* (2012) included some delivery through sport organisations (Luepker *et al.* 1994, Kumpusalo *et al.* 1996, Brown *et al.* 2003, Elley *et al.* 2003, Lupton *et al.* 2003, Wendel-Vos *et al.* 2009), but some did not include sport. For example, Brown *et al.* (2003) reported on a walking programme, partially delivered through sport clubs, and Elley *et al.* (2003) reported on a home-based exercise and walking intervention with telephone support from an exercise specialist employed by a local sports foundation. Five studies showed no statistically significant increases in physical activity, and four were rated by a previous Cochrane review (Baker *et al.* 2011) as having a high risk of bias. One in ten participants in the home-based exercise and walking intervention (Elley *et al.* 2003) increased their physical activity to over 150 min per week after 12 months, but this study was assessed low quality by a previous Cochrane review (Foster *et al.* 2005), and that the exercise specialist was employed by a 'sports foundation' did not provide a meaningful sport element.

The remaining four studies considered by Cavill *et al.* (2012) focused on exercise prescription or referral in which sport was mentioned (Cunningham *et al.* 1987, Harland *et al.* 1999, Fujita *et al.* 2003, Petrella *et al.* 2003). Only one (Harland *et al.* 1999) explicitly included sport, but only as part of a wider motivational interview focused on 'all walking, cycling and other sports or leisure activities', which was ineffective in raising physical activity levels and was judged low quality by a previous Cochrane review (Foster *et al.* 2005). The remaining three interventions focused on older retired adults. Fujita *et al.* (2003) reported on exercise classes, but the only sport-related element was the use of a static cycling machine. While this intervention demonstrated large increases in physical activity, the intervention was very prescriptive, there was no real sport element, and the study was judged low quality by a previous Cochrane review (Foster *et al.* 2005). The two remaining interventions focused on walking and jogging (Cunningham *et al.* 1987) and a stepping fitness test together with self-selected physical activities, 'mostly walking in local parks and malls' (Petrella *et al.* 2003, p. 318). While both studies showed significant increase in fitness levels, neither included a post-intervention follow-up measure of physical activity, although Petrella *et al.* (2003), despite being assessed high quality by a previous Cochrane review (Foster *et al.* 2005), assumed that '[i]mplicit in the achievement of higher levels of fitness is a greater participation rate in exercise sessions during the intervention' (p. 321). Cunningham *et al.* (1987) had a semi-sporting focus on jogging, but was assessed low quality by a previous Cochrane review (Foster *et al.* 2005) and did not include a physical activity measure.

Consequently, despite Cavill, Richardson, and Foster's (2012) conclusions that well-designed studies provide evidence for the effectiveness of sporting interventions, the discussions above clearly show that any studies showing a significant positive outcome variously did not include a meaningful sport element, were judged to be of low quality or high risk of bias, and/or did not measure physical activity levels. Cavill, Richardson, and Foster (2012, pp. 47–48) did acknowledge studies 'tend to use measures of physical activity that mix sport with other types of physical activity including walking and cycling. This makes it very difficult to untangle the specific contribution of sport'. However, this caveat does not justify the conclusion that there is 'evidence for the effectiveness of sporting interventions' (Cavill *et al.* 2012, p. 47). Rather, based on the studies Cavill *et al.* (2012) considered, the opposite is true: there are no well-designed studies of interventions with a meaningful sport element that can provide evidence to underpin the effectiveness logic model for sport as a public health intervention. Furthermore, a search of Google Scholar and the Cochrane Reviews Library, conducted on 10 December 2015 using the search terms <health>, <sport>, and <participation> and the date parameters 2010–2015, identified only one additional source utilising a controlled design to assess the effectiveness of a sport intervention to improve physical health in non-disabled adults. However, this source contained only a report of the method, and a follow up paper containing results could not be located. This suggests that the evidence base has not developed significantly since the Cavill *et al.* (2012) review, and there remains no top-tier evidence to underpin the effectiveness logic model for sport as a public health intervention.

The UK Government's theory of change is that sport can be used as a public health intervention to increase physical activity among the less and least active to deliver improvements in the physical health of the population. The discussions above show that the credibility of this theory of change is dependent not on the efficacy logic model, for which there is good evidence that sport participation leads to physical health benefits, but on the effectiveness logic model which details the processes by which it is assumed that sport participation can be increased among the less and least active. Unfortunately, it appears that there is no existing top-tier evidence from controlled designs available to underpin the assumptions of the effectiveness logic model.

Method

Given the lack of existing top-tier evidence from controlled designs, this paper develops two time-series analyses of data from current and historical national surveys of sport participation in the UK to explore the extent to which they provide evidence to underpin the effectiveness logic model for sport as a public health intervention for physical health. In the absence of top-tier evidence from controlled designs, such time-series designs have become accepted as second-tier evidence that can contribute to informing policy (Canadian Task Force on the Periodic Health Examination 1979, Sackett 1989, Barton 2000, Burns *et al.* 2011).

The first analysis comprises a review and reanalysis of current English national survey data to understand the size and the propensity to change of the less and least active that are not currently engaged with sport. Three recent and current national surveys provide repeated cross-section time-series data on sport participation: the Active People survey provides data between 2007 and 2015, the Health Survey for England provides data between 1998 and 2012, and the Taking Part survey provides data between 2006 and 2012. Taking Part is an interviewer completed survey, undertaken in the home, of participation in a range of cultural and recreational activities, and has an annual sample size of around 15,000. From 2013, results from the sport element of the Taking Part survey were integrated with the Active People survey. However, from 2011 the Taking Part survey also included a repeated measures cohort, and this provides the basis for this analysis.

Cohort data from the Taking Part survey collected from 6227 adults at two time points approximately a year apart between 2011 and 2014 were reanalysed to derive four broad population groups according to levels of sport participation and changes made in sport participation. These data were triangulated with cross-sectional data from the Active People Survey (2012/2013) and the Health Survey for England (2012) relating to both sport participation and wider levels of physical activity.

The second analysis comprises a review and reanalysis of six surveys that have provided official national statistics for sport participation or physical activity levels between 1977 and 2015. The reanalysed and harmonised data from these surveys were compared to the implementation of changing sport participation policies and practices in England since 1977 to explore any links with shifts in sport participation and physical activity levels. The six surveys comprised the General Household Survey (old method[4]) (1977, 1980, 1983, 1986), General Household Survey (new method[5]) (1987, 1990, 1993, 1996, 2002), Health Survey for England (1997, 1998, 2003, 2004, 2006, 2008, 2012), Active People Survey (old method[6]) (2006), Active People Survey (new method[7]) (2008–2015), and Taking Part (2006–2012). The reanalysis focused on changes in sport and physical activity levels rather than absolute levels of participation, and used an approach outlined by Gratton and Tice (1994) to develop a continuous measure of participation change across the six surveys. Gratton and Tice (1994) projected forward the trend for participation changes in the General Household Survey (old method), and projected backward the trend in the General Household Survey (new method) to establish a continuation point for a harmonised continuous measure of participation change. This approach was applied in this analysis to provide a continuous measure of sport participation change (in population percentage points) between 1997 and 2015. Changes in physical activity levels,[8] measured by the Health Survey for England, were also available between 1997 and 2012, and these are presented alongside the analysis of sport participation.

These data were compared to the policies and priorities outlined in six national sport strategies spanning 1972–2015. Changes in emphases and objectives, and resulting changes in programmes, practices, and funding, since 1977 were compared with the harmonised data to identify trends in sport participation and, where available, physical activity levels, that might be associated with changes in policy and practice.

Results

Review and reanalysis of current English national survey data

Data on current participation in sport in England, and how that has recently changed, particularly among the less and least active, can be provided by three surveys: Active People, Taking Part, and the Health Survey for England. Each survey suggests relative stability in sport participation: Active People shows participation at least once a week varying between 35.6% and 36.9% across 2007–2015; Taking Part shows participation at least once a month varying between 53.0% and 55.2% across 2006–2012; Health Survey for England shows participation at least once a month varying between 45.9% and 48.5% across 1998–2012.

However, the stability in population-level sport participation shown in these repeated cross-sectional surveys masks considerable changes in individuals' sport participation over time. Between 2011 and 2014, the Taking Part survey included a repeated measures element, with 6227 adults asked about their sport participation at two time points approximately a year apart. These data can be presented in multiple ways, but the analysis for this paper (Figure 4) shows current sport participation activity or change stratified by previous participation. The data show that 43.6% of the population DID NOT change their participation (or their non-participation) in sport during the previous year, with the participation of 56.4% of the population varying as follows:

- 39.2% did some sport in the previous year but had not participated in the previous month at one of the measurement points.
- 8.0% are doing less sport than a year ago.
- 8.9% are doing more sport than a year ago.

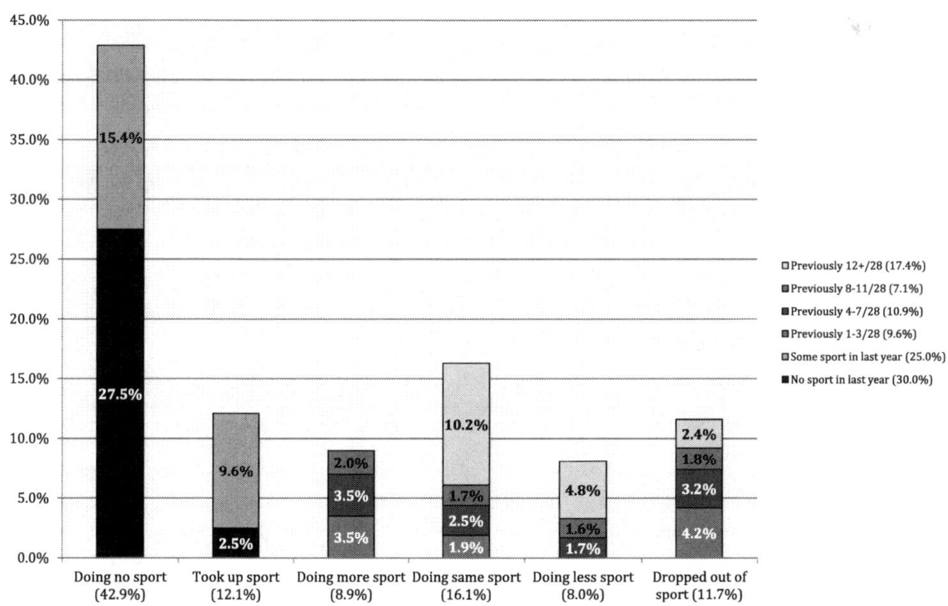

Figure 4. Current sport participation activity or change stratified by previous participation. Source: Taking Part Survey (2011–2014), $n = 6227$.

The Taking Part repeated measures data allow a more sophisticated categorisation of the population than a single cross-sectional measure, which can only show current participation. Based on current sport participation, previous sport participation, and likelihood to change, the repeated measures data suggest four categories: the sporty, the semi-sporty, the not sporty, and those who dislike sport. The sporty population (24.7%) have consistently participated in sport once a week or more throughout the previous year, and while their participation frequency has varied, they have maintained regular sport participation. The semi-sporty (22.3%) have participated in sport once a week or more at some point in the previous year, but have not consistently done so, thus their participation has been irregular. The not sporty (25.5%) have participated at some point in the previous year, but never once a week or more – they have tried sport, but not been engaged. Finally, the dislike sport group (27.5%) have not participated in any sport for 2 years.

This analysis is broadly consistent with cross-sectional results from other surveys. Active People (2013) shows that 52% of the population did sport less than once a month, including 30% of the population who had not participated at all in the previous year. Health Survey for England (2013) showed 52% of the population do no sport, defined as not having participated in sport for more than 10 min in the last month. These data suggest that around half of the population – the not sporty and those who dislike sport – are unlikely to move through the steps of the effectiveness logic model for sport as a public health intervention. The latter group has not engaged with sport for at least 2 years, while the former group has tried very low levels of sport participation, but not been engaged. Consequently, there is no reason to believe that sport as a public health intervention will be effective with these groups. Interestingly, though, the Health Survey for England shows that around a quarter of the 52% of the population doing no sport (13% of the population) would not be categorised as the less and least active because they do meet government physical activity guidelines. Therefore, if this active group is removed, the data presented in this section collectively indicate that the less and least active 40% of the population are consistently not doing sport, do not meet government physical activity guidelines, and show no inclination to change their sport participation habits. Given this profile, and particularly the lack of inclination to change, evidence from current national survey data suggest that the assumptions of the effectiveness logic model may not hold for the less and least active, and thus that the UK Government's theory of change for sport as a public health intervention may not be credible.

Analysis of shifts in sport participation and physical activity levels and the changing implementation of sport policy (1977–2015)

Following the establishment of the Sports Council[9] as a quasi-automous UK government agency in 1971, the first national sports strategy, *Sport in the Seventies* (Sports Council 1972) was published. Since then, there have been a further five documents that might meaningfully be called national sport strategies, published by either the Sports Council or its successors or by government: *Sport in the Community – The Next Ten Years* (Sports Council 1982), *Sport: Raising the Game* (DNH 1995), *Game Plan* (Cabinet Office 2002), *Grow, Sustain, Excel* (Sport England 2008), *Sporting Future: A New Strategy for an Active Nation* (Cabinet Office 2015). Across this period, commencing with the 1977 General Household Survey, official national statistics for sport participation have been available. This presents an opportunity to explore the impact of changing UK sport policy since the 1970s on sport participation.

Figure 5 shows the percentage of the population participating in sport at least once a month according to six surveys between 1977 and 2015. In addition, data from the Health Survey for England (1998–2012) for the percentage of the population achieving the CMOs' pre-2011 recommendation for physical activity (at least 30 min of moderate to vigorous activity on at least 5 days a week) is shown. However, more useful than the raw data in Figure 5 are data for the change in sport participation, harmonised across surveys, and smoothed using a 5-year average. This is shown in Figure 6 as change in population percentage points alongside similarly smoothed data for

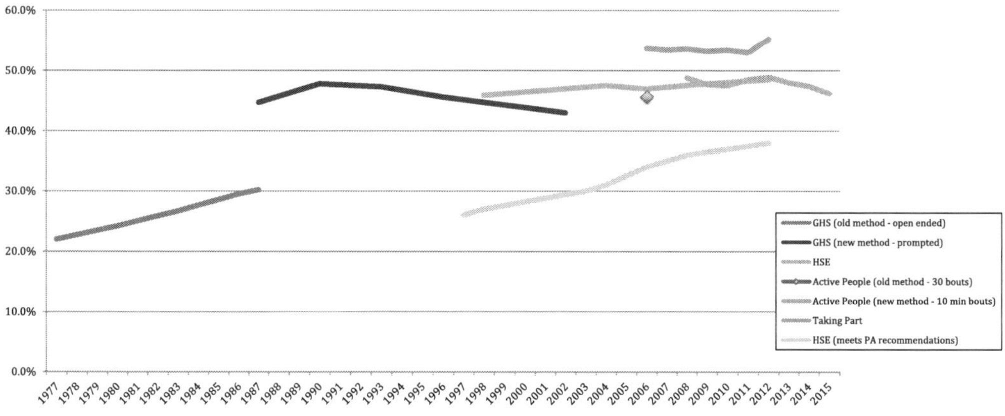

Figure 5. Sport participation and physical activity data from six surveys (1977–2015).

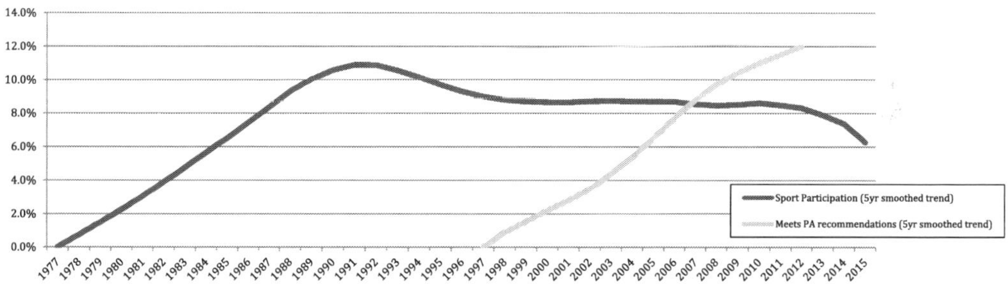

Figure 6. Sport participation change (harmonised across surveys) and physical activity change, smoothed by 5-year averages.

physical activity levels. These data show continuous growth in sport participation between 1977 and 1991 totalling an additional 11% of the population, followed by a 2% fall between 1992 and 1997, a period of stagnation between 1998 and 2012 (0.5% fall), and a further fall of 2% between 2012 and 2015. Across the period of stagnation in sport participation, an additional 10% of the population achieved CMO recommendations for physical activity. Of course, this is the harmonised data, but the raw data comparing sport participation and physical activity from the same survey (Health Survey for England) between 1998 and 2012 show an increase in sport participation of 2.6% of the population, but an increase in physical activity of 11% of the population. These data broadly show two things: first, an increase in sport participation between 1977 and 1990, and falling or stagnating sport participation since 1990; second, a considerable increase in physical activity during a time (1998–2012) when sport participation was stagnating.

Sport participation policy in the 1970s, as expressed in *Sport in the Seventies* (Sports Council 1972), was focused on significantly increasing the stock of sport facilities, while in the 1980s, *Sport in the Community: The Next Ten Years* (Sports Council 1982) largely focused on increasing access to those sport facilities (Coghlan and Webb 1990). Exploring these approaches in the context of the effectiveness logic model shown earlier (Figure 3), it appears that between 1977 and 1990 a range of provision focused sport participation policies catered for a level of unsatisfied latent demand for sport participation among those interested in sport by making available a greater supply of sport facilities and removing structural barriers to the use of those facilities to create effective demand. As noted earlier, these are the easiest and most convenient steps in the effectiveness logic model for policymakers to address, as the success of interventions is largely dependent on resources to increase and ensure access to provision. However, since 1990, a range of sport participation policies focusing on, at various points in time, continued facility investment, addressing both structural and psychological barriers to participation, stimulating motivation and interest in sport, and increasing awareness of sport participation opportunities, have had no long-term impact on sport participation. This suggests two things: first, that latent demand had become exhausted by 1990; second, that sport participation interventions targeting awareness, interest, and psychological barriers to encourage movement between the earlier steps of the effectiveness logic model have been largely ineffective in the long term. This, therefore, seems to undermine the credibility of the UK Government's theory of change that sport can be used as a public health intervention to increase physical activity among the less and least active.

Of course, sport stakeholders, policymakers, practitioners, and providers might argue that the fall or stagnation in sport participation since 1990 is related to societal and technological changes which have resulted in the population becoming less active, more sedentary, and more obese (c.f., Crouch 2015). However, the growth, by circa 10% of the population, in those achieving CMO recommendations for physical activity between 1998 and 2012 provides clear evidence that more people are finding ways to be physically active that do not include sport. Once again, this appears to undermine the government's theory of change that sport can be used as a public health intervention to improve physical health because it suggests that investing in sport may not be the most effective intervention to increase physical activity levels among the less and least active.

Discussion

The results above call into question the credibility of the UK Government's theory of change that sport can be used as a public health intervention to increase physical activity among the less and least active to deliver improvements in the physical health of the population. There is good top-tier evidence from controlled designs to show that sport participation can improve physical health, thus supporting the efficacy logic model underpinning this theory of change. However, there is no top-tier evidence from controlled designs which shows that sport participation can be increased among the less and least active, and the analysis presented in this paper provides second-tier time-series evidence that shows that it has not yet been possible to increase sport participation among the less and least active, thus potentially undermining the UK Government's theory of change for sport as a public health intervention.

The evidence discussed, analysed, and presented in this paper shows that there is no top-tier evidence to support, and some second-tier evidence to undermine, the effectiveness logic model that underpins the UK Government's theory of change. At the very least, this means that the theory of change that sport can be used as a public health intervention to increase physical activity among the less and least active to deliver improvements in the physical health of the population is not proven. By the standards of evidence that the UK Government sets for itself (HM Treasury 2011a, 2011b, 2013, National Audit Office 2013), sport as a public health intervention for physical health should therefore not be supported and implemented. Such standards were set out by the then newly appointed UK Secretary of State for Health in 2010, Andrew Lansley, who was clear that 'public health services must meet tougher tests of evidence and evaluation ... We must only support effective interventions that deliver proven benefits' (Lansley 2010, para. 104, 106). Similarly, the House of Commons Select Committee on Health stated in its report on health inequalities that unproven public health interventions '... are experiments on the public and can be as damaging (in terms of unintended effects and opportunity cost) as unevaluated new drugs or surgical procedures' (House of Commons Health Committee 2009, p. 115). In addition the report states that '[s] uch wanton large-scale experimentation is unethical, and needs to be superseded by a more rigorous culture of piloting, evaluating and using the results to inform policy' (House of Commons Health Committee 2009, p. 115).

Why, then, if the effectiveness of sport as a public health intervention is unproven, does the UK Government continue to invest in it? The answer may lie in a further element that can determine the effectiveness of interventions: provider acceptance (Singal *et al.* 2014). Provider acceptance is the extent to which policymakers, practitioners, and providers accept the evidence and the resulting need, or not, to intervene. For sport as a public health intervention, the issue appears to be that providers and practitioners do not accept that there is no top-tier evidence to support, and some second-tier evidence to undermine, the effectiveness logic model. This was illustrated by a survey of over 200 sport stakeholders undertaken by Cavill *et al.* (2012) to inform their report to Sport England on the links between sport and health. Of the 151 responses (circa 75% response rate), almost half (48%) answered that 'there is good evidence that sport can reach inactive people', while a further 44% answered 'I believe sport can reach inactive people, but there is not much evidence'. As such, almost half of respondents were either unaware of, or did not understand, the evidence base, and a further 44% believed that sport could be effective as a public health intervention with the less and least active despite the lack of evidence. In total, 92% of sport stakeholders supported sport as a public health intervention with the less and least active.

The prevalence of a belief that sport can be effective as a public health intervention among sport stakeholders may be interpreted by policymakers and politicians in government as 'expert opinion'. However, in almost all evidence hierarchies (e.g., Canadian Task Force on the Periodic Health Examination 1979, US Preventative Services Task Force 2008), expert opinion is considered to be the lowest quality evidence; and in some UK evidence hierarchies for social policy (e.g., Social Exclusion Task Force 2008), it is not even listed. Furthermore, Leigh (2009), in suggesting an evidence hierarchy for Australian policymakers to the Australian Treasury, lists expert opinion as the lowest quality evidence alongside 'theoretical conjecture'. Nevertheless, for politicians 'expert opinion' can be compelling, and because both sport stakeholders and politicians often conflate evidence of efficacy with evidence of effectiveness (Beedie *et al.* 2015), it can appear that such opinion is supported by evidence. In relation to sport as a public health intervention, the conflation is that the good evidence that underpins the efficacy logic model that sport participation can improve physical health is sufficient to assume that there is evidence to support the effectiveness logic model that sport participation can be increased among the less and least active, which there is not. There are clear examples of this conflation in the government's recent sport strategy, in which the then Prime Minister states (Cameron 2015, p. 6): 'Sport is also good for us' (for which there is good efficacy evidence)... 'It encourages us all to lead healthier and more active lives' (for which there is no effectiveness evidence). Similarly, the Minister for Sport, in the same document, states (Crouch 2015, p. 9): 'The impact that sport has on physical and mental health' (for which there is good efficacy evidence), '... shows the power to transform people's wellbeing and create a fitter, healthier and happier nation' (for which there is no effectiveness evidence).

Taken together, the recourse to what appears to be misguided expert opinion, and the conflation of efficacy and effectiveness evidence, show that there is a problem in terms of provider acceptance when it comes to considering the credibility of the government's theory of change for sport as a public health intervention. Specifically, that sport stakeholders, policymakers, practitioners, and providers either do not appreciate, or do not accept, that there is no top-tier evidence to support, and some second-tier evidence to undermine, the effectiveness of sport as a public health intervention to increase physical activity among the less and least active.

However, the implications do not end with the conclusion that the UK Government's theory of change that sport can be used as a public health intervention to increase physical activity among the less and least active to deliver improvements in the physical health of the population is not proven because investing in sport for this purpose has opportunity costs. Such opportunity costs relate to the possibility that resources currently allocated to promoting sport may deliver greater physical health benefits at a population level if they were reallocated to initiatives to promote physical activities other than sport to the less and least active. Certainly, the resources involved are considerable. In 2014/2015, Sport England invested over £200 million in sport participation initiatives and over £50 million in facilities (Sport England 2015), with its Chief Executive noting it will have spent over £1 billion trying to raise sport participation over the government's most recent 5-year investment cycle (Bitel 2015). Given that this paper has shown that there is no top-tier evidence to support, and some second-tier evidence to undermine, the effectiveness of sport as a public health intervention to increase physical activity among the less and least active, a consideration of the *comparative effectiveness* of investing in sport as a public health intervention to improve physical health is clearly warranted. Comparative effectiveness evidence is concerned with the relative benefits and harms of alternative interventions (Sox and Greenfield 2009). This includes the relative or net harm of interventions in comparison with the opportunity cost of not implementing alternatives (House of Commons Health Committee 2009). In other words, a consideration of the possibility that investing in sport as a public health intervention to improve physical health will cause net harm if investing in alternative ways of becoming active that do not privilege sport is more effective in improving population physical health than investing in sport. The UK Government strategy, 'Sporting Future: A New Strategy for an Active Nation' (Cabinet Office 2015) sets a clear outcome to increase the percentage of the population in England meeting the CMO's guidelines for physical activity and to achieve a decrease in those physically inactive. But the key question for a consideration of comparative effectiveness is: why should a 'new strategy for an active nation' be linked to sport? Are there other ways that the strategic goal of a more active nation might be achieved?

The effectiveness logic model for sport as a public health intervention, illustrated earlier in Figure 3, can be extended to include a comparative effectiveness dimension that does not privilege sport and considers alternative ways of becoming active. In doing so, the first step is no longer to increase awareness of sport because sport is no longer privileged as the route to improving physical health. The first step becomes promoting the desire to improve physical health by becoming physically active (which assumes a focus on the less and least active). Once this desire exists, the next step is to increase awareness of a wide range of ways to become active that will include, but not privilege, sport. With awareness raised, the remaining steps for sport are mirrored for other ways of becoming physically active (Figure 7). As the analysis in this paper suggests that latent demand for sport became saturated around 1990, the key steps in the effectiveness logic model for sport are to either increase interest in sport or create effective demand by removing psychological barriers. However, there is no top-tier evidence from controlled studies with a meaningful sport element that can underpin the assumptions of the effectiveness logic model that sport participation can be increased among the UK Government's target group, the circa 40% of the population who are less and least active and who do not participate in sport. Furthermore, second-tier evidence utilising national time-series data suggest that the less and least active are long-term non-participants with little or no interest in engaging with sport. Additional second-tier evidence from the longitudinal analysis of sport participation and physical activity levels shows that, while sport participation stagnated or fell from1990, since 1997 a significant proportion of the population (circa 10%) have become physically active in ways that do not include sport. While these data do not provide granular evidence at each step of the effectiveness logic model, it does strongly suggest that there is a chain of effectiveness evidence to support the promotion of ways of becoming physically active other than sport as a public health intervention to improve physical health. This suggests that a theory of change should be developed that explicitly does not privilege sport. Consequently, first, the credibility of the UK Government's theory of change for investment in sport as a public health intervention is undermined by a lack of evidence for its effectiveness. However, second, and more importantly, in comparison with the opportunity cost of not implementing potentially effective alternatives that promote wider physical activity choices that do not privilege sport, investment in sport as a public health intervention may be causing net harm to the physical health of the population.

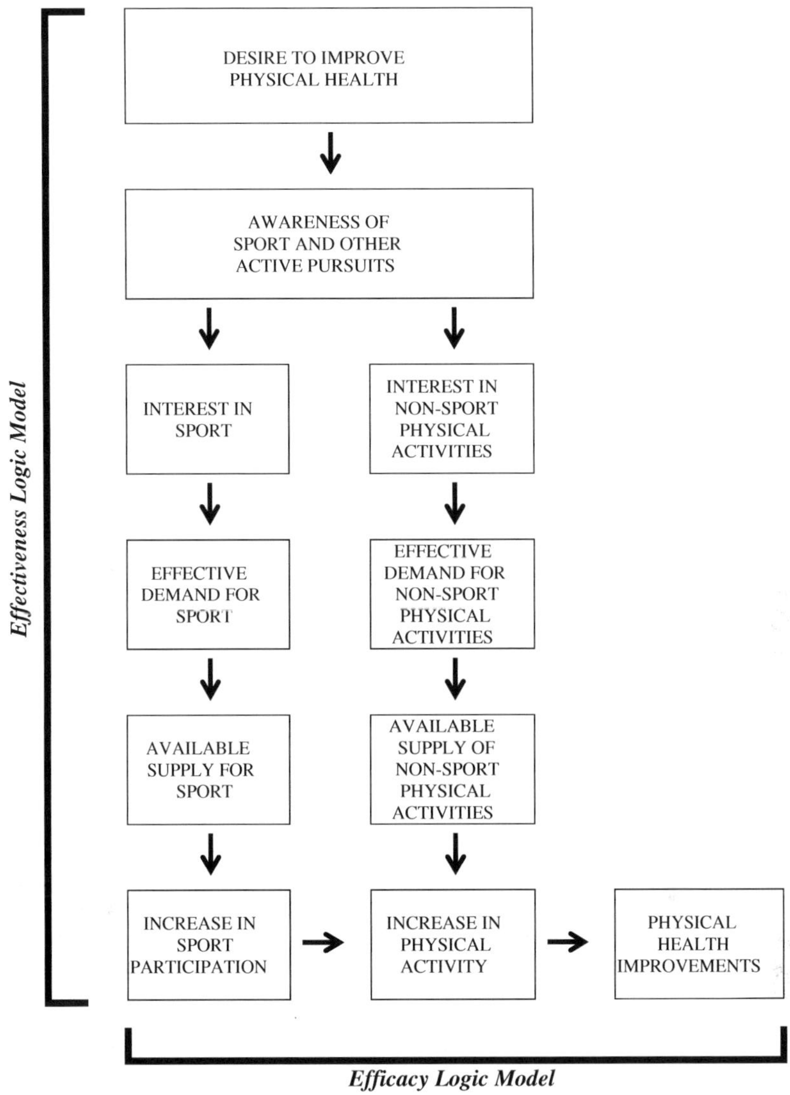

Figure 7. Effectiveness and efficacy logic models for sport and for non-sport physical activity as public health interventions to improve physical health.

Conclusion

This paper has shown that the UK Government's theory of change that sport can be used as a public health intervention to increase physical activity among the less and least active to deliver improvements in the physical health of the population is not credible. This is because, although there is top-tier evidence from controlled designs to support the efficacy logic model that sport participation can improve physical health, there is no top-tier evidence to support, and some second-tier time-series evidence to undermine, the assumptions of the effectiveness logic model that sport participation can be increased among the less and least active. By the standards that the UK Government sets for itself (House of Commons Health Committee 2009, Lansley 2010, HM Treasury 2011a, 2011b, 2013, National Audit Office 2013), sport as a public health intervention for physical health should therefore not be supported and implemented. However, because there is no provider acceptance of this lack of evidence, and because policymakers and politicians appear to privilege misguided expert opinion while also conflating evidence of efficacy with evidence of effectiveness, UK Government investment in sport as a public health intervention seems set to continue. This, despite the possibility that, in comparison with the opportunity cost of not implementing potentially effective alternatives that do not privilege sport, UK Government investment in sport as s public health intervention may be causing net harm to the physical health of the population.

Of course, UK Government policymakers and politicians may argue that the recently published Sporting Future strategy (Cabinet Office 2015) brings together sport and physical activity because it recognises that 'projects that feature activities such as dance, utility cycling and walking can be extremely effective in reaching inactive people, who might not consider themselves at all "sporty"' (p. 27). However, their practical response to implementation is to broaden Sport England's role to include 'certain kinds of physical activity, including cycling, dancing and walking … which can [now] be subject to Sport England measurement and support' (p. 28). Clearly, making certain kinds of physical activity subject to Sport England measurement and support is an approach that continues to privilege sport by bringing together sport and physical activity in a way that subsumes physical activity within sport. As this paper has shown, sport is least relevant to the less and least active, and it would seem unlikely that supporting, delivering, and measuring certain kinds of physical activities under the auspices of sport will help in this respect, rather, it would seem to be more likely to hinder. A slightly modified theory of change that sport, *and certain kinds of physical activity supported and measured under the auspices of sport*, can be used as a public health intervention to increase physical activity among the less and least active to deliver improvements in the physical health of the population, seems no more credible than the original. Rather than tinkering around the edges of what constitutes sport, the conclusion suggested by this paper is that investment in promoting sport as the route to improving physical health should be dropped in favour of an alternative that does not privilege sport and focuses investment on promoting the desire to improve physical health by becoming physically active. Such investment should explicitly promote choice as to what such activities might be, and there should be no role for sport other than to be one among many activity providers.

Notes

1. Although claims are made for the impact of sport on mental health, and while mental well-being is one of the sought outcomes of the UK Government's new strategy, for simplicity and clarity the focus of the paper is limited to physical health.
2. https://www.gov.uk/guidance/case-programme (accessed 26 January 2016).
3. http://www.thisgirlcan.co.uk (accessed: 26 January 2016).
4. Respondents were asked open-ended unprompted questions about sports and activities.
5. A list of sports and activities was used to prompt respondents answers to questions.
6. Respondents were asked about sports and activities done in at least 30-min bouts.
7. Respondents were asked about sports and activities done in at least 10-min bouts.
8. Measured by the percentage of the population meeting the pre-2011 Chief Medical Officers' (CMOs) guidelines of 30 min moderate to vigorous physical activity on at least 5 days in a week.
9. The Sports Council was granted Royal Charter in 1971 with a UK wide remit. Since then, there have been a number of reorganisations and restructures to create agencies for the UK home nations. There are now five agencies: the UK sport has responsibility for elite sport pathways and development across the UK, whereas the four UK home country agencies, *Sport England, sportscotland*, the *Sports Council for Wales,* and *Sport Northern Ireland*, have responsibility for community sport and sport participation.

Disclosure statement

No potential conflict of interest was reported by the author.

References

Baker, P.R., *et al*. 2011. Community wide interventions for increasing physical activity. *Sao Paulo Medical Journal*, 129 (6), 436–437. doi:10.1590/S1516-31802011000600013

Barton, S., 2000. Which clinical studies provide the best evidence? *BMJ*, 321, 255. doi:10.1136/bmj.321.7256.255

Beedie, C., *et al*., 2015. Death by effectiveness: exercise as medicine caught in the efficacy trap!. *British Journal of Sports Medicine*, 50, 323–324.

Bitel, N., 2015. *Strategic report: chair's foreword. In sport England, annual report and accounts for the year ended 31 March 2015*. London: Sport England, 2.

Brown, W., *et al*., 2003. 10,000 steps Rockhampton: establishing a multi-strategy physical activity promotion project in a community. *Health Promotion Journal of Australia*, 14 (2), 96–101.

Brown, W.J., *et al*., 2012. *Development of evidence-based physical activity recommendations for adults*. Canberra: Department of Health.

Burns, P.B., Rohrich, R.J., and Chung, K.C., 2011. The levels of evidence and their role in evidence based medicine. *Plastic and Reconstructive Surgery*, 128 (1), 305–310. doi:10.1097/PRS.0b013e318219c171

Cabinet Office, 2002. *Game plan*. London: Cabinet Office.

Cabinet Office, 2015. *Sporting future: a new strategy for an active nation*. London: Cabinet Office.

Cameron, D., 2015. Foreword by the prime minister. *In*: Cabinet Office, eds. *Sporting future: a new strategy for an active nation*. London: Cabinet Office, 6–7.

Canadian Task Force on the Periodic Health Examination, 1979. The periodic health examination. *Canadian Medical Association Journal*, 121 (9), 1193–1254.

Cavill, N., Richardson, D., and Foster, C., 2012. Improving health through participation in sport: a review of research and practice. *Report to Sport England*. Available from: http://www.sportengland.org/media/103075/full-report-inactivity-sport.pdf [Accessed 20 December 2015].

Coghlan, J.F. and Webb, I.M., 1990. *Sport and British politics since 1960*. London: Routledge.

Collins, M.F., 2014. *Sport and social exclusion*. 2nd ed. London: Routledge.

Crouch, T., 2015. Foreword by the minister for sport. *In*: Cabinet Office, eds. *Sporting future: a new strategy for an active nation*. London: Cabinet Office, 8–9.

Cunningham, D., *et al*. 1987. Exercise training of men at retirement: a clinical trial. *Journal of Gerontology*, 42 (1), 17–23. doi:10.1093/geronj/42.1.17

DCMS (Department for Culture, Media and Sport), 2002. *Game plan: a strategy for delivering government's sport and physical activity objectives*. London: DCMS.

DCMS (Department for Culture, Media and Sport), 2010. *Plans for the legacy from the 2012 Olympic and Paralympic games*. London: DCMS.

DNH (Department for National Heritage), 1995. *Sport: raising the game*. London: DNH.

DoH (Department of Health), 2011. *Start active, stay active: a report on physical activity from the four home countries' chief medical officers*. London: DoH.

Elley, C.R., *et al*. 2003. Effectiveness of counselling patients on physical activity in general practice: cluster randomised controlled trial. *BMJ*, 326 (7393), 793. doi:10.1136/bmj.326.7393.793

Foster, C., *et al*., 2005. Interventions for promoting physical activity. *Cochrane database of systematic reviews*: CD003180

Fujita, K., *et al*., 2003. Effects of exercise training on physical activity in older people: a randomized controlled trial. *Journal of Epidemiology*, 13 (2), 120–126. doi:10.2188/jea.13.120

Gratton, C. and Tice, A., 1994. Trends in sports participation in Britain: 1977–1987. *Leisure Studies*, 13 (1), 49–66. doi:10.1080/02614369400390041

Harland, J., *et al*. 1999. The Newcastle exercise project: a randomised controlled trial of methods to promote physical activity in primary care. *BMJ*, 319 (7213), 828–832. doi:10.1136/bmj.319.7213.828

Haynes, L., *et al*., 2012. *Test, learn, adapt: developing public policy with randomized controlled trials*. London: Cabinet Office.

HM Treasury, 2011a. *The green book: appraisal and evaluation in central government*. London: HM Treasury.

HM Treasury, 2011b. *The magenta book: guidance for evaluation*. London: HM Treasury.

HM Treasury, 2013. *Managing public money*. London: HM Treasury.

House of Commons Health Committee, 2009. *Health inequalities: third report of session 2008-09 – volume I*. London: The Stationary Office.

Kumpusalo, E., *et al*. 1996. Finnish healthy village study: impact and outcomes of a low-cost local health promotion programme. *Health Promotion International*, 11 (2), 105–115. doi:10.1093/heapro/11.2.105

Lansley, A., 2010. *Secretary of state for health speech to the UK faculty of public health conference: a new approach to public health*. London: Department of Health. Available from: http://webarchive.nationalarchives.gov.uk/+/www.dh.gov.uk/en/MediaCentre/Speeches/DH_117280 [Accessed 16 Sep 2016).

Leigh, A., 2009. What evidence should social policymakers use? *Australian Treasury Economic Roundup*, 1 (1), 27–43.

Luepker, R.V., *et al.*, 1994. Community education for cardiovascular disease prevention: risk factor changes in the Minnesota heart health program. *American Journal of Public Health*, 84 (9), 1383–1393. doi:10.2105/AJPH.84.9.1383

Lupton, B.S., Fonnebo, V., and Sogaard, A.J. 2003. The Finnmark intervention study: is it possible to change CVD risk factors by community-based intervention in an arctic village in crisis? *Scandinavian Journal of Public Health*, 31 (3), 178–186. doi:10.1080/14034940210134077

Marsh, K., *et al.*, 2010. *Understanding the drivers of engagement in culture and sport*. London: Culture and Sport Evidence Programme. Available from: https://www.gov.uk/government/publications/case-programme-understanding-the-drivers-impacts-and-value-of-engagement-in-culture-and-sport [Accessed 12 December 2015].

National Audit Office, 2013. *Evaluation in government*. London: NAO Communications.

Petrella, R.J., *et al.* 2003. Can primary care doctors prescribe exercise to improve fitness? The step test exercise prescription (STEP) project. *American Journal of Preventive Medicine*, 24 (4), 316–322. doi:10.1016/S0749-3797(03)00022-9

PricewaterhouseCoopers, 2009. *London 2012 Olympic and Paralympic games impacts and legacy evaluation framework*. London: DCMS.

Priest, N., *et al.*, 2008a. Interventions implemented through sporting organisations for increasing participation in sport. *Cochrane database of systematic reviews*: CD004812.

Priest, N., *et al.*, 2008b. Policy interventions implemented through sporting organisations for promoting healthy behaviour change. *Cochrane database of systematic reviews*: CD004809.

Rogers, P.J., 2008. Using programme theory to evaluate complicated and complex aspects of interventions. *Evaluation*, 14 (1), 29–48. doi:10.1177/1356389007084674

Sackett, D.L., 1989. Rules of evidence and clinical recommendations on the use of antithrombotic agents. *Chest*, 95 (2S), 2–4. doi:10.1378/chest.95.2_Supplement.2S

SDPIWG (Sport for Development and Peace International Working Group), 2008. *Harnessing the power of sport for development and peace*. Geneva: Right to Play.

Singal, A.G., Higgins, P.D.R., and Waljee, A.K., 2014. A primer on effectiveness and efficacy trials. *Clinical and Translational Gastroenterology*, 5, e45. doi:10.1038/ctg.2013.13

Social Exclusion Task Force, 2008. *Think research: using research evidence to inform service development for vulnerable groups*. London: Cabinet Office.

Sox, H.C. and Greenfield, S., 2009. Comparative effectiveness research: a report from the institute of medicine. *Annals of Internal Medicine*, 151 (3), 203–205. doi:10.7326/0003-4819-151-3-200908040-00125

Sport England, 2008. *Grow sustain excel: sport England strategy 2008–2011*. London: Sport England.

Sport England, 2010. Places people play – delivering a mass participation sporting legacy from the 2012 Olympic and Paralympic games. Available from: http://www.sportengland.org/about_us/places_people_play_-_deliverin.aspx [Accessed 10 January 2015].

Sport England, 2015. *Annual report and accounts for the year ended 31 March 2015*. London: Sport England.

Sports Council, 1972. *Sport in the seventies*. London: Sports Council.

Sports Council, 1982. *Sport in the community – the next ten years*. London: Sports Council.

Taylor, P., *et al.*, 2015. *A review of the social impacts of culture and sport*. London: Culture and Sport Evidence Programme. Available from: https://www.gov.uk/government/publications/a-review-of-the-social-impacts-of-culture-and-sport [Accessed 22 December 2015].

US Preventive Services Task Force, 2008. *Procedure manual (AHRQ Publication No. 08-05118-EF)*. Rockville: Agency for Healthcare Research and Quality.

Weed, M., *et al.*, 2015. The Olympic games and raising sport participation: a systematic review of evidence and an interrogation of policy for a demonstration effect. *European Sport Management Quarterly*, 15 (2), 195–226. doi:10.1080/16184742.2014.998695

Wendel-Vos, G.C., *et al.*, 2009. Lifestyle factors of a five-year community-intervention program: the Hartslag Limburg intervention. *American Journal of Preventive Medicine*, 37 (1), 50–56. doi:10.1016/j.amepre.2009.03.015

WHOROE (World Health Organisation Regional Office for Europe), 2011. *Promoting sport and enhancing health in European Union countries*. Copenhagen: WHOROE.

The State and management of partnership arrangements in France: an analysis of the implementation of the 'Sport, Health and Well-being' plan

Marina Honta

ABSTRACT

In France, the national 'Sport, Health, and Well-being' programme (*Programme sport, santé, bien-être* – PSSBE) aims to develop an active way of life in a country where physical inactivity is becoming increasingly prevalent. While its implementation is based on an inter-ministerial approach whereby responsibility is given to the local government personnel of the Ministry of Sport and the Ministry of Health, numerous studies have shown that the complexity of the State machine and the compartmentalisation of its departments may have a negative impact on the success of this process. In addition, due to recent State reforms, government agents are also faced with numerous changes which affect their working conditions. Based on the results of a survey conducted in a French region via semi-structured interviews held with the agents of these two ministerial bodies, we demonstrate that although the implementation of the PSSBE has helped to institutionalise the inter-ministerial partnership, it also exacerbates the difficulty caused by these reforms: that of reconciling the missions of territorial departments with the resources allocated to them. These observations reflect the risk that the work of the network built around sport and health issues may be brought to a standstill.

The growing recognition that physical activity is a determinant of health stems from the seriousness of health issues, a factor that has been demonstrated as knowledge of the subject has developed (Smith *et al.* 2004, Toussaint 2008, Bossy 2010). Available data indicate that this kind of activity prevents excess weight and obesity, that it can reduce cases of heart disease and type-2 diabetes by half, and that it can significantly bring down the risk of high blood pressure and certain forms of cancer (Hillsdon *et al.* 2005, Hardman et Stensel 2009, Bazex *et al.* 2012). It also helps to reduce stress, anxiety and depression. Conversely, physical inactivity is said to be responsible for one death out of ten throughout the world, or 3 million people (World Health Organization 2013).

In France various international studies show that the French population's level of physical activity is among the lowest in Europe (Cavill *et al.* 2006, Sisson and Katzmarzyk 2008). French children feature in the category of the least active in the world, although they have several opportunities to reach the recommended minimum level of physical activity throughout their day (Oppert *et al.* 2005, 2010, Guinhouya 2010, Institut national de prévention et d'éducation pour la santé 2011).

The need to contain the risks linked to physical inactivity has led to the set-up of several prevention and health education programme in France. The most recent is the 'Sport, Health, and

Well-being' (*Programme sport, santé, bien-être* – PSSBE) programme, launched in October 2012 by the French Ministries of Health and Sport. This strategy, which is part of a more general process to institutionalise the State's position as leader in this field, aims both at controlling the substantial costs (social and financial) of chronic illness and at ensuring the cohesion of a system in which the stakeholders in the conception and/or implementation of public health policies (associations, schools and universities, healthcare networks, local authorities and businesses) are becoming more diverse.

In this context of a pluralisation of the public sphere, the regional level has gradually become identified as the appropriate level for coordination, so that the State can retain the general governance of the health system. To this end, the local government agents of the Ministry of Sport and the Ministry of Health, the DRJSCS (Regional Directorates for Young People, Sport and Social Cohesion) and the ARS (Regional Health Agencies) have the joint mission of relaying the objectives, principles and milestones of the programme in the regions in order to encourage the mobilisation of local stakeholders.

While the implementation of this plan is based on an inter-ministerial, transverse approach, many studies have shown that its structure is by no means clear. The complexity of the State machine, the compartmentalisation of its services and the dispersion of its areas of competence have a decidedly negative impact on the success of this process (Moquay 2005, Lagroye *et al.* 2006). It would be wrong to place too much emphasis on this fragmentation and the potential conflicts which make up this 'piecemeal State' (Dupuy and Thoenig 1985, Epstein 2013), as they do not hide the essential issue of the reconciliation of interests that State agents may experience in the implementation of public policies. Although these agents occupy positions as major players (Sabatier 1986, Hill and Hupe 2002), they are exposed to numerous changes affecting their practises and working conditions because of the reforms that have profoundly reconfigured the regional administration of the French State (Honta and Julhe 2015). Following on from research that has examined the actions of the State, and without becoming bogged down in the specifics of each of its administrative bodies, the present analysis aims to understand the main effects of the implementation of the PSSBE.

After presenting the strategic priorities of this programme and the principles that have guided State reform in France, we will aim to show that while the programme's implementation incontestably contributes to the institutionalisation of the inter-ministerial partnership, it also exacerbates the difficulties, engendered by the State reforms, in reconciling the missions of departments with the resources allocated to them. As such, several regimes of coordination are shown – a notion that makes reference to the very widespread concern over mutual agreement between different protagonists on actions to be taken (Dodier 1993, p. 67) – which do not always blend well with each other. These observations reflect the risk that the work of the network built around sport and health issues may be brought to a standstill.

1. Physical activity, public health and state reform in France

The fight against physical inactivity as a result of its categorisation as a health risk is today related to social realities which are significant of its political scope. Against this backdrop, and echoing the all-encompassing definition adopted by the World Health Organization whereby 'health describes a complete state of physical, mental and social well-being, not characterised only by the absence of illness or infirmity', various international and national programmes have highlighted the benefits of physical and sporting activities (the Global Strategy on Diet, Physical Activity and Health (WHO 2004), Patchett *et al.* 2014, Van Hoek *et al.* 2016). In France as elsewhere, these programmes promote a positive view of health and self-empowerment, leading to the emergence of the rational and responsible individual who, thanks to suitable information, can change their lifestyle in order to optimise their health capital (Berlivet 2005). Their aim is to boost the independence of individuals and make them accountable so that they adopt 'healthy lifestyles'. These 'body governance' measures also require collective stakeholders to help deal with this public problem (Bergeron *et al.* 2014).

1.1. *The PSSBE as a measure to manage the risks linked to sedentary lifestyles*

In France, the cost of treating the consequences of physical inactivity is systematically highlighted in the preamble of the countless reports written on this topic. For example, the foreword of the 2008 report by the French Health and Medical Research Institute states that 'Physical activity has become a new public health challenge.' (Institut National de Santé et de Recherche Médicale 2008, p. 13). This report and the National Plan for Prevention by Physical or Sport Activity (since 2008), the National Nutrition and Health Plan (PNNS, since 2002) and the Obesity Plan (since 2011) are all built on overlapping diagnostics and all promote the adoption of an active lifestyle via guidelines and recommendations communicated to the population (Toussaint 2008).

The problem with framing the definition of physical inactivity as a public problem and a risk factor, after many years in which physical and sporting activity was widely seen as conducive to accidents (Génolini and Clément 2010), is that there is the direct risk of pre-empting certain solutions and hence also the configurations of the legitimate stakeholders who devise and implement them (Gusfield 1981). It was with this in mind that the Ministry of Sports and the Ministry of Health jointly engaged in a policy to promote the practise of physical and sporting activity as a public-health factor. Their Council of Ministers[1] paper and their inter-ministerial instruction on the methods for implementing the plan[2] specify its strategic priorities and target audience. As well as being constructed on the basis of scientific expertise demonstrating the positive health effects of engaging in physical and sporting activities (Bazex *et al.* 2012), provided that the levels recommended by the World Health Organization are observed, the PSSBE is also legitimised by social justice objectives. Indeed, this framing of physical inactivity as a public problem also contributes to the acknowledgement of other risk categories and their inclusion among the priorities of the public authorities. In this respect the inter-ministerial instruction states that despite several national public health programmes (the PNNS, the obesity plan, the cancer plan, etc.) incorporating the promotion and development of physical and sporting activities as a health factor, and despite the existence at local level of various projects designed and implemented through the involvement of the State, local authorities and the associative sports sector, many categories of people are still alienated from physical activity, and this merely exacerbates health inequalities. State of health, disability, age, socioeconomic level and place of residence are explicitly presented as potential 'obstacles' to access for all to the practise of physical activity.

The PSSBE, which also takes account of the socio-economic and environmental determinants of access to physical and sporting activities and more broadly speaking to health (Wilkinson and Marmot 2003, Gordon-Larsen *et al.* 2006, WHO 2013), avoids becoming bogged down in individualistic and astructural tropism (Hall and Larmont 2009). It must therefore target populations referred to as 'special needs' (the disabled, the chronically ill, the ageing) but also people in a situation of poverty living in urban districts referred to as 'disadvantaged' and whose state of health has been weakened by the difficulties they encounter in accessing healthcare systems. This fight against physical inactivity thus becomes a part of public action, or better, a social space, at the meeting point between several pre-existing political problems (public health, healthcare, education, poverty, isolation, local planning and development, etc.), with as many stakeholders as there are specific measures.

In this context, DRJSCS and ARS agents have been asked to jointly roll out this plan at regional level in order to improve access to physical and sporting activity as a non-medicinal therapy, with the aim of preserving this 'health capital'. Entrusted with organising the implementation and management of the PSSBE alongside the public and private protagonists concerned and/or motivated, the agents of these government bodies are at the same time exposed to a transformation of their working context due to various State reforms.

Greatly inspired by private-sector precepts and stimulated by New Public Management, the reforms have attempted to boost State credibility via better management of its public policies (Aucoin 1990, Pollitt and Bouckaert 2004, Bezes 2005). Embodying the shift from a culture of means to a culture of results, the two most recent of these reforms have also been accompanied by particularly significant cutbacks in civil service staff: the General Review of Public Policies (RGPP since 2007) and the Modernization of Public Action (since 2012).

The local State administration reform is one of the decisions made to this end. After the increasing marginalisation of local government departments due to the greater power given by the decentralisation laws to territorial authorities in various areas of public action (Epstein 2013), the reform has reorganised these departments by merging them together in order to encourage a new 'inter-ministeriality' that will strengthen the unity of State action at local level.

With regard to the Ministry of Sport, its former departments have been incorporated into those for social affairs through the creation of new operational departments since January 2010: the DRJSCS at regional level and the DDCS (Departmental Directorates for Social Cohesion) at local (*départemental*) level.

In the health sector, the 'Hospital-Patients-Health-Territories' law adopted in 2009 confirmed that the regional level was the most suitable for the definition and implementation of health policies, and created the ARS. Through these public institutions, the objectives of regionalisation are once again the de-compartmentalised management of health policies in the medical, social, healthcare and health promotion sectors. The law also provides for the creation of a territorial delegation (DT) per *département* entrusted with the implementation of regional health policy, without however specifying the respective missions and the relationships they must have with the ARS head office.

1.2. *Methods*

These factors are key to understanding the working environment of the local agents of these two ministerial bodies entrusted with rolling out the PSSBE in the regions. Their role may also be made more difficult by the structure of local State administration, which is not generally conducive to the integration of the sectoral concerns of public departments and institutions (Moquay 2005). Indeed, these departments and institutions remain anxious to protect their position, their autonomy of action and their network in the regions. The institutionalisation of the expected forms of governance negotiated for the implementation of the PSSBE therefore involves a local confrontation of practises and interests which may be divergent (Lagroye *et al.* 2006). An 'in-depth' analysis of these complex modalities of inter-ministerial co-production of action in the field of public health is part of the theoretical and empirical debates on the 'State in concrete form' (Jobert and Muller 1987, Hooghe and Marks 2003). By the same token it is also essential to examine what these administrative reforms are doing to State professionals and most particularly to the policymakers tasked with the implementation of public policies (Laffin 1998, Clarke *et al.* 2000, Ackroyd *et al.* 2007). Like all professional groups, these policymakers are not in a position of stability but instead permanently faced with change, as they directly bear the cost of these transformations (Lipsky 1980, Dent *et al.* 1999, Farrell and Morris 2003, Ferlie and Geraghty 2005, Bezes *et al.* 2011).

Based on an exploration of the meaning that actors assign to their practises and representations, the survey was conducted in the French region of Aquitaine, via semi-structured interviews with agents (14) from the two ministerial bodies charged with the implementation of this plan (Table 1): agents from the DRJSCS/DDCSs and ARS/DTs networks, with various statuses (State civil servants, contracted policy officers, both private and public sector) and from various professional corps (health and social inspectors, public healthcare physician-inspectors and technical and educational personnel – PTP from the Ministry of Sport).

Two interviews were also conducted with representatives of the Sport, Health and Well-being national resources centre. It was created in 2013 and tasked with promoting physical and sporting

Table 1. List of network advisory members interviewed.

	ARS and DTs
ARS	Public healthcare physician-inspector, centre for health promotion, prevention
ARS	'Nutrition' policy officer, centre for health promotion, prevention – regional advisor responsible for regional management of the programme
ARS-DT1	Nurse, centre for Monitoring, health safety and environmental risks
ARS-DT2	Nurse of public healthcare
ARS-DT3	Nurse of public healthcare
ARS-DT4	Inspector of health and social affairs, public healthcare and health action
ARS-DT5	Public healthcare physician-inspector
	DRJSCS and DDCSs
DRJSCS	Consultant physician
DRJSCS	Technical and educational personnel (PTP), regional advisor responsible for regional management of the programme
DDCS1	PTP, CNDS advisor
DDCS2	PTP, CNDS advisor
DDCS3	PTP, CNDS advisor
DDCS4	PTP, CNDS advisor
DDCS5	PTP, CNDS advisor

activity as a health factor. It is presented as a 'national tool' available to the departments of the Ministry for Sport and partners and stakeholders who work in this field. The purpose of these two interviews was to collect data on the manner in which the PSSBE plan is being rolled out in other regions, in order to better position Aquitaine and thus to avoid focusing on a single case.

The content of the interviews was analysed manually in order to identify constants. Coding was performed based on a grid containing the various themes of the interview guide: 1) the respective intervention rationales of the various actors, 2) the (individual and/or collective) working mode adopted, 3) the representations of partnership action involving the operations to combat physical inactivity, 4) the way the agents feel about the role they have been given, its potential transformations and, more generally, their status as civil servants.

These sources were supplemented by data from brochures, charters, annual reports and tools produced by local stakeholders, and by treatment of the academic literature and public and press reports (Appendix) on the fight against inactivity.

2. The workings of mutual recognition

By establishing the regional level as the correct one for implementation of the PSSBE, the State has made the region a place of adjustment, appropriation, mobilisation and learning of inter-ministerial cooperation. Although State intervention may pose problems as long as that State is riddled with internal contradictions between its different administrative bodies, all keen on preserving their position in the game, the agreement on a joint plan and the formalisation of rules in order to reconcile the interests present remains possible. In Aquitaine, the implementation of the PSSBE has given rise to previously unheard of encounters between stakeholders who, until that point, did not know each other.

2.1. *The institutionalisation of the partnership action*

The PSSBE is not the first prevention programme that has sought to encourage partnerships between the regional agents of the Ministries of Sport and Health. The PNNS, which was launched in France more than 10 years before the PSSBE, inaugurated a public health prevention policy whose general aim was to improve the state of health of the population by focusing on one of its major factors, nutrition. Justified by the desire to reduce the risks associated with unbalanced food consumption and sedentary lifestyles (Cavill *et al.* 2006), it relies on a broad definition of nutrition, incorporating diet and energy expenditure via physical activity, the increase of which is an aim of the programme in its own right.

Although steered by the Ministry of Health, it has an inter-ministerial and inter-sectoral dimension. As such, it offered the former Regional Departments for Health and Social Affairs, and now the ARS, the opportunity to incorporate sports policies into their regional health strategy. Entrusted, here again, with the implementation of this programme, they were invited right from its launch to liaise with the local departments of the Ministry of Sports in the initiative. The mobilisation of these departments has proved to be very disparate, as various studies (Honta and Haschar-Noé 2011), have demonstrated and as an officer from the Ministry of Health regrets:

> *They are wondering what they are doing here, on the PNNS steering committee. When we talk to them about the PNNS so that they can help us to incorporate this physical activity aspect correctly, they can't see how . . .It's true that they look after sports clubs, but at the moment they come to meetings and listen, and that's it, they just listen. . .*

Having 'historically' a public policy scope which was restricted in terms of public health, the actions of the Ministry of Sport have long been limited to anti-doping measures and the safety of sportsmen and women. This path dependence (Pierson 2000) has thus hindered the adoption and support of other health promotion programmes and explains why the PNNS was initially seen as an unimportant issue for this ministry. In this regard, one of its officers says, *'Sports medicine as a whole is very much behind in France. We get declarations of intent but few resources are allocated to the implementation of the PNNS. It's not a priority for the Sports Directorate'.*

After this awkward, or even tense, launch of the PSSBE, which enshrines the importance of physical activity as a public-health factor and therefore legitimises the role of the Ministry of Sport in the definition of a policy on the subject, the personnel of the two ministerial bodies, under the leadership of two advisers responsible for regional management of the programme after publication of the circular, have managed to organise themselves and to gradually institutionalise concerted rules for action. The adoption by these professionals of the viewpoints, ways of working and constraints of their interlocutors along with the design and implementation of this plan required a learning curve which those interviewed now consider as 'successful': *'What I am most proud of is this ARS-DRJSCS partnership. I think it is a real strength that we can work together, have a common view of things and exchange ideas and opinions. Sometimes it is strained, but at the same time we are building something'.*

According to the agents, this success is directly attributable to the extensive integration work they are carrying out, a task with varied dimensions, intended to promote flexible forms of regulation.

These aim first to add to or replace the rationales behind national public health programmes, which have often been defined on the basis of public action categories (sport, health, food), pathologies (cancer, obesity, etc.) or target audiences (the elderly, the young, the disabled, those living in poverty). These forms of regional regulation, which are complex to operationalise and primarily concern the pivotal role of the health policies entrusted to the ARS, need their programmes to be reworked in order to make them more comprehensible before being publicised to the territorial partners, as an ARS policy officer points out:

> *From 2009, it was all about the set-up of the ARS: in terms of national programming, a national food* program *arrived; then there was the wait for a third PNNS with its little friend, the obesity plan. And then, at the end of 2012, an order came to set up a sport, health and well-being* program *at regional level. All that from national level! And in Aquitaine, the region is also full of initiatives. Plenty of initiatives on the ground, plenty of national* programs *to be deployed at regional level, all inter-ministerial, but led by different ministries. In this unclear context, we have tried to pool energies and establish an unusual framework together, with objectives we can all get behind and which could then activate the tools we have available. There is a desire to work on de-*compartmentalization*. This is what we are endeavoring to do, but there's a long way to go.*

In this regard and in order to avoid the multiplication of uncoordinated initiatives, the programme *'Manger mieux, bouger plus en Aquitaine'* [Eat better and do more exercise in Aquitaine] was conceived as the 'integrated and transverse' version of the PNNS, the obesity plan, the national food programme and the SSBE plan, the latter forming its 'physical activity' component. Leaving aside this fragmentation of ministerial programmes which only the territorial personnel appear able to articulate, everyone is getting organised around steering bodies, schedules and specific financing methods. In the framework of the PSSBE, it consists, first, in a 5% levy on the local government share of funds from the National Center for the Development of Sport (*Centre National pour le Développement du Sport* – CNDS) allocated to each DRJSCS. The CNDS is a public institution under the administrative supervision of the Ministry of Sport, and its resources are used to promote growth in the practise of sport for as broad a population as possible, especially people who have become alienated from sport. For the ARS-DTs network, funding is allocated from the Regional Intervention Fund (FIR) which supports prevention projects and health promotion.

The instruction specifying the methods for its implementation invites DRJSCS and ARS agents to opt for the call for projects system in order to promote local initiatives, support innovative approaches and spread good practise. This is the option adopted in Aquitaine (Box 1), but its operational side has presented agents with difficulties due to the inconsistency of rules and financing schedules within each ministry. Here again, while in other French regions this constraint has brought an end to the joint examination of bids by DRJSCS and ARS agents, in Aquitaine the creation of 'rules on rules' has allowed these constraints to be circumvented, at least partially:

> *Calls for projects were the first collaboration tool for the ARS and the DRJSCS, and therefore a way of saying: we are going to pool our finances and see how we can improve things. We soon realized that we were dealing with fixed financial criteria and so we could not create a 'common fund'. In fact, each one provides separate funding because, in our case, we can only fund approved sports clubs. The ARS can fund anything and it also has greater interchangeability of credits which means that it can sometimes draw on other financial budgets. There are organizations whose project we agree to finance but which are funded by ARS prevention loans and not by those related to the call for projects. That's how we have to work!'*

Box 1. Specifications for the Aquitaine call for projects (extracts)

The aim of the call for projects is to promote the development of physical and sporting activities for leisure and well-being among those who do not practice sport, thus excluding those who currently practice sport on an individual basis, or in a sports association. The project should aim to attract new potential sportsmen and women, especially among those who are most alienated from physical and sporting activity (adolescents, sedentary adults, women, the elderly, the disabled, the chronically ill and/or those who are weakened socioeconomically). This call for projects encourages the pooling of skills and resources across the region.

It is aimed at sports associations, health and medico-social establishments (hospitals, care establishments for the elderly and disabled), local authorities, educational institutions and associations, training centers. It is based on the following selection criteria:

- project justified by the context (territorial analysis),
- relevance of the proposed project to the targeted aims: choice of public, area of action, locations and types of action
- quality of the partnership: partners' actions should be complementary, ensuring that aims and actions can be achieved and sustained throughout the region
- implementation of the project: organization, management, schedule, planned budget
- quality of project assessment: planned assessment and indicators adapted specifically to the nature of the project.

2.2. *Operations in common and overlapping interests*

This partnership learning curve, or this 'taming process' to quote a stakeholder, has been achieved through the organisation of working seminars bringing together the agents from the two ministries. Because each administrative body has a perception of public problems which are specific to it depending on its history, its routines and its expertise (Muller and Surel 1998), the first aim of these seminars was to bring an end to the ambiguity surrounding the categories employed. With this in mind, the sharing of knowledge and information judged to be relevant, including the definitions of physical activity, sport and health proposed by the World Health Organization, has proved to be an indispensable stage in establishing a common reference point, one which is necessary in particular for the joint examination of applications for subsidies sent in by operators in response to the call for projects:

> *A colleague from the DRJSCS led a seminar on "how health and sport can learn to work together". So we spent a half day comparing our definitions. For us, the definition we might have of health, and for them, their definition of sport. And we compared our cultures like that. We spent a really fruitful day, as by comparing our cultures, we found divergences but also bridges which will allow us to work together. It was also interesting to note that we are dealing with a win-win strategy. We know the added value that can be gained from working together. As people on the ground, we are more often in contact with different organizations than they are. We have even more flexibility in our missions and therefore we have an expertise which interests them greatly. They are surrounded by the entire medical field. We need this knowledge, and this network. It's a win-win situation.*

The interactions produced by the seminars, and the meetings of the steering committee bringing together the two regional bodies and the sports-health representatives from the five DDCSs (PTP, CNDS advisor) and DTs, also allowed these two regional bodies to get to know each other's networks.

An essential step in order to avoid these players undertaking potentially similar actions at local level without being aware of it, the ARS 'Nutrition' policy officer confirmed what had been said previously, adding that working together in this way had gradually opened up different avenues for future collaboration from those put forward within the framework of the call for projects:

> *The most technical and the most interesting aspect of the partnership is being able to combine our points of view and our expertise. In the first year, work started in great haste and the deadlines were very tight, but since then we have been able to take advantage of this initial experience, and make improvements. For the first call for projects, we worked much more on formalizing the network by holding joint meetings of 'Young people and Sports' and ARS teams, bringing in the local (département) level. We are not experts in physical activity, but at the Ministry for Young People and Sports, there are agents who are still working in the field and who, for this reason, have a very much clearer vision of what happens than we do. Thus there is clearly a benefit in working together. The reason I say that things have improved is that last year, everyone just gave out their opinion, but with no real framework, and we found it difficult to agree. This year, after the joint DRJSCS and ARS seminars, we found we were in agreement on almost all the projects that required funding. There were 2 on which we were not in total agreement. By sharing expertise and working together, other ideas emerged. We started to consider the question of training, in order to qualify "sport-health" educators.*

Finally, the two advisers from the DRJSCS and the ARS in charge of managing and leading the programme drew up a framework document presenting its target audience (sedentary persons or persons alienated from the practise of physical or sporting activity, persons living in poverty, the disabled, those suffering chronic illness and the elderly), its aims, directions and the series of definitions on which all DRJSCS/DDCSs and ARS/DTs network personnel had agreed (DRJSCS and ARS Aquitaine 2015).

Although the content of this document largely adopts the national positions of the PSSBE, it does not only aim at giving the State departments an explicit and shared guideline determining and ranking its actions, but also at formalising and announcing clear strategic directions to local operators. This guideline is also regionalised in that it highlights the particular issues of 'deprived regions', in other words 'difficult' neighbourhoods in urban areas and rural revitalisation zones.

These integrational behaviours, which help actors learn how to conduct action in a partnership, cannot hide the fact that the actions of these professionals also come up against many obstacles caused by the recent reforms of the local State administration. However, there was a distinct disconnect, of varying intensity depending on the locations, between the forms of regional coordination that were adopted and which could be described as maximalist – i.e. able to be transposed in time and space and producing agreements that were probably going to be long-lasting (Dodier 1993) – and the coordination observed at the level of the five *départements*. In this context, the question of the sustainable implementation of the PSSBE and the dynamic of the network on which it is based needs to be fully addressed.

3. Multi-level coordination still in its infancy

Although the reform of the local State administration had the aim of simplifying the administrative structure, its implementation has given rise to modalities that have not all proved their relevance. In this regard, the Court of Auditors (2013) distinguishes the regional directorates, described as 'well established', from those like the DRJSCS, which 'pose more problems'. As for the ARS, they appear as 'fabulous cars with empty tanks' (Rolland and Pierru 2013). These organisations are faced with multiple difficulties which the personnel we met expressed in great detail. The effects of these reforms are experienced as a weakening of public services as they influence the frequency, or even the very existence, of their relations with their local partners, and as a threat to their professionalism. When these factors were added to the different levels of individual commitment to this programme, the internal regulations and balance of power of the two bodies (health and sports) and the priorities set by the hierarchy in both the DDCS and the DT, the result was multi-level coordination – first at the local (*department)* level, then between local, regional and national levels – which was difficult to merge into a whole.

3.1. *Differentiated mobilisations*

Whether at the Ministry of Sports or the Ministry of Health, the reduction in headcount has made working conditions far more fragile, particularly at local level. In doing so it also led to 'a moral hierarchisation of work' (Hughes 1971). The tasks of the DDCS or the DT are perceived and/or experienced as being the least rewarding due to the tensions that now exist between the sheer number of these tasks and the ever more limited resources available. With the reduction in staff in particular, the resources set aside to implement the policies are meagre, while the scope of the missions set by the State has remained the same (Kada 2012, Pierru 2012, Rolland and Pierru 2013). Such a diversity of tasks, albeit less so in regional directorates due to larger teams, undermines the capacities of agents to perform them[3]:

> *I was the adviser for 6 projects last year! Our national directives contain innumerable different measures! So you try to find a link between them in your mind. I tried to link missions together because if you disconnect them, it becomes very complicated. Unfortunately, due to the staff numbers in the departments, at any given point in time you are in a hurry, so you don't have the time to make this link and anticipate the future.*

This lack of resources destabilises the formation or upkeep of strong working collectives. As the ensuing individualisation of tasks is not particularly conducive to social cooperation, it is above all through individual strategies that the agents in charge of several projects adjust their professional involvement according to their interest in, and taste for, such-and-such a task. A nurse, who was a programme advisor in one of the DTs, stated, *'for my part, I have not followed the local* program *on a regular basis as I was often called away for other missions and topics when no physician-inspector was available'*, however, an agent in one of the DDCSs disagreed:

> *As a sports-health adviser to the DDCS, when I took charge of the case, I had my nose to the grindstone for one year and invested a lot of time in it. Why? Because it was a project that interested me and I had never had the opportunity to work with my colleagues on these issues. It was great. So I spent a lot of time on it. I had been on disabled sport for two years, so I could let it tick over for a bit. I could make time for sport and health. So I went all out. Personally I believe one thing, which is that first you should decide on the importance you want to attach to a project, what position you give to it, both for yourself and for our directorate. How much time you want to spend on it, and if you want to spend time on it.*

Apart from the fact that for some agents the programme makes their work interesting and agreeable, for others it enables them to (re)gain recognition and a feeling of social utility. When the services were merged, this disrupted the resource allocation processes, changed the nature of missions and jobs, interfered with professional identities, affected the distribution of tasks and thus affected so many aspects that helped make sense of this work. Insisting firmly that 'she did not want to be recognised, but was willing to be identified', a nurse working in one of the DTs added:

> *Before working here, I completed a two-year mission in the humanitarian sector and I am still deeply affected by that. There have been no complications since. After this experience, I came here. At first, I found it difficult as I had arrived in a world that was very administrative, very surprising, and I was not at all – this is just an observation, not a criticism – I was not put forward to demonstrate my own skill set. My strength lies in my interpersonal skills and my desire to get things done. My problem is that I am in a medical center where I work with 4 or 5 physicians, so in their eyes, I am ... what? For the physicians, it's not clear what I am. In the eyes of others, I don't necessarily bring something of my own to the table. When the ARS reform came along, the Nutrition policy officer at head office asked for one adviser per DT, and so the inspector who works on prevention and with whom I get on very well said, "That's for you!" It's linked with the humanitarian work I was doing before. I don't feel that I am in any way a specialist in other subjects like poverty or sport, and I have no ambition to become a specialist. However, since this is my job at the moment, I say, "Anything that's nutrition, I'll have it", even sport-health because this campaign is going on and we have the call for projects. So, I'm being perfectly open about this because it's still what I feel, I'm talking about my job, I do lots of things.*

The agents that we met showed varying degrees of commitment to implement the PSSBE, according to how interested they were and/or how much time they could devote to it. Indeed, the forms of coordination observed at local level were variable, and can even be described as minimal (Dodier 1993) in certain locations, in other words, they consisted of barely formalised arrangements between agents, and seemed to lack stability. Consequently, the range of regional orientations of the PSSBE varies greatly from one DDCS and one DT to another.

The two advisors tasked with managing the programme stressed how difficult it had been for them to successfully combine all the various initiatives at regional level:

> *I am at the ARS, I only manage the nutrition file, but still, I can spend a lot of time on it. In the DTs, nutrition is only one topic among many others in prevention and prevention is far from being the most important mission for the DTs. Since the RGPP, there is no longer a hierarchical relationship between the DRJSCS and the DDCSs. Colleagues are under the direct authority of both their head of section and the Prefect of the département and when these two parties say 'go to the right', our colleagues go right and when they say go left, they go off to the left. Meanwhile, we are waiting for them to be available to spend time on this* program*!*

The dangers of certain representatives and departments becoming disinterested in health-sports issues and more generally in education and health promotion missions, viewed as the poor relations of health policies in France so dominated by the healthcare sector, are also very significant. However, although the aims of the 'Hospital, Patients, Health, Territories' law were to promote a view of health that is not limited simply to the absence of illness and to create an ARS-DTs network capable of implementing a general regional health policy, funding for public health programmes through the FIR remains limited. The path dependence that was referred to previously in the case of the Ministry for Sport can also be clearly seen here. This public health inspector remarked:

> *We have the feeling, in our ARS-DTs network at least, that there is a movement towards developing prevention and health promotion step by step, using the means that we have available. This has a lot to do with our Director General, as he is convinced of the advantage of implementing a global approach to health. If we consider the question from a theoretical point of view, for prevention and the promotion of health our first port of call should not necessarily be the health establishment. I think we're moving in the right direction; in any case, we're starting from so far away that things can only get better!*

3.2. *Increasing difficulties reconciling missions with resources*

This lack of resources also weakens the professional legitimacy of the agents, as the implementation of the PSSBE invites them to 'recruit' public and private sector stakeholders likely to participate in this public health programme. Because they feel less available for their respective partner networks, the agents are afraid that they will produce 'down-market' (Belorgey 2011, p. 33) services themselves, and thus that their difficulties will be highlighted as performance problems for which they alone would be responsible. An agent in one of the DDCSs added in the same vein:

> *'The issue of resources has become a real problem. Most of the funded projects have only been able to carry on since the call for projects first began because of our CNDS/FIR funding. The duration of these projects was an important criterion for their eligibility. We are blocked somewhat at present because our credits have not increased from year to year in the present economic climate... the original projects, at least the majority of them, will come to an end if we no longer subsidize them. The main concern is that if we continue to finance them, the available resources will not be sufficient to allow us to support any new projects we may be offered'.*

In addition to the disparities mentioned above in coordination between regional and local levels, there are other inequalities that may arise as a result of this lack of resources, with consequences not only for access to aid provided through the PSSBE by new operators, but also for the continuity of care offered to beneficiaries by the structures that are currently receiving support. As a result, it is as if, in light of the public resources that can be mobilised to promote sustainable actions and encourage the development of new projects, it is preferable here that the ability and/or willingness of local stakeholders to commit to this programme should remain insufficient.

Against this backdrop of tensions between missions and resources, department heads have also gradually prioritised the intervention of departments in the traditional government prerogatives of inspection and control (institutions, leisure centres, profession of sports educator), presented by the agents interviewed as being the main or even the only focus of senior management in this field:

> *The fear is that ultimately, our mission will be exclusively limited to traditional government roles and therefore control. And that ties in with the importance our directors want to attach to this sports-health mission. For them it's not crucial. We're not dealing with the safety of the sportsman. These inspection tasks are basically short-termism, because we are dealing with the safety of the user and not taking the longer view which would consist in acting to protect their health.*

This polarisation, which they also say they understand because of the meagre resources allocated, is however detrimental to territorial coordination, support to local operators and appraisals. Faced with these situations which devalue and undermine the scope of their work, they consider that their skills are now underused. The missions prioritised by their superiors are therefore likely to be of out of step not only with their description but also with the content of ministerial policies. And so, just like the agents of other ministerial bodies, they fear that the activities that form their professional identity may disappear. This feeling of decline is accentuated by the fact that in several departments, some projects are only managed by contract staff. The absence of any prospect of these contracts being renewed exacerbates the malaise, as it generates a sense of inability to take the projects on after they have gone.

More generally, the agents interviewed considered that the PSSBE would also benefit from proactive national management which would remind the directors of the DRJSCS and ARS of their responsibilities in the matter. They also highlight the need for networking based on a national pooling of experiences on the ground; a dynamic which they say does not exist despite the existence of a national resources centre:

> *Colleagues have had three months to put together the regional* program, *that's practically nothing. They've done what they can. I blame the Ministry for that and the State departments almost daily. It means that we are never working for the long term, we're always rushing around, it is a real problem. And then there is a problem with the data we have. There is a national resources center for sport-health which existed, then stopped existing and then arose from the ashes. Personally, I get the impression that it's mainly used for passing on statistics on the number of people with type-1 or type-2 diabetes, rather than for good initiatives. It should be offering more, it should be a control room of good initiatives, it should work on modeling and toolboxes that we could subsequently make use of. At the moment, it's rather poor.*

Reinforcing the observation that the State is not a uniform whole with a unified will, such contradictions between the official view and the actual experience, between policies that have to be applied and the practical conditions in which they have to be implemented (Dubois 2012), create the impression that, in the framework of this programme too, governments are using and abusing media hype and other processes in 'symbolic politics' (Edelman 1985).

4. Conclusion

The regional roll-out of the PSSBE produces paradoxical effects, marked by the deepening of the inter-ministerial partnership, and by the disparate and fragile involvement of the territorial departments of the two ministerial bodies in this programme. The learning of collective action is particularly perceptible in the organisational work undertaken to tackle this public problem of physical inactivity. It mainly consists in making it intelligible enough to allow action to be taken in the area. This has involved agreeing on the definitions and thus aligning this problem with the internal divisions, missions, routines and value systems of the two ministerial bodies.

This learning process has hit several obstacles, however. They are not only caused by the usual tension between decision and implementation so regularly described in public policy analysis, just as they cannot solely be put down to the fact that the ARS and the DRJSCS are young entities. The merger carried out at breakneck speed against a tense budgetary backdrop, and the requirements to reduce the number of posts, have led to a 'sham' territorialisation of this programme, a product of the complex interplay between national, regional and infra-regional regulation processes. Because the combination of material, institutional and cognitive factors generated by the implementation of the PSSBE represents additional costs for the staff, especially at local level, this may lead ultimately to its deterioration. Consequently, while public policies exist in concrete terms because of the activities of agents on the ground, whose work is so much an integral part of the ongoing process of creating public action, it is clear that, given their current working conditions, they will struggle in future to perform what has for so long been described as a decisive role (Lipsky 1980).

While the difficulties expressed by the agents we met mainly reflect the uncertainties in which public authorities are immersed, another big programme has been launched in France. It includes a review of the missions which the State would keep after the new regional reform reducing from 22 to 13 the number of regional authorities as of 1 January 2016. This reform will lead to a new series of DRJSCS/ARS mergers and the restructuring of the DDCSs and the DTs in order to fit in with these new regional boundaries.

This first analysis of the effects of the PSSBE implementation may finally be properly completed. As the body is a favourite focus of the exercise of power and an object of government for the State and a number of other stakeholders (Turner 1992, Fassin and Memmi 2004, Foucault 2004), a further study should look at the way this public problem of physical inactivity has been taken on board by organisations in the sports, medico-social and health sectors, in their registers and categories of action. By extending the focus to the operators themselves and to the manner in which they adopt the guidelines institutionalised by the DRJSCS/ARS network, we will be able to examine how the adoption of these guidelines allows these protagonists to establish (or not) their credibility in a sector (sport and health) where power struggles can be significant (Abbott 1988).

Notes

1. Council of Ministers paper, 10 October 2012.
2. Instruction on the operational implementation of the measures to promote and develop the practise of physical and sporting activity as a public health factor, announced in the Council of Ministers of 10 October 2012.
3. These aspects confirm a situation presented by the Court of Auditors in 2013: the continued staff cutbacks in 2013 actually expose departments to great inequalities with regard to their intervention capacity: the technical and educational staff of the Ministry of Sport, although on average four in number in each DDCS, do not tally with the indicative staff numbers. In this context and regarding the DDCS in the Orne for example, only seven

inspections of institutions out of the reported 915 were carried out with one member of staff. Inspection of equipment is even further reduced.

Disclosure statement

No potential conflict of interest was reported by the author.

References

Abbott, A., 1988. *The system of professions. An essay on the division of expert labor.* Chicago, IL: The University of Chicago Press.

Ackroyd, S., Kirkpatrick, I., and Walker, R., 2007. Public management reform and its consequences for professional organisation: a comparative analysis. *Public administration*, 85 (1), 9–26. doi:10.1111/j.1467-9299.2007.00631.x

Aucoin, P., 1990. administrative reform in public management: paradigms, principles, paradoxes and pendulums. *Governance*, 3, 115–137. doi:10.1111/gove.1990.3.issue-2

Bazex, J., Pène, P., and Rivière, D., 2012. Physical activities and sport. Implications for health and society. *Bulletin de l'Académie Nationale de Médecine*, 196 (7), 1429–1442.

Belorgey, N., 2011. Réduire le temps d'attente et de passage aux urgences. Une entreprise de « réforme » d'un service public et ses effets sociaux. *Actes de la recherche en sciences sociales*, 4 (189), 16–33. doi:10.3917/arss.189.0016

Bergeron, H., Castel, P., and Dubuisson-Quellier, S., 2014. Gouverner par les labels. Une comparaison des politiques de l'obésité et de la consommation durable. *Gouvernement et action publique*, 3 (3), 7–31. doi:10.3917/gap.143.0007

Berlivet, L., 2005. Uneasy prevention: the problematic modernization of Health Education in France after 1975. *In*: V. Berridge and K. Loughlin, eds. *Medicine, the market and mass media: producing health in the twentieth century*. London: Routledge, 95–122.

Bezes, P., 2005. Le renouveau du contrôle des bureaucraties. L'impact du New Public Management. *Informations sociales*, 126, 26–37.

Bezes, P., *et al.*, 2011. New Public Management et professions dans l'État : au-delà des oppositions, quelles recompositions? *Sociologie du travail*, 53, 293–348. doi:10.1016/j.soctra.2011.06.003

Bossy, T., 2010. *Poids de l'enjeu, enjeu de poids. La mise sur agenda de l'obésité en Angleterre et en France*. Thèse de doctorat en science politique. IEP de Paris. Paris.

Cavill, N., Kahlmeier, S., and Racioppi, F., 2006. *Physical activity and health in Europe: evidence for action*. Copenhague Ø: World Health Organization.

Clarke, J., Gewirtz, S., and Mc Laughin, E., 2000. *New managerialism: new welfare?* London: Sage.

Dent, M., O'Neill, M., and Bagley, C., 1999. *Professions: new Public Management and the European Welfare State*. Staffordshire: University Press.

Dodier, N., 1993. Les appuis conventionnels de l'action. Eléments de pragmatique sociologique. *Réseaux*, 11 (62), 63–85. doi:10.3406/reso.1993.2574

DRJSCS, ARS Aquitaine. 2015. *Plan d'action « Sport, Santé Bien-Etre » en Aquitaine*. Bordeaux: janvier.

Dubois, V., 2012. Ethnographier l'action publique. Les transformations de l'État social au prisme de l'enquête de terrain. *Gouvernement et action publique*, 1 (1), 83–101. doi:10.3917/gap.121.0083

Dupuy, F. and Thoenig, J.C., 1985. *L'administration en miettes*. Paris: Fayard.

Edelman, M., 1985. *The symbolic uses of politics*. Chicago, IL: University of Illinois Press.

Epstein, R., 2013. *La rénovation urbaine. Démolition-reconstruction de l'État*. Paris: Presses de Sciences Po.

Farrell, C. and Morris, J., 2003. The `Neo-Bureaucratic' state: professionals, managers and professional managers in schools, general practices and social work. *Organization*, 10, 129–156. doi:10.1177/1350508403010001380

Fassin, D. and Memmi, D., eds, 2004. *Le gouvernement des corps*. Paris: Editions de l'Ehess.

Ferlie, E. and Geraghty, K.J., 2005. Professionals in public service organizations. Implications for public sector reforming. *In*: E. Ferlie, L. Jr., and C. Pollitt, eds. *The Oxford handbook of public management*. Oxford: Oxford University Press, 422–445.

Foucault, M., 2004. *Sécurité, territoire et population. Cours au collège de France. 1977–1978*. Paris: Gallimard-Seuil.

Génolini, J.-P. and Clément, J.-P., 2010. Lutter contre la sédentarité: l'incorporation d'une nouvelle morale de l'effort. *Sciences sociales et sport*, 3 (1), 133–156. doi:10.3917/rsss.003.0133

Gordon-Larsen, P., *et al.*, 2006. Inequality in the built environment underlies key health disparities in physical activity and obesity. *Pediatrics*, 117 (2), 417–424. doi:10.1542/peds.2005-0058

Guinhouya, B.C., 2010. Activité physique de l'enfant scolarisé en France. Le paradoxe d'une priorité de santé publique ! *Revue d'Épidémiologie et de Santé Publique*, 58, 255–267. doi:10.1016/j.respe.2010.02.111

Gusfield, J., 1981. *The culture of public problems: drinking-driving and the symbolic order*. Chicago, IL: The University of Chicago Press.

Hall, P.A. and Lamont, M., 2009. Introduction. *In*: P.A. Hall and M. Lamont, eds. *Successful societies: how institutions and culture affect health*. New York: Cambridge University Press, 1–22.

Hardman, A.E. and Stensel, D.J., 2009. *Physical activity and health: the evidence explained*. 2nd ed. London: Routledge.

Hill, M. and Hupe, P., 2002. *Implementing public policy: governance in theory and practice*. London: SAGE.

Hillsdon, M., *et al.*, 2005. *A review of the evidence on the effectiveness of public health interventions for increasing physical activity amongst adults: a review of reviews*. London: Health Development Agency.

Honta, M. and Haschar-Noé, N., 2011. Les politiques préventives de santé publique à l'épreuve de la territorialisation: l'introuvable gouvernance régionale du Programme national nutrition santé en Aquitaine. *Sciences sociales et santé*, 29 (4), 33–62. doi:10.3917/sss.294.0033

Honta, M. and Julhe, S., 2015. Serving the state and the private sector: the paradoxical effects of the reconstruction of public action on the career paths of Sports Ministry agents in France. *International review for the sociology of sport*, 50 (2), 179–195. doi:10.1177/1012690213478253

Hooghe, L. and Marks, G., 2003. Unraveling the central state, but how ? types of multi – level governance. *American political science review*, 97 (2), 233–243.

Hughes, E.C., 1971. *The sociological eye. Selected papers*. Chicago, IL: Adline-Atherton.

Institut national de prévention et d'éducation pour la santé. 2011. *Promouvoir l'activité physique des jeunes. Élaborer et développer un projet de type Icaps*. Paris: INPES.

Institut National de Santé et de Recherche Médicale. 2008. *Activité physique, contextes et effets sur la santé*. Paris: La Documentation Française.

Jobert, B. and Muller, P., 1987. *L'État en action. Politiques publiques et corporatismes*. Paris: Presses Universitaires de France.

Kada, N., 2012. La réforme de l'État territorial ? *Revue française d'administration publique*, 141 (1), 109–120. doi:10.3917/rfap.141.0109

Laffin, M., Ed., 1998. *Beyond bureaucracy? the professions in the contemporary public sector*. Aldershot: Ashgate Publishing.

Lagroye, J., Sawicki, F., and François, B., 2006. *Sociologie politique*. Paris: Presses de Sciences Po.

Lipsky, M., 1980. *Street-level bureaucracy: dilemmas of the individual in public service*. New York, NY: Russel Sage Foundation.

Moquay, P. 2005. L'Etat territorialisé, ou l'arroseur arrosé: les ambiguïtés de l'Etat face aux recompositions territoriales en France. *In*: Breher, L., *et al.* eds. *Jeux d'échelle et transformation de l'Etat. Le gouvernement des territoires au Québec et en France*. Laval: PUL, 85–116.

Muller, P. and Surel, Y., 1998. *L'analyse des politiques publiques*. Paris : Montchrestien.

Oppert, J.-M., Charreire, H., and Simon, C., 2010. Activité physique et santé: remettre les enfants d'aujourd'hui en mouvement. *Revue d'Épidémiologie et de Santé Publique*, 58, 235–236. doi:10.1016/j.respe.2010.06.005

Oppert, J.M., *et al.*, 2005. *Activité physique et santé. Arguments scientifiques, pistes pratiques. Les synthèses du Programme national nutrition santé*. Paris: Ministère de la Santé, de la Jeunesse, des Sports et de la Vie Associative.

Patchett, A.D., Yeatman, H.R., and Johnson, K.M., 2014. Obesity framing for health policy development in Australia, France and Switzerland. *health promotion international*, August 21, doi:10.1093/heapro/dau066

Pierru, F., 2012. La santé en fusions. L'accouchement des agences régionales de santé au forceps institutionnel. *In*: G. Castaing, ed. *La territorialisation des politiques de santé*. Bordeaux: Editions hospitalières, 77–108.

Pierson, P., 2000. Increasing returns, path dependence, and the study of politics. *The American political science review*, 94 (2), 251–267. doi:10.2307/2586011

Pollitt, C. and Bouckaert, G., 2004. *Public management reform. a comparative analysis*. 2nd ed. Oxford: Oxford University Press.

Rolland, C. and Pierru, F., 2013. Les Agences Régionales de Santé deux ans après? Une autonomie de façade. *Santé Publique*, 4 (25), 411–419.

Sabatier, P.A., 1986. Top-down and bottom-up approaches to implementation research: a critical analysis and suggested synthesis. *Journal of public policy*, 6 (1), 21–48. doi:10.1017/S0143814X00003846

Sisson, S.B. and Katzmarzyk, P.T., 2008. International prevalence of physical activity in youth and adults. *Obesity reviews*, 9 (6), 606–614. doi:10.1111/obr.2008.9.issue-6

Smith, A., Green, K., and Roberts, K., 2004. Sports participation and the 'Obesity/Health Crisis': reflections on the case of young people in England. *International review for the sociology of sport*, 39 (4), 457–464. doi:10.1177/1012690204049081

Toussaint, J.F., 2008. *Retrouver sa liberté de mouvement – PNAPS: plan national de prévention par l'activité physique et sportive*. Paris: Rapport au Ministère de la Santé, de la Jeunesse, des Sports et de la Vie associative.

Turner, B.S., 1992. *Regulating bodies: essays in medical sociology*. New York, NY: Routledge.

Van Hoek, E., *et al.*, 2016. Development of a Dutch intervention for obese young children. *Health promotion international*, first published online January 10, 2016 doi:10.1093/heapro/dav115

Wilkinson, R.G. and Marmot, M.G., eds., 2003. *Social determinants of health: the solid facts*. Copenhague Ø: World Health Organization.

World Health Organization. 2004. *Global Strategy on Diet, Physical Activity and Health*. Genève: WHO Publications.

World Health Organization Regional Office for Europe. 2013. *Physical activity promotion in socially disadvantaged groups: principles for action*. Copenhague Ø: World Health Organization Regional Office for Europe.

Appendix: Public reports on the fight against inactivity and obesity

Bourdillon, F., Cano, N., Delarue, J., Turck, D., 2010. *Propositions pour le PNNS 2011–2015 des sociétés savantes et d'experts en nutrition*, novembre.

Boyer, V., 2008. *La prévention de l'obésité*. Rapport d'information de la Commission des affaires culturelles, familiales et sociales, Assemblée nationale, septembre.

Castetbon, K., Hercberg, S., 2007. *Etude Nationale Nutrition Santé. Situation nutritionnelle en France en 2006 selon les indicateurs d'objectif et les repères du Programme national nutrition santé (PNNS)*. Institut national de veille sanitaire, décembre.

Deriot, G., 2005. *La prévention et la prise en charge de l'obésité*. Rapport de l'Office parlementaire d'évaluation des politiques de santé, octobre.

De Danne, A., 2009. *Commission pour la prévention et la prise en charge de l'obésité*. Rapport au Président de la république, décembre.

Haschar-Noé, N., Basson, J.C., Julhe, S., Malric, L., Merlaud, F., Rolland, C., Terral P., 2010. *Activité physique, nutrition et santé: la mise en oeuvre du Programme national nutrition santé en Midi-Pyrénées*. Rapport de recherche pour le Conseil régional Midi-Pyrénées, Toulouse.

Hercberg, S., Tallec, A., 2000. *Pour une politique nutritionnelle de santé publique en France*. Rapport pour le Haut comité de Santé publique.

Institut national de prévention et d'éducation pour la santé, 2011. *Promouvoir l'activité physique des jeunes. Élaborer et développer un projet de type Icaps*. Paris: INPES.

Inspection générale des affaires sociales, 2003. *Santé, pour une politique de prévention durable*. Rapport annuel. Paris: La Documentation française.

Inspection générale des affaires sociales et Conseil général de l'alimentation, de l'agriculture et des espaces ruraux, 2010. *Rapport sur l'évaluation du programme national nutrition santé PNNS2, 2006–2010*. Paris.

Ministère de la Santé, de la Jeunesse, des Sports et de la Vie associative, 2008. *Activité physique et obésité de l'enfant. Bases pour une prescription adaptée*, novembre, Paris.

Ministère de la Santé et des Solidarités, 2005. *Activité physique et santé. Arguments scientifiques, pistes pratiques*. Paris.

Ministère de la Santé et des Solidarités, 2006. *Deuxième Programme national nutrition santé, 2006–2010, Actions et mesures*, septembre.

Ministère du Travail, de l'Emploi et de la Santé, 2011, *Programme National Nutrition santé, 2011–2015*. Paris.

Ministère du Travail, de l'Emploi et de la Santé, 2011. *Plan obésité, 2010–2013*. Paris.

A political spectator sport or policy priority? A review of sport, physical activity and public mental health policy

Andy Smith, Jon Jones, Laura Houghton and Tom Duffell

ABSTRACT

In the context of policy and political claims about the benefits of encouraging participation in sport, physical activity (PA) and exercise for physical and mental health, and for improving the effectiveness of prevention, early intervention and treatment services for people with mental illness, this article provides, for the first time, a critical overview of policy related to community sport, PA and public mental health (PMH). Focusing on England, the article analyses 18 key policy documents published between 1995 and May 2016. We explain that the promotion of PMH and prevention and treatment of mental illness through participation in PA or exercise, as a formal goal of mental health policy, has been generally absent from the public health policy landscape. Until very recently, PMH and illness are also shown to be neglected as core priorities of community sport and PA policy in England. Even where PMH is discussed explicitly in national policy, a clear definition of specific and measurable goals, which can be used to determine the efficacy, effectiveness and comparative effectiveness of policy in addressing PMH outcomes, is notably absent. The article concludes by suggesting that, at present, the improvement of PMH and tackling mental illness through community sport and PA appears to be more of a political spectator sport than a clearly thought-out, sustained and long-term commitment of public policy.

Introduction

There is increasing global concern about the substantial health problems that arise from mental, neurological and substance (MNS)[1] disorders (Whiteford *et al.* 2015), and especially about the association of these mental illnesses with the scale of social (especially relative income and wealth) inequalities in different countries (e.g. Wilkinson and Pickett 2010; Marmot 2015, Pickett and Wilkinson 2015). Data from Wilkinson and Pickett's (2010) *The spirit level: why equality is better for everyone* suggest that the prevalence of mental illness is higher in more unequal rich countries such as the USA, Australia, the UK, Canada and New Zealand (where around one-in-four people will at some point in any given year experience mental illness), and much lower in more equal countries such as Germany, Italy, Japan and Spain (where fewer than one-in-ten experience mental illness each year).

Despite the skewed social distribution of mental illness, MNS disorders are the leading cause of the global disease burden (Whiteford *et al.* 2015), and exceed the burdens associated with each of four other major categories of non-communicable diseases (NCDs): cardiovascular diseases, chronic respiratory diseases, diabetes, and cancer (Bloom *et al.* 2011). The findings of the Global Burden of

Disease Study 2010 (GBD 2010) conducted in 187 countries revealed that mental and substance disorders accounted for 183.9 million disability adjusted life years (DALYs), a rise of 37.6% since 1990 (133.6 million), which is associated with the long-term shift in burden from communicable to non-communicable diseases (Whiteford *et al.* 2013). In 2010, mental and substance disorders represented 7.4% of the world's measurable burden of disease (and the fifth leading cause of DALYs) and included 8.6 million years of life lost due to these disorders. The highest proportion of DALYs was reported by 10–29-year-olds, and depressive disorders were the most prevalent in all regions represented in the study, followed by anxiety, illicit drug use and alcohol use (Whiteford *et al.* 2013). Particularly significant was the almost three-fold increase in DALYs for depressive disorders for age 5–9 and 10–14, and nearly four-fold increase for age 5–9 and 20–24 (the peak age band for depressive disorders) (Whiteford *et al.* 2013).

Globally, depression is experienced by an estimated 350 million people, and is predicted to make one of the greatest contributions to global disease burden by 2020 (WHO 2015). Depression is also a significant risk factor for suicide, which accounts for approximately 800,000 global deaths annually and is currently the second leading cause of death among 15–29-year-olds (WHO 2015). Although important national variations exist (see NCISH 2015), data from the UK – where mental illness is the single largest cause of disability and costs approximately £105 billion annually (roughly the cost of the entire National Health Service budget) (Davies 2014, Mental Health Taskforce 2016) – also indicate that suicide is a significant public health problem. In 2014, there were 6109 suicides in the UK of which 76% were by men (n = 4623) (CALM 2015). This means approximately 12 men in the UK die every day by suicide, making it the single biggest cause of death by men under the age of 45 (CALM 2015). Mental illness is also common among children and young people, with one-in-ten 5–16-year-olds in England having a mental health disorder, 5.6% are estimated to have a conduct disorder, and 3.6% experience emotional disorders (Public Health England [PHE] 2015). Half of all adult mental illnesses (excluding dementia) are also first experienced by age 14, and approximately 75% of mental illnesses experienced by adults were first present by the age of 18 (HMG/Department of Health [DH] 2011, DH 2015).

These introductory remarks represent the starting point for this article, the central objective of which is to provide, for the first time, a critical overview of policy related to community sport, physical activity (PA) and public mental health (PMH)[2] and illness in England. It does so in the context of policy and political claims about the benefits of encouraging participation in sport, PA and exercise for physical and mental health, and for improving the effectiveness of prevention, early intervention and treatment services for people with mental illness. The next section examines PMH and illness as global policy problems and some of the major policy responses to those problems by the World Health Organization (WHO). We then focus particularly on national PMH policy priorities in England before reviewing the content of over 20 years of community sport and PA policy, which, as we shall discuss, have until very recently largely ignored PMH and illness as key policy priorities.

Mental health and illness as a global policy problem

Despite policy and political claims that PMH is equally as important as physical health (WHO 2001, 2008, HMG/DH 2011, Social Care, Local Government and Care Partnership Directorate 2014), in very many countries there remains a considerable lack of parity of esteem between physical and mental health policy (Becker and Kleinmann 2013, Davies 2014, All Party Parliamentary Group on Mental Health 2015). Indeed, the lack of parity of esteem between physical and mental health policy and associated failure of many countries to integrate PMH sufficiently into all aspects of health care, policy, and practice, has resulted in a global neglect and marginalisation of mental health (Becker and Kleinmann 2013).

This having been said, since 2000, there have been several important milestones in the development of an alleged global commitment to improving PMH, enhancing mental health care provision, and addressing the costs of mental illness. The *World Health Report* (WHR) 2001, for example, focused on public health approaches to mental health, the burden of mental and behavioural disorders, solving mental health problems, and PMH policy and service provision (WHO 2001). Its purpose was to enhance public and professional awareness of the actual burden and human, social and economic costs of mental disorders (WHO 2001), and help break down barriers such as stigma, discrimination and inadequate services that prevent many people worldwide from receiving treatment (WHO 2001). The report made 10 recommendations for international action, which included: the provision of treatment in primary care and communities; educating the public about mental health to tackle stigma and discrimination; establishing national policies, programmes and legislation for mental health; and involving communities, families and consumers in the development and decision-making of policies, programmes and services (W 2001).

In 2002, the WHO mental health Global Action Programme (*mhGAP*) was endorsed by the 55th World Health Assembly, which emphasised the need for Member States to improve their health care systems to deliver better quality and standards of care to people with MNS disorders. While this formal commitment strengthened the position of PMH on the global public health agenda, the *mhGAP* was only introduced in 2008 to: (i) reinforce all stakeholders' commitment to increasing the financial and human resources needed to support the care of MNS disorders; and (ii) to enhance the coverage of MNS interventions, particularly in low and lower middle income countries where large proportions of the global burden of MNS disorders are found (WHO 2008). These interventions focused on those mental illnesses (e.g. depression, schizophrenia, suicide, dementia, disorders due to alcohol and illicit drug use, and mental disorders in children) that cause the greatest burden in terms of morbidity, mortality and disability, and have the highest economic costs and human rights violations (WHO 2008).

The WHO commitment to addressing PMH and illness was further articulated in *Investing in Mental Health: Evidence for Action* (WHO 2013a) and *Mental Health Action Plan 2013–2020* (WHO 2013b). In the first of these, the WHO outlines the clear socio-economic case and supporting evidence base for investing in PMH, while the second provided guidance for national plans and sought to avoid duplicating the work of the *mhGAP* programme (WHO 2013b). More particularly, in adopting a comprehensive and multisectoral approach to PMH with an emphasis on promotion, prevention, treatment, rehabilitation, care and recovery, the action plan has at its heart the 'globally accepted principle that there is "no health without mental health"' (WHO 2013b, p. 6). In doing so, it identifies a series of actions for Member States and associated partners as well as numerous indicators and targets that can be used to evaluate the success of implementation, progress and impact of PMH policy (WHO 2013b).

The comprehensive and multi-sectoral approach described by the WHO is intended to achieve the main goal of the plan, namely: to 'promote mental well-being, prevent mental disorders, provide care, enhance recovery, promote human rights and reduce the mortality, morbidity and disability for persons with mental disorders' (WHO 2013b, p. 9). This theme was further addressed in the *Social Determinants of Mental Health* (WHO 2014), which built upon previous work on the social determinants of health (e.g. Commission on the Social Determinants of Health 2008, WHO 2013c), and introduced the principle of *proportionate universalism* and the importance of adopting a *life course approach* to mental health. As Allen *et al.* (2014) and Marmot (2010, 2015) have noted, these seminal (and other) investigations into the social determinants of health make clear how the conditions in which people lead their lives are the main influences on their health. These conditions are, however, unequally distributed and the clear social gradient in health they produce are seen as avoidable, unjust and require sustained social action and political will to reduce them (Wilkinson and Pickett 2010; Allen *et al.* 2014, Marmot 2015, Pickett and Wilkinson 2015). In relation to mental illness, which becomes progressively more common further down the social class structure, the impact of the social determinants of PMH become especially significant because people with mental illness typically have a life expectancy between 10 and 20 years shorter than those who do not have mental illness (Marmot 2015). For Marmot (2015), this reduced life expectancy is associated with a complex interaction of physical, psychological and social processes that are, in turn, related to the significant inequities people experience in the conditions in which they are born, grow, live, work and age, and in the inequities in power, money and resources that influence them.

Given the global burden posed by the increased incidence of mental illness in many population groups, it is perhaps not surprising that the promotion of positive PMH was recently included as one of the Sustainable Development Goals of the United Nations (UN) (UN 2015). In particular, the UN (2015) now seeks to promote mental well-being and reduce by one-third premature mortality from NCDs through improved prevention and treatment by 2030. An additional goal is the prevention and treatment of drug abuse (including alcohol and narcotic drugs) as part of the UN's broader commitment to promoting physical and mental health, and to extending life expectancy for all (UN 2015).

Public mental health policy in England: no health without mental health?

The global policy landscape for mental health and illness outlined above provides the context for PMH policy in England where one of the most recent population-based mental health policies to have been introduced is *No Health Without Mental Health: A Cross-Government Mental Health Outcomes Strategy for People of All Ages* (HMG/DH 2011). In addition to the rising incidence of mental illness, the strategy was introduced to build resilience, promote mental health and well-being, and tackle health inequalities. It also sought to prevent mental illness, intervene early when it develops, and improve the quality of life of people with mental illness and their families (HMG/DH 2011).

In this regard, the promotion of PMH was described as being 'everyone's business' that could be achieved only through multisectoral and multi-partner working oriented towards the achievement of six objectives, locally and nationally. These objectives, intended to improve the mental health of individuals and the whole population, are: (i) more people will have good mental health; (ii) more people with mental health problems will recover; (iii) more people with mental health problems will have good physical health; (iv) more people will have a positive experience of care and support; (v) fewer people will suffer avoidable harm; and (vi) fewer people will experience stigma and discrimination (see HMG/DH 2011). The promotion of community sport was identified as being important to the achievement of Objective 1 – More people will have good mental health – for which the Department for Culture, Media and Sport (DCMS) was to be responsible. More specifically, it was suggested that improving the proportion of people with good mental health could be achieved through the creation of a School Games event to promote competitive sport and by developing a mass participation/community sport legacy programme from the London 2012 Olympic Games (HMG/DH 2011). While not explicitly stated, the use of exercise also appeared to be endorsed as part of the Improved Access to Psychological Therapies programme, and the percentage of adults meeting the recommended PA guidelines (5 × 30 minutes per week) was cited as an indicator of progress made in relation to the promotion of PMH (HMG/DH 2011).

No Health Without Mental Health is supported by an implementation framework intended to bring about long-term change in mental health (Centre for Mental Health *et al.* 2012), and by the recommendations of *Closing the Gap: Priorities for Change in Mental Health* (hereafter, '*Closing the Gap*') (Social Care, Local Government and Care Partnership Directorate 2014). *Closing the Gap* identified 25 aspects of mental health care and support as policy priorities for shorter-term action, which were clustered into the following categories of activity: increasing access to public mental health services, integrating physical and mental health care, starting early to promote mental well-being and prevent mental health problems (e.g. focusing on mothers and children), and improving the quality of life of people with mental health problems (Social Care, Local Government and Care Partnership Directorate 2014). To help improve the quality of life of people with mental illness,

Closing the Gap noted – albeit in passing – the role that might be played by PA by emphasising the role mental health support workers and carers can play in encouraging people to reduce and stop smoking, and become more physically active (Social Care, Local Government and Care Partnership Directorate 2014).

The need for structural change leading to improved efficiency and effectiveness (among other outcomes) in public health, including PMH, was also emphasised in the 2014 *NHS Five Year Forward View* (NHS 2014). The *Forward View* argued that there needs to be a closer integration of patient-focused health and social care, primary and specialist care, and physical and mental health care, to meet the increasingly complex health problems presented by the population (NHS 2014). A number of 'ambitions' (e.g. improved access to services, new waiting times for mental health, increased number of beds for young people) were stated to achieve by 2020 a genuine parity of esteem between physical and mental health (NHS 2014). Although significant challenges remain (see The King's Fund 2016), the ambition to integrate physical and mental health care was endorsed by the Mental Health Taskforce in its *Forward View for Mental Health*, the purpose of which was to ensure a cross-system commitment to improving mental health outcomes throughout the health and care system, which had yet to be achieved despite the introduction of *No Health Without Mental Health* (Mental Health Taskforce 2016). The Taskforce made a series of recommendations (requiring an additional £1 billion investment) to achieve parity of esteem between mental and physical health, including: the need for better prevention and early intervention services, improved access to crisis care, and better integration of mental and physical health care.

Unlike the broader *NHS Five Year Forward View* (NHS 2014), which made no mention of sport, PA or exercise, *Forward View for Mental Health* noted that people with mental illness (who are at greater risk of poor physical health) should get access to primary and secondary prevention and screening programmes, including interventions for PA and other health conditions (e.g. obesity, diabetes, heart disease, and cancer) (Mental Health Taskforce 2016). In light of what the Chief Executive of the NSPCC, Peter Wanless, has described as the impending 'time bomb of mental health problems' in young people (NSPCC 2015), the Mental Health Taskforce (2016) also identified children and young people as priority groups for PMH promotion, prevention and early intervention. It also recommended the full implementation of policy reforms suggested by the Children and Young People's Mental Health and Wellbeing Taskforce in its publication, *Future in Mind: Promoting, Protecting and Improving Our Children and Young People's Mental Health and Wellbeing* (hereafter, '*Future in Mind*') (DH 2015). *Future in Mind* made a whole series of recommendations, including the need to build resilience, promote good mental health, and adopt prevention and early intervention strategies during childhood (DH 2015). In doing so, *Future in Mind* emphasised – in its only reference to sport (PA and exercise are not mentioned) – the scope available for general practitioners and other professionals to offer social prescribing of activities such as sport to improve well-being and mental health in children and young people (DH 2015).

Physical activity and exercise: neglected features of mental health policy

Having reviewed some of the major recent mental health policy pronouncements in England, it is clear that few systematic attempts have been made to consider the potential contribution that sport, PA and exercise might make to the promotion of good PMH and the prevention and treatment of conditions such as depression and anxiety. The general absence of PA and exercise, in particular, from the mental health policy landscape in England is especially noteworthy for conditions such as depression, which is the first and only mental illness for which PA is recommended as an evidence-based treatment (Ekkekakis 2015). Indeed, for depression, PA has been regarded as an efficacious intervention that has global accessibility, few adverse side-effects, is relatively low cost, and represents an attractive cost-effective option for health care systems and organisations (Ekkekakis 2015).

In some countries (including England) that adopt 'stepped care' models of health care, PA is also 'recommended in clinical practice guidelines as one of the options that should be offered to patients with subthreshold depressive symptoms or mild to moderate levels of depression' (Ekkekakis 2015, p. 21). This is because there is now strong evidence linking PA and exercise (particularly of low to moderate intensity) to many elements of PMH (Callaghan 2004, Rosenbaum *et al.* 2015), and to the prevention and treatment of mental illness. For adults, in particular, there is substantial evidence that exercise (particularly aerobic exercise) is as effective in reducing depressive symptomology as pharmacotherapy and psychotherapy (Smith and Blumenthal 2013), and that being physically active is preventive in the onset of, and contributes to reductions in, mild to moderate depression (Mammen and Faulkner 2013; Rosenbaum *et al.* 2014, Ekkekakis 2015, Schuch *et al.* 2016). PA has also been shown to make a significant reduction to symptom severity among people with schizophrenia (Faulkner and Biddle 1999, Faulkner *et al.* 2013, Rosenbaum *et al.* 2015), and is thought to be more effective compared to control conditions at decreasing Post-Traumatic Stress Disorder (PTSD) and depressive symptoms in people with PTSD (Rosenbaum *et al.* 2015).

The evidence base for exercise and PA as an intervention for anxiety in adults is more mixed and less developed than for depression, though a review of cross-sectional, longitudinal and randomised studies concluded that both exercise and PA can reduce risk factors for the development of anxiety disorders and symptoms for specific and generalised anxiety (Utschig 2013). The study also concluded that anxiety disorders are associated with lower levels of PA, and that the relationship between PA and anxiety may be bi-directional (Utschig 2013, see also Stonerock *et al.* 2015). A more recent systematic review of 12 randomised control trials and five meta-analyses found that exercise, as a treatment for elevated anxiety or anxiety disorders, can be as beneficial as established treatments including medication, but noted that most studies suffered from a range of significant methodological limitations (Stonerock *et al.* 2015). In this regard, the authors noted that the evidence base for exercise is not of sufficient scientific rigor to recommend it as a form for treatment for people with clinically elevated anxiety (Stonerock *et al.* 2015).

In comparison to adults, the impact of exercise and PA on the mental health of children and young people has received considerably less attention, with depression, anxiety, self-esteem and cognitive functioning being the most widely studied conditions in the limited evidence that exists (Larun *et al.* 2006, Biddle and Asare 2011, Brown *et al.* 2013, Smith and Blumenthal 2013). In a review of reviews, Biddle and Asare (2011) concluded that PA: (i) has potentially positive effects for reduced depression; (ii) has small beneficial effects for reduced anxiety; (iii) can improve self-esteem, at least in the short-term; and (iv) can be associated with improved cognitive functioning, including academic performance, but these associations are usually small and inconsistent. In each case, however, the evidence was reported to be limited, and many studies were mainly cross-sectional and regarded as involving low quality intervention designs (Biddle and Asare 2011).

A follow-up systematic review and meta-analysis found a small, but significant, treatment effect for PA on depression in children and adolescents, which suggests that PA may play a role in the prevention and treatment of depression (Brown *et al.* 2013). Greater treatment effects were observed in studies where reductions in depression was the only programme outcome, where a PA intervention was complemented by an educational component, and where programmes targeted key participant characteristics (e.g. males or females, overweight or obese populations). The authors concluded that more outcome-focused studies are needed to inform the implementation of programmes that seek to reduce depression in young people (Brown *et al.* 2013). Investigations of Dutch adolescents have also found that the intensity, frequency duration or nature of PA does not predict a major depressive episode onset among males and females (Stavrakakis *et al.* 2013), and that declines in PA over a one-year period does not predict changes in depressive symptoms and self-esteem (Van Dijk *et al.* 2016). In this regard, changes in mental health were more likely to be affected by baseline levels of mental health, rather than declines in PA, and PA was thus considered as being particularly beneficial for adolescents with moderate to severe depression (Van Dijk *et al.* 2016).

While it is important to remain mindful of the limitations of the existing evidence base, PA and exercise are now often recommended by researchers as important components of interventions for people with mental illness (especially adults). They are also frequently identified as having a dual benefit for physical and mental health in the general population, as well as those with specific mental illnesses (Callaghan 2004, Rosenbaum *et al.* 2014, Ekkekakis 2015, Schuch *et al.* 2016). However, as Callaghan (2004) has noted, despite its potential effectiveness exercise appears to be a largely neglected intervention in mental health care, is rarely recognised by those in mainstream mental health services, and together with PA, exercise remains largely absent from the mainstream PMH policy landscape. The next section indicates that PMH and mental illness have also – until very recently – been largely overlooked in policy related to community sport and PA in England.

Public mental health and community sport and physical activity policy in England

Given the long-standing, and now routinely and uncritically expressed, ideology that links sport and PA with good health (Waddington 2000), we might have expected PMH and mental illness to feature prominently in community sport and PA policy in England. In this section, we provide a critical overview of the content of 18 key documents related to national community sport and PA policy published in England between 1995 and May 2016, a time frame that begins with the publication of only the second ever sport policy released by a British government (the other was in 1975) and when PA promotion began to be considered a government responsibility (Milton and Bauman 2015) (see Table 1). While there are some clear overlaps between the policies analysed, for ease of presentation we shall divide the documents into two broad kinds of policy: PA and sport.

Community physical activity policy

Not surprisingly, during the review period, PA policy was primarily oriented towards public health concerns and most commonly published by the DH. Perhaps the most substantial discussions of PMH and illness were to be found in policies authored by the Chief Medical Officer (CMO), including *At Least Five a Week: Evidence on the Impact of Physical Activity and its Relationship to Health* (hereafter, *'At Least Five a Week'*), published by the DH (DH 2004). *At Least Five a Week* devoted a whole chapter to PA, psychological well-being and mental illness in adults, and noted the benefits of PA for the mental health of older people, children and adolescents. Overall, the

Table 1. Key documents related to national physical activity and community sport policy in England, 1995–May 2016.

Policy or policy-related document	Organisation
Sport: Raising the Game, 1995	DNH
Strategy Statement on Physical Activity, 1996	DH
A Sporting Future for All, 2000	DCMS
Game Plan, 2002	DCMS/Strategy Unit
At least Five a Week, 2004	DH
The Framework for Sport in England, 2004	Sport England
Before, During and After: making the Most of the London 2012 Games, 2008	DCMS
Healthier Communities, 2008	Sport England
Healthy Weight, Healthy Lives, 2008	DH
Playing to Win, 2008	DCMS
Be Active, Be Healthy, 2009	DH
Start Active, Stay Active, 2011	DH
Creating a Sport Habit for Life, 2012	DCMS/Sport England
Everybody Active, Every Day, 2014	PHE
Moving More, Living More, 2014	HMG/Mayor of London
Sporting Future, 2015	HMG
What Works in Schools and Colleges to Increase Physical Activity? 2015	PHE, Youth Sport Trust and Association of Colleges Sport
Towards an Active Nation, 2016	Sport England

evidence review concluded unambiguously that PA and exercise are effective in promoting mental health in the general population, in both the prevention and treatment of some mental illnesses such as depression, and as an adjunctive measure in lifestyle interventions. For adults, PA was said to be effective in the treatment of mild, moderate and severe clinical depression and can be as successful as psychotherapy or medication, particularly in the longer term. PA was also cited as being beneficial for people with generalised anxiety disorder (by reducing state and trait anxiety), those who experience phobias, panic attacks and stress disorders (via reducing physiological reactions to stress), and can have a positive effect on psychological well-being in people with schizophrenia as well as improving self-esteem, particularly in those with initial low self-esteem. Improved sleep and – in older people – aspects of cognitive function were among the other cited benefits of PA (DH 2004).

Despite the positive endorsement of PA and exercise in *At Least Five a Week*, it was activity of a particular kind and intensity that was cited as being particularly beneficial to the promotion of PMH and prevention and treatment of mental illness. In particular, it was claimed that:

> Regular moderate intensity activity can improve psychological well-being. Evidence is strongest for activity which lasts between 20 and 60 minutes. However, shorter bouts (10–15 minutes) of moderate intensity walking can induce significant positive changes in mood. Rhythmic aerobic forms of exercise – such as brisk walking, jogging, cycling, swimming or dancing – appear to be most consistently effective. Resistance exercise may be useful for enhancing self-perceptions, as it can have rapid effects on how the body feels and functions. (DH 2004, p. 6)

Competitive sport and vigorous exercise were also regarded as important sources of psychological well-being for people who are already accustomed to those activities (DH 2004), while group recreational sports were said to bring social and mood benefits for participants. In children and adolescents, the then evidence was described as indicating that PA interventions can have a generally positive impact on mental health but a weak effect on reducing stress, anxiety and depression in adolescents. Sport and exercise were also regarded as important contexts for young people to experience positive effects on self-esteem and self-perceptions of competence and body image, with a stronger effect being noted for those already low in self-esteem (DH 2004).

Five years later, in *Be Active, Be Healthy* (DH 2009), the former CMO, Professor Sir Liam Donaldson, re-emphasised the aforementioned benefits of regular moderate intensity PA for mental health. The report further noted, however, that these benefits are frequently overlooked and that in some cases PA can be offered to patients with mild to moderate depression as an alternative to pharmaceutical treatment (DH 2009). The National Institute for Health and Care Excellence (NICE) clinical guidelines for depression were also endorsed, with the report recommending that all patients with mild depression should be advised of the benefits of following an exercise programme that is structured and supervised (DH 2009).

The third CMO-authored report included in the review period was the 2011 publication *Start Active, Stay Active: Report on Physical Activity in the UK* (DH 2011), which superseded *At Least Five a Week* and included – for the first time – a common set of PA recommendations across the UK. Among other things, it was suggested that, for adults, 30 minutes of at least moderate intensity PA on at least 5 days each week plays an important role in preventing mental illness, promoting mental health and well-being, and improving the quality of life of those with mental illness (DH 2011). In particular, participating in this kind of PA was described as beneficial for reducing the risk of depression, dementia and Alzheimer's disease, as well as enhancing psychological well-being via improvements in self-perception and self-esteem, mood and sleep quality, and reductions in levels of anxiety and fatigue (DH 2011).

The promotion of PA in helping to reduce the prevalence and incidence of dementia in older adults (specifically 65–74-year-olds) was identified in *Everybody Active, Every Day* (PHE 2014) as one of seven public health priorities for 2014–2024. This was prompted by the estimate that approximately 800,000 people in the UK currently experience dementia and evidence that being physically active can help reduce the risk of vascular dementia as well as having a positive impact on non-vascular dementia (PHE 2014). Once again, it was moderate PA lasting 30 minutes each day (such as taking a brisk walk, swimming, gardening, or cycling to the shops or to work), which was regarded as being particularly effective for promoting PMH. While no specific strategies for enhancing PMH, or preventing or treating mental illness are mentioned, another report published by PHE – which focused on PA promotion in schools and colleges – suggested that improved mental well-being, self-esteem and reduced levels of anxiety and stress are amongst some of the benefits of PA for children and young people (PHE 2015). None of the other documents that focused on PA mentioned PMH or mental illness.

Community sport policy

In contrast to policy broadly oriented towards PA, reference to PMH and the prevention and treatment of mental illness has very rarely been the focus of community sport policy in England. Indeed, despite regularly extolling the alleged health benefits of sport participation, neither mental health nor mental illness were mentioned in *Sport: Raising the Game* (DNH 1995), *A Sporting Future for All* (DCMS 2000), *Before, During and After: Making the Most of the London 2012 Games* (DCMS 2008a), *Playing to Win: A New Era for Sport* (DCMS 2008b), or *Creating a Sporting Habit for Life: A New Youth Sport Strategy* (DCMS/Sport England 2012). Even in what has been regarded as one of the more comprehensive government statements on sport and PA in England – *Game Plan: A Strategy for Delivering Government's Sport and Physical Activity Objectives* (DCMS/Strategy Unit 2002) – only two references were made to mental health. First, it was claimed that research has 'found a consistent link between exercise and anxiety reduction; and protection against the development of depression' (DCMS/Strategy Unit 2002, p. 45), and second, Professor William Haskell of Stanford University Medical School was quoted as saying that 'Exercise isn't a panacea, but it has consistently been shown to relieve both depression and anxiety' (DCMS/Strategy Unit 2002, p. 51).

Over a decade of Sport England policy has similarly produced just a handful of references to mental health, including in 2004, when it was claimed that 'participation in sport and physical activity contributes positively to overall personal health and fitness levels, and also to mental health with a positive effect on anxiety, depression, mood and emotion, self-esteem, and cognitive functioning' (Sport England 2004, p. 29). Four years later, in *Healthier Communities: Improving Health and Reducing Health Inequalities through Sport*, the claim that sport can contribute to improved mental health and well-being (Sport England 2008) was the only direct reference made to mental health.

It is clear, then, that throughout almost all of the review period there has been a near complete absence in published community sport policy of the mental health of children, young people and adults, and of mental illness in these population groups. However, between the end of 2015 and May 2016, two significant policy documents – *Sporting Future: A New Strategy for a Sporting Nation* (hereafter, '*Sporting Future*') (HMG 2015) and *Towards an Active Nation* (Sport England 2016) – identified 'mental well-being' (rather than PMH, which is not identified but conflated with 'mental well-being') as one of five outcomes to be addressed as part of the Conservative Government's concern with delivering social outcomes through participation in sport and PA, as well as increasing the proportion of physically active and inactive people.

Published by the DCMS in December 2015, *Sporting Future* makes clear how the enhancement of mental well-being and the other four outcomes will 'define who we [government] will fund, what we fund and where our priorities lie in the future' (HM Government 2015, p. 9). To provide evidence of sport's contribution to each overall outcome, various other 'high-level outcomes' (measured at a national level) are identified alongside three broad 'outputs', which are to be assessed by a number of population-level 'Key Performance Indicators' (KPIs) (HMG 2015). In relation to mental well-being, the high-level outcome is 'improved subjective well-being' (HMG 2015, p. 74), which consists of four key elements: feelings of life satisfaction, worthiness, happiness and anxiety. The main output is 'more people taking part in sport and physical activity' (HMG 2015, p. 77), which is aligned to KPI 3 – 'Increase in the percentage of adults utilising outdoor space for exercise/health reasons' (HMG 2015, p. 78).

While the increased attention paid to mental well-being in *Sporting Future* is notable, this part of the strategy is also characterised by some significant confusion and contradiction. Not only is mental *well-being* treated synonymously and misleadingly as being the same as mental *health*, it is also unclear – because no supporting evidence is cited – why increasing only adults' (and, interestingly, not children's and young people's) use of particular settings (i.e. outdoor space), for particular motivations (i.e. exercise/health reasons), is prioritised over participation in other settings and other motivations. Claims made about the respective evidence bases for sport, PA and exercise are similarly confused and lacking in internal coherence. On the one hand, it is suggested that the 'evidence for sport's impact on physical and mental health, building social capital, educational attainment and employability and economic growth is *well-established*' (HMG 2015, p. 72; emphases added), and that it is in each of these five areas 'where sport can make its greatest contribution' (p. 72). In addition, a variety of other benefits to mental health and illness are simultaneously claimed for *sport* (i.e. 'Sport is, for many people, a hugely enjoyable experience'), *PA* (i.e. 'Physical activity can reduce stress and anxiety'), and *exercise* (i.e. 'Research has shown that exercise can be as effective as anti-depressants for those with mild clinical depression') (HMG 2015, p. 74). Collectively, these positive outcomes are regarded as being 'every bit as important as the physical benefits from taking part in sport, and evidence is clear on the mental as well as physical health benefits of meeting the CMO [physical activity] guidelines' (HMG 2015, p. 74).

On the other hand, despite claims of the clear and well-established evidence base for sport's contribution to positive mental well-being, *Sporting Future* suggests that the links between them are not well understood. Indeed, it is suggested that in comparison to the benefits of meeting *PA* guidelines, 'less is known about the precise links between mental wellbeing and sporting behaviours' (HMG 2015, p. 74). Together with individual development and social and community development, it is also claimed that 'more work will be needed over the coming years to understand and evidence the exact impact that sport and physical activity can make' (HMG 2015, p. 72) on mental well-being. Another more cautious assessment of the evidence base made clear that 'where causality is *less well understood* or the evidence base *does not yet exist* (*mental wellbeing*, individual development, social and community development) we will work to develop a robust understanding of how sport contributes that will then form the basis for how impact is measured in the future' (HMG 2015, p. 73; emphases added).

In response to *Sporting Future*, Sport England – which in 2015 collaborated with the mental health charity, Mind, to launch the three-year *Get Set to Go* programme to promote sport participation in 75,000 people with mental illness (Sport England 2015) – published its own 2016–2021 strategy, *Towards an Active Nation* (Sport England 2016). Not surprisingly, since *Sporting Future* made very clear the expectations the DCMS now have of Sport England, *Towards an Active Nation* sets out how Sport England will work to help achieve the key outcomes and policy trajectory identified in *Sporting Future*. In doing so, Sport England suggest that it will need to 'develop new ways of evaluating the broader outcomes of sport, especially mental wellbeing, individual development and social and community development' (Sport England 2016, p. 7) to enable it and other organisations to show how they are contributing to the Government's policy priorities, thus helping to strengthen the rationale for continued public investment in sport (Sport England 2016).

At first glance, the claims made in *Sporting Future*, in particular, might seem to indicate that the benefits to mental well-being from engaging in sport, PA and exercise are overwhelming, but it is important to note that the available evidence – including the findings of the studies reviewed earlier – refer not to sport, but to PA or exercise. But these are not the same thing, and while there is certainly widespread acceptance of the idea that 'sport is good for health' (Waddington 2000), the conflation of sport with PA and exercise (and their respective evidence bases) in *Sporting Future* is significant in policy and public health terms. As noted elsewhere (Waddington 2000, Mansfield and Malcolm 2015), sport varies in several important ways from PA and exercise, including in the degree to which sport: (i) is inherently more competitive and institutionalised; (ii) can be associated with higher rates of injury and violence (especially at higher levels of sport); (iii) is characterised by different kinds of social relationships that make the intensity, frequency and timing of participation more difficult to control; (iv) and is more commonly associated with a whole range of values and behaviours that may compromise (mental) health. At the very least, a recognition of these important differences – which are contested, historically dynamic and culturally variable (Mansfield and Malcolm 2015) – sound a clear warning against accepting without question the presumed and inherently positive relationship between PMH and sport, PA and exercise as articulated in *Sporting Future* and associated policies.

It is also clear that while the scientific evidence may provide a strong case for promoting PMH through engagement in PA and exercise, and including these in the routine delivery of interventions to people with mental illness (Callaghan 2004, Rosenbaum *et al.* 2014), the evidence base for sport is presently much less developed and robust than is assumed in *Sporting Future*. Indeed, until recently comparatively less emphasis has been placed on exploring sport participation and its association with PMH outcomes (Faulkner and Tamminen 2016). According to Faulkner and Tamminen (2016), there are several reasons for this, including the propensity for researchers investigating the links between PA and PMH to be primarily concerned with controlling the dose of exercise undertaken by participants while eliminating any potentially confounding variables (such as social interaction) to explore potential associations, which is considerably difficult in sporting contexts. Researchers have also frequently devoted more attention to examining the health compromising behaviours (some of which relate to mental illness) associated with sport, and investigated the PMH benefits of PA and exercise, which, by comparison to traditional forms of sport, become progressively more popular over the life course for a larger proportion of the population (Faulkner and Tamminen 2016).

Since the current evidence base in this area is more complex and nuanced than is perhaps commonly assumed, policy-makers and practitioners face a number of challenges in seeking to provide government with evidence of the contribution made by sport participation (though the same applies to PA and exercise) to PMH. Central among these is the tendency for different kinds of sports participation to generate different mental health outcomes, among different groups of participants, in different social contexts where sports-based community-focused projects are delivered. A closer attention will thus need to be paid to understanding the contexts, mechanisms and processes (see Coalter 2007, 2016, Whitelaw *et al.* 2010, Mansfield *et al.* 2015) that are associated with sport participation and the differential PMH outcomes generated by it. An understanding of the problem of self-selection in sport participation, the quality of participation experiences, and the other constraints that impact on mental health are among the other complex issues that need to be considered by bodies such as Sport England (2016) if they are to develop more robust and consistent evaluation practices that help identify the progress they make towards the government's outcomes. In this regard, on the basis of the current evidence, it is perhaps more balanced and realistic to suggest that participating in sport *may* make a positive contribution to aspects of mental health (or mental well-being, in *Sporting Future* parlance), and *may* be a helpful component in preventing and treating mental illness, but this is likely *only to occur under specific circumstances which as yet are not well understood* (Whitelaw *et al.* 2010).

Conclusions

In this article we have sought to provide, for the first time, a critical overview of sport, PA and PMH policy via an analysis of key policy documents published in England between 1995 and May 2016. It was clear that there has been increased but gradual interest (however rhetorical) among those in key policy communities in the contribution that sport, PA and exercise might make to PMH and mental illness. While some of the policy documents contained (often rather vague) references to the importance of sport, PA and exercise for PMH and illness, the clear definition of specific and measurable goals that can be used to determine the efficacy, effectiveness and comparative effectiveness of national policy in addressing PMH outcomes was notably absent. Even in the most explicit discussion of PMH in community sport policy – namely, *Sporting Future* – reference was made only to 'mental well-being' as a desired outcome without identifying any clearly defined targets or policy goals against which to judge progress. In this regard, the absence of any discussion about what constitutes policy effectiveness, about how progress is to be monitored and evaluated, and about how to identify the differential contribution participation in different kinds of sports, physical activities and exercises might make to any observed changes in mental well-being are significant oversights. Similarly, while making more regular, detailed and systematic reference to the evidence base that exists for the impact of PA and exercise on PMH and illness, community PA policy in England has also failed to include specific and measurable population targets, which can be used to determine the progress made by policy in which PA and exercise are used to affect positive change in PMH and illness through community-based programmes and interventions.

It is unclear why these details were absent from the various policy documents analysed, but claims made about the need to encourage population level engagement in community-based sport, PA and exercise for mental health benefit need to be balanced against real term reductions in funding and services for PMH in England. This may be particularly significant for those in community sport who, in the battle for public funding and support, appear willing to present sport as an important contributor to overall PA, and as a vehicle for addressing current concerns about PMH and illness. Attempts to do so, as revealed very clearly in *Sporting Future*, provides further evidence of the marginal status of community sport as a policy sector relative to other, generally more secure and powerful (e.g. health and medicine), policy communities. Indeed, that those in the sport policy community appear so keen to generalise their interests to other policy areas that bolster their legitimacy in the eyes of others, and helps justify their work as a legitimate area of activity worthy of political support and funding, may be seen as further evidence of the status anxiety and marginality experienced by those in the sector. While there may be genuine interest in addressing concerns about PMH and illness through community sport and PA, might the association with PMH also be a vague, convenient and largely symbolic one unlikely to stimulate any long-lasting and real change in policy and practice? Or will the allegiance between those in community sport and PA on the one hand, and PMH on the other, help strengthen considerably their ability to lobby more effectively for resources, legitimacy and status within the political and policy hierarchy? These are questions for which there are as of yet very few answers.

Finally, the policy developments examined in this article may be indicative of the gradual (and as yet partial) convergence of the community sport and PA policy communities, and a growing intersection between the fields of sport, health and medicine, which supports the increasingly decentralised, and locally determined, approach to the delivery of public services. However, as developments in the provision of health care services indicate, the devolvement of responsibility for policy decisions to local government and services in contexts of austerity is more likely to increase, rather than help breakdown, local variations in mental health service provision and use, and skew even further the unequal social distribution of (mental) health outcomes across communities. It is also likely to strengthen the dominant but largely ineffective neo-liberal approach towards policy in which disproportionate emphasis is placed on exercising independence and personal choice, individual behaviour change, self-responsibilisation, and self-governance. For reasons explained elsewhere (e.g. Marmot 2010, Wilkinson and Pickett 2010, Marmot 2015, Pickett and Wilkinson 2015), such an approach not only detracts attention from the very significant social processes associated with unequal health outcomes, but most often contributes to widening socially structured inequalities in PMH. Many of the inequalities associated with poor PMH outcomes also typically precede inequalities in sport and PA participation in many countries (Coalter

2007, 2016), so the simple promotion of sport and PA – whether on their own or in combination with other activities – is considerably unlikely to tackle effectively the increasing prevalence of mental illness, or promote good PMH, unless the deep-seated roots of corrosive forms of social inequality are tackled first. Regardless of whether one accepts these conclusions, they at the very least merit more serious attention by those with a genuine commitment to better understanding and tackling the inequalities that contribute to the global burden of mental illness and the considerable human costs associated with it. Recognising the importance of these issues may be a first step in ensuring that the improvement of PMH and tackling mental illness through community sport and PA becomes less of a political spectator sport, and more of a clearly thought-out, sustained and long-term commitment of public policy.

Notes

1. MNS disorders exist in all countries, but are often underpinned by Western-based definitions that take insufficient account of the importance of cultural contexts in understanding their development, presentation and treatment. The Global Burden of Disease Study 2010 is not immune from these weaknesses and the data presented below should be interpreted accordingly (see Whiteford *et al.* 2015).
2. Following the UK's Chief Medical Officer (Davies 2014), we have adopted the term 'public mental health' where appropriate to refer to those 'mental health variations of importance exhibited by populations' and which consists of 'mental health promotion', 'mental illness prevention' and 'treatment and rehabilitation' (Davies 2014, p. 12), for which there is a good deal of persuasive evidence compared to the vaguer notion of 'well-being' as it relates to mental health.

Disclosure statement

No potential conflict of interest was reported by the authors.

References

All Party Parliamentary Group on Mental Health, 2015. *Parity in progress? The all party parliamentary group on mental health's inquiry into parity of esteem for mental health.* London: Author.

Allen, J., *et al.*, 2014. Social determinants of mental health. *International review of psychiatry*, 26, 392–407. doi:10.3109/09540261.2014.928270

Becker, A. and Kleinmann, A., 2013. Mental health and the global agenda. *The new England journal of medicine*, 369, 66–73. doi:10.1056/NEJMra1110827

Biddle, S.J.H. and Asare, M., 2011. Physical activity and mental health in children and adolescents: a review of reviews. *British journal of sports medicine*, 45, 886–895. doi:10.1136/bjsports-2011-090185

Bloom, D.E., *et al.*, 2011. *The global economic burden of noncommunicable diseases.* Geneva: World Economic Forum.

Brown, H., *et al.*, 2013. Physical activity interventions and depression in children and adolescents. *Sports medicine*, 43, 195–206. doi:10.1007/s40279-012-0015-8

Callaghan, P., 2004. Exercise: a neglected intervention in mental health care? *Journal of psychiatric and mental health nursing*, 11, 476–483. doi:10.1111/j.1365-2850.2004.00751.x

Campaign for Living Miserably (CALM)., 2015. Suicide stats and research. Available from: https://www.thecalmzone.net/about-calm/suicide-research-stats/.

Centre for Mental Health, *et al.*, 2012. *No health without mental health: implementation framework.* London: Authors.

Coalter, F., 2007. *A wider social role for sport.* London: Routledge.

Coalter, F., 2016. Youth and sport-for-change programmes: What can you expect? *In*: K. Green and A. Smith, eds. *The Routledge handbook of youth sport.* London: Routledge.

Commission on the Social Determinants of Health, 2008. *Closing the gap in a generation: health equity through action on the social determinants of health.* Geneva: World Health Organization.

Davies, S.C., 2014. *Annual report of the chief medical officer 2013. Public mental health priorities: investing in the evidence.* London: Department of Health.

Department for Culture, Media and Sport, 2000. A sporting future for all. London: Department for Culture, Media and Sport.

Department for Culture, Media and Sport/Strategy Unit, 2002. Game plan: a strategy for delivering government's sport and physical activity objectives. London: Department for Culture, Media and Sport/Strategy Unit.

Department for Culture, Media and Sport, 2008a. *Before, during and after: making the most of the London 2012 games.* London: Author.
Department for Culture, Media and Sport, 2008b. *Playing to win: a new era for sport.* London: DCMS.
Department of Health, 1996. *Strategy on physical activity.* London: Department of Health.
Department of Health, 2004. At least five a week: evidence of the impact of physical activity and its relationship to health. London: Department of Health.
Department of Health, 2009. Be active, be healthy. A strategy to get the nation moving. London: Department of Health.
Department for Culture, Media and Sport/Sport England, 2012. Creating a sporting habit for life: a new youth sport strategy. London: Department for Culture, Media and Sport/Sport England.
Department of Health, 2011. *Start active, stay active. A report on physical activity for health from the home countries' chief medical officers.* London: Department of Health.
Department of Health, 2015. *Future in mind: promoting, protecting and improving our children and young people's mental health and wellbeing.* London: Department of Health.
Department of National Heritage, 1995. Sport: raising the game. London: Department of National Heritage.
Ekkekakis, P., 2015. Honey, I shrunk the pooled SMD! Guide to critical appraisal of systematic reviews and meta-analyses using the Cochrane review on exercise for depression as example. *Mental health and physical activity*, 8, 21–36. doi:10.1016/j.mhpa.2014.12.001
Faulkner, G. and Biddle, S., 1999. Exercise and schizophrenia: a review. *Journal of mental health*, 8, 441–457. doi:10.1080/09638239917157
Faulkner, G. and Tamminen, K., 2016. Youth sport and mental health. In: K. Green and A. Smith, eds. The routledge handbook of youth sport. London: Routledge.
Mammen, G. and Faulkner, G., 2013. Physical activity and the prevention of depression: a systematic review of prospective studies. *American journal of preventive medicine*, 45, 649–57.
Her Majesty's Government/Department of Health, 2011. *No health without mental health: a cross-government mental health outcomes strategy for people of all ages.* London: Author.
HM Government, 2015. *Sporting future: a new strategy for an active nation.* London: Cabinet Office.
Larun, L., *et al.*, 2006. Exercise in prevention and treatment of anxiety and depression among children and young people. *Cochrane database of systematic reviews*, 3. Art. doi:10.1002/14651858.CD004691.pub2
Mansfield, L., *et al.*, 2015. The Health and Sport Engagement (HASE) Intervention and Evaluation Project: protocol for the design, outcome, process and economic evaluation of a complex community sport intervention to increase levels of physical activity. *BMJ open*, 5, e009276. doi:10.1136/bmjopen-2015-009276
Mansfield, L. and Malcolm, D., 2015. The olympic movement, sport and health. *In*: J. Baker, P. Safai, and J. Fraser-Thomas, eds. *Health and elite sport: is high performance sport a healthy pursuit?* London: Routledge.
Marmot, M., 2010. *Fair society healthy lives (the marmot review): strategic review of health inequalities in England post 2010.* London: Marmot Review.
Marmot, M., 2015. *The health gap: the challenge of an unequal world.* London: Bloomsbury.
Mental Health Taskforce, 2016. *The five year forward view for mental health.* Leeds: NHS England.
Milton, K. and Bauman, A., 2015. A critical analysis of the cycles of physical activity policy in England. *International journal of behavioral nutrition and physical activity*, 12, 8. doi:10.1186/s12966-015-0169-5
National Confidential Inquiry into Suicide and Homicide by People with Mental Illness (NCISH), 2015. *Annual report: England, Northern Ireland, Scotland and Wales July 2015.* Manchester: University of Manchester.
National Health Service (NHS), 2014. NHS Five Year Forward View. London: NHS.
National Society for the Protection of Cruelty to Children, 2015. 1 in 5 children are rejected mental health treatment. Available from: https://www.nspcc.org.uk/fighting-for-childhood/news-opinion/1-in-five-5-children-referred-to-local-mental-health-services-are-rejected-for-treatment/.
Pickett, K. and Wilkinson, R., 2015. Income inequality and health: a causal review. *Social science & medicine*, 128, 316–326. doi:10.1016/j.socscimed.2014.12.031
Public Health England, 2014. Everybody active, every day. London: Public Health England.
Public Health England, Youth Sport Trust and Association of Colleges Sport, 2015. *What works in schools and colleges to increase physical activity?* London: Authors.
Rosenbaum, S., *et al.*, 2014. Physical activity interventions for people with mental illness: a systematic review and meta-analysis. *The journal of clinical psychiatry*, 75, 964–974. doi:10.4088/JCP.13r08765
Rosenbaum, S., *et al.*, 2015. Physical activity in the treatment of post-traumatic stress disorder: a systematic review and meta-analysis. *Psychiatry research*, 230, 130–136. doi:10.1016/j.psychres.2015.10.017
Schuch, F., *et al.*, 2016. A critical review of exercise as a treatment for clinically depressed adults: time to get pragmatic. *Acta neuropsychiatrica*. doi:10.1017/neu.2016.21
Smith, P. and Blumenthal, J., 2013. Exercise and physical activity in the prevention and treatment of depression. *In*: P. Ekkekakis, ed. *The routledge handbook of physical activity and mental health.* London: Routledge.
Social Care, Local Government and Care Partnership Directorate, 2014. *Closing the gap: priorities for change in mental health.* London: Author.

Sport England, 2004. *The framework for sport in England. Making England an active and successful sporting nation*. London: Sport England.
Sport England, 2008. *Healthier communities: improving health and reducing health inequalities through sport*. London: Sport England.
Sport England, 2015. *Help to get active for those with mental health problems*. Available from: http://www.sportengland.org/media-centre/news/2015/july/13/help-to-get-active-for-those-with-mental-health-problems/.
Sport England, 2016. *Towards an active nation*. London: Sport England.
Stavrakakis, N., *et al*., 2013. Physical activity and onset of depression in adolescents: a prospective study in the general population cohort TRAILS. *Journal of psychiatric research*, 47, 1304–1308. doi:10.1016/j.jpsychires.2013.06.005
Stonerock, G., *et al*., 2015. Exercise as treatment for anxiety: systematic review and analysis. *Annals of behavioral medicine*, 49, 542–556. doi:10.1007/s12160-014-9685-9
The King's Fund, 2016. *Bringing together physical and mental health: a new frontier for integrated care*. London: Author.
United Nations, 2015. *Transforming our world: the 2030 agenda for sustainable development*. New York: Author.
Utschig, A.,, *et al*., 2013. The relationship between physical activity and anxiety and its disorders. *In*: P. Ekkekakis, ed. *The Routledge handbook of physical activity and mental health*. London: Routledge.
Van Dijk, M.L., *et al*., 2016. Decline in physical activity during adolescence is not associated with changes in mental health. *BMC public health*, 16, 300. doi:10.1186/s12889-016-2983-3
Waddington, I., 2000. *Sport, health and drugs*. London: T&FN Spon.
Whiteford, A., *et al*., 2015. The global burden of mental, neurological and substance use disorders: an analysis from the global burden of disease study 2010. *PLoS ONE*, 10 (2), e0116820. doi:10.1371/journal.pone.0116820
Whiteford, H., *et al*., 2013, Global burden of disease attributable to mental and substance use disorders: findings from the global burden of disease study 2010. *The lancet*, 382 (9904), 1575–1586. doi:10.1016/S0140-6736(13)61611-6
Whitelaw, S., *et al*., 2010. The physical activity-mental wellbeing association in young people: a case study in dealing with a complex public health topic using a 'realistic evaluation' framework. *Mental health and physical activity*, 3, 61–66. doi:10.1016/j.mhpa.2010.06.001
Wilkinson, R. and Pickett, K., 2010. The spirit level: why equality is better for everyone. London: Penguin.
World Health Organization, 2001. *The world health report. Mental health: new understanding, new hope*. Geneva: Author.
World Health Organization, 2008. *mhGAP: mental health gap action programme: scaling up care for mental, neurological and substance use disorders*. Geneva: Author.
World Health Organization, 2013a. *Investing in mental health: evidence for action*. Geneva: Author.
World Health Organization, 2013b. *Mental health action plan 2013–2020*. Geneva: Author.
World Health Organization, 2013c. *Review of social determinants and the health divide in the WHO European region: final report*. Geneva: Author.
World Health Organization, 2014. *Social determinants of mental health*. Geneva: Author.
World Health Organization, 2015. *2014 mental health atlas*. Geneva: Author.

Olympic sport and physical activity promotion: the rise and fall of the London 2012 pre-event mass participation 'legacy'

Paul Bretherton, Joe Piggin and Guillaume Bodet

ABSTRACT

The legacies of Sport Mega Events (SMEs) such as the Olympic Games are increasingly regarded as significant opportunities to increase sport and physical activity (PA) participation. Major sport/PA legacy objectives may even be pursued before the event takes place. This article examines a specific pre-event sport/PA policy target of the London 2012 Olympic Games: the aim of increasing overall participation by two million between June 2008 and the Games in 2012 (a target that was abandoned in 2011).

Within a governmentality analytical framework, this research examined how London 2012's pre-event sport/PA participation legacy targets were constructed by organisations responsible for their delivery. Three specific themes are discussed: the inconsistency between how sport/PA participation was constructed in terms of both 'risk' and 'reward' by different organisations; the reliance upon intangible concepts such as 'inspiration' and the status of the Olympic Games to increase participation; and the rationales given for the subsequent abandonment of the pre-event PA participation targets in 2011.

The abandonment of the pre-Games participation targets holds two overarching policy implications for future SME host governments and organisers. First, host governments cannot rely on the unique status or 'inspiration' of the Games alone to increase participation and must pursue this more proactively. Second, the ultimate failure of these policies should not be attributed exclusively to their intrinsic limitations, but also to a range of external environmental factors. Pre-event SME legacies must therefore be planned with sufficient awareness of the social and political contexts in which the event takes place.

For the UK government, the 'first priority' of the London 2012 Olympic Games was 'to make the UK a world-leading sporting nation' (DCMS 2008, p. 3). Seeking to capitalise upon the 'inspiration' of the Games in the years leading up to the event, the UK public were encouraged to become 'increasingly active, with a goal of seeing two million people more active by 2012' (DCMS 2008, p. 3). Within this overall pre-event target of two million, one million more people were to begin participating in sport and another million were to take up PA by 2012. These aims were ambitious. Had the target of one million more people taking up sport by 2012 been met, it would have represented a 15% increase in participation following two decades without progress (Bullough 2012).

Despite the optimism with which these targets were announced, three years of limited progress saw the UK government acknowledge their abandonment by 2011 (Kelso 2011, Weed 2013). Several months before the Games began, a new sport participation legacy strategy was published with a narrowed focus upon youth participation (DCMS 2012). On one level, this shift of emphasis represented a quantifiable failure of an Olympic host government attempt to fulfil a published pre-event legacy objective. More broadly, this policy change must be understood within a broader context that witnessed both economic instability and a change of UK government in May 2010. This fluid political environment saw extensive debates around sport policy issues such as funding for School Sport Partnerships (SSPs) and a perceived UK government shift towards 'sport for sport's sake' (Devine 2013, p. 257) instead of mass participation sport.

Since 2012, sport has been further prioritised as a vehicle for increasing PA and public health, as demonstrated by Sport England's Get Healthy Get Active funding stream as well as a change in government policy emphasis from the measurement of participation to that of physical and mental health alongside individual, community and economic development (HM Government 2015). Although further measurement and evaluation will be required to determine if these approaches – and the participation legacy of London 2012 – ultimately prove successful, the abandonment of the DCMS's pre-event participation legacy targets merits specific attention. With aspiring Olympic hosts increasingly required to demonstrate how the event will bring about long-term social benefits (Fussey *et al.* 2011), the abandonment of these pre-event participation targets has important implications for future SME hosts.

The current research aimed to understand more about how the proposed London 2012 sport/PA participation legacy was constructed and adjusted by key policy actors between 2003, when the UK government confirmed that London would bid for the 2012 Games, and 2012, when the event took place. This is not to say that the year 2012 represented the end of policy attempts to realise a sport/PA participation legacy from London 2012, but that this research focuses specifically on both the rhetoric of the bidding stage and the pre-event sport/PA targets published in 2008. Drawing upon a governmentality analytical framework (Foucault 1994), policy material published by four organisations (UK government, Greater London Authority, Sport England, London 2012 Bid Team/LOCOG) was analysed in order to better understand the challenges that domestic sport/PA policy must overcome in seeking to better implement pre-event social legacies around SMEs.

Olympic legacies

Research on SME and Olympic legacies has increased as the concept has become more formalised over time (Cashman 1999, Leopkey and Parent 2012a). Notable trends include the consideration of tangible/intangible, hard/soft and physical/spiritual legacies as well as broader legacy areas such as transport, infrastructure, volunteering, employment, sport policy and sport participation (Chappelet 2012). The Olympic Games in particular has been associated with the notion of long-term benefit from its modern revival onwards, but in recent years these benefits have 'evolved from general benefits and impacts of the Games to sustainable long-term legacies, which have been strategically planned from the time of the bid' (Leopkey and Parent 2012a, p. 938).

This reference to intended legacy 'benefits' is important, as it is in these positive terms that Olympic legacies are primarily articulated by organisers and host governments. For example, Gratton and Preuss (2008) identify how Olympic legacies may be understood as positive or negative, planned or unplanned and tangible or intangible. Beyond the recognition that legacy is not inherently positive, the possibility that legacies may be unplanned or intangible also illustrates the social complexity faced by policy makers who may seek to use the Games to bring about desirable changes in the host nation. As the scope and formality of potential Olympic legacies have increased over time, these legacies have also been shown to be increasingly shaped by discursive construction (MacAloon 2008). Furthermore, Agha *et al.* (2011) describe how the fact that an Organising Committee of the Olympic Games (OCOG) disbands within two years of the event gives rise to 'a series of broad legacy claims' (p. 126) that are further complicated by the multitude of different organisations involved in the event's delivery (Chappelet and Kübler-Mabbott 2008).

A milestone event in the development of Olympic legacy planning was the 2002 amendment of the Olympic Charter to include the statement that one of the IOC's official roles is 'to promote a positive legacy from the Olympic Games to the host cities and host countries' (IOC 2013a, p. 17). Fussey *et al.* (2011) describe how recent Games of the twenty-first century have seen the IOC set OCOGs the requirement to 'adopt more environmentally and socially responsible approaches to planning' (p. 29) for the Games, which has seen heightened importance attached to considerations of legacy and regeneration in evaluations of the Games. The IOC (2013b) present these 'social responsibilities' in five thematic categories: 'cultural/social/political', 'environmental', 'economic', 'urban' and 'sporting', and although each OCOG must consider all five within its planning and delivery of the Games, it was the 'sporting' legacy of London 2012 that was described as '"first among equals" in the minds of the IOC, LOCOG, the government and the UK media' (Weed 2013, p. 95). Within this overall sporting legacy, London 2012's pre-event sport/PA participation targets represented a clear example of a contemporary Olympic legacy policy in terms of both their proactive timescale and as a proclaimed attempt to use the event to positively influence individual behaviour.

There is a clear link between the positive phrasing which accompanies host governments' and policy makers' claims about the overall legacy of the event and the specific area of sporting legacies and sport more broadly. For Kay (2012), the underlying commitment of the Olympic Games to social change manifests itself in how it is 'captured in the notion of legacy', which is in turn based upon a 'powerful advocacy' (Kay 2012, p. 899) of sport's inherent social potential. These positive assumptions are evident in academia (e.g. Smith and Westerbeek 2007) as well as contemporary UK sport policy. For example, Grix and Carmichael's (2012) conceptualisation of a 'virtuous cycle of sport' articulates how elite success, increased participation and the widening of a national 'talent pool' are suggested to work together in cyclical fashion. But despite the enthusiasm with which sport's social potential may be advocated, there remains a lack of consistency in how it can be defined and understood. For example, Grix and Carmichael (2012) note that UK government policy discourse 'does not always clearly distinguish between participation in "PA" or a more formal "sport"' (p. 84), and such a lack of clarity can make it difficult to understand precisely which form of activity is being referred to in public statements that may conflate sport and PA in both competitive and non-competitive settings, as well as their intended implications for health.

The sport and PA participation legacy of London 2012

London 2012's legacy visions sought distinction 'from both previous editions of the Games and from its bid competitors' (Weed 2013, p. 87). Within this overall vision, London 2012's unprecedented commitments to health promotion (Commission for a Sustainable London 2012 2011) were a central component. In relation to the DCMS's (2008) pre-event mass participation targets, the announcement of these objectives highlighted the 'general health benefits' (p. 22) of completing five 30-minute sessions of PA per week, thus setting out the presumed positive correlation between this level of sport/PA participation and health promotion. However, before the publication of London 2012's pre-event participation targets, research on previous editions of the Olympic Games had demonstrated only a negligible increase in adult participation both in the host nation (Bauman *et al.* 2001, Veal 2003, Tsuoros *et al.* 2007) and in other countries (Hindson *et al.* 1994) following the event. These conclusions are consistent with the results of several reviews of the evidence base for the effect of major sporting events upon sport/PA participation (Murphy and Bauman 2007, Weed *et al.* 2009, McCartney *et al.* 2010, Mahtani *et al.* 2013).

This evidence does not necessarily prove that any attempt to increase participation using the Games is impossible (Weed *et al.* 2009, McCartney *et al.* 2010), but there are a range of factors that make both achieving and measuring (Wellings *et al.* 2011) a participation increase particularly problematic. For example, there is no evidence that the staging of the event alone is sufficient to inspire a 'trickle down' or 'demonstration' effect that encourages participation automatically (Weiler and Stamatakis 2010), and legacy planners must also recognise that efforts to capitalise upon the presumed inspiration of the Games require the systematic cooperation of numerous domestic sport organisations (Coalter 2004) and effective leadership at local level (Charlton 2010). For Girginov and Hills (2008), the UK government's attempt to use London 2012 to increase sport/PA participation represented 'the most ambitious project in the history of the Olympic Games' given both its scope and its task in addressing 'not only people's behaviour but also deeply rooted social structures' (p. 2092). Weed *et al.* (2012) advise that because of the need for a sport/PA participation legacy to be brought about proactively – given concerns around a demonstration effect in relation to the least active adults – policy makers would be best advised to emphasise participation in PA ahead of sport, such as by generating a festival effect around the Games that emphasises its reach beyond sport alone and into local communities.

Beyond these technical issues, the need to address certain social structures and relations also depends upon wider political dynamics. For Murphy and Bauman (2007), the successful use of SMEs to increase mass participation depends upon successful cooperation between the health and sport sectors – who can potentially find themselves in direct competition with one another (Weiler and Stamatakis 2010). Furthermore, the role of social and political factors in shaping the sport/PA participation legacy of London 2012 is noted by Girginov and Hills (2009), for whom Olympic legacy features 'contested and complex aspects' that may be 'defined and operationalised according to multiple interests and objectives' (p. 165). These accounts of how Olympic legacies must be understood within broader political processes are consistent with both the growth of sport as a public policy concern (Green and Houlihan 2006) and the increasing social responsibilities expected of Olympic hosts (Fussey *et al.* 2011). With this understanding of Olympic legacy established, this research's theoretical perspective is presented next.

Research approach: governmentality perspective

This research is guided by Foucault's (1994) conceptualisation of governmentality. For Foucault, governmentality could be understood as follows.

> The ensemble formed by the institutions, procedures, analyses, and reflections, the calculations and tactics that allow the exercise of this very specific albeit complex form of power, which has as its target population, as its principal form of knowledgepolitical economy, and as its essential technical means apparatuses of security. (p. 219)

In the second and third parts of this definition, Foucault describes how in the West, a form of power known as 'government' has gradually gained pre-eminence, leading to 'a whole series of specific governmental apparatuses' and 'a whole complex of knowledges' (p. 220), a process that can be traced to the 'state of justice of the Middle Ages' (p. 220). Here it is worth noting Markula and Pringle's (2006) observation that significant parallels can be drawn between Foucault's original work and contemporary sport and exercise – despite Foucault not addressing these areas directly. This research uses Foucault's original work as a starting point but focuses primarily upon more recent sources that have both advanced the concept of governmentality and applied it in the contexts of modern sport/PA policy.

A governmentality analytical approach examines the way that power is shared among 'a whole variety of authorities' that 'govern in different sites, in relation to different objectives' (Rose *et al.* 2006, p. 85) and is never absolute or exclusive. For Dean (1999), government refers to 'any more or less calculated and rational activity' and can be performed by 'a multiplicity of authorities and agencies' that may use 'a variety of techniques and forms of knowledge' in order to shape conduct (p. 18). Dean's articulation is directly applicable to the London 2012 sport/PA participation legacy, which represents an explicit attempt to influence individual behaviour that is coordinated by a range of different public (and private) organisations. This author's reference to 'shaping conduct' also resonates with the way that governmentality research is typically applied to 'neoliberal' societies in which conduct cannot be controlled explicitly. On this note it has been levelled that 'neoliberalism has been increasingly used in a pejorative sense as dismissive shorthand by critics' (Heynen *et al.* 2007, p. 3) – to which Ferguson (2009) argues that 'if we can go beyond seeing in "neoliberalism" an evil essence or an automatic unity' it is possible to 'see a field of specific governmental techniques' (p. 183) that may be used more constructively by researchers. This research approaches and deploys governmentality in line with both Dean (1999) and Ferguson (2009), taking the view that, although ideologically-driven, 'governing' represents a set of techniques or tactics that can be performed or resisted by multiple entities as opposed to the inherently dystopian or 'evil' essence described by Heynen *et al.* (2007).

For Osborne (1997), 'governments can at best provide the conditions' to encourage people to adopt healthy lifestyles but 'cannot guarantee health as such' (p. 179). This impossibility of 'guaranteeing' health is consistent with more recent accounts of 'steering' (Vallentin and Murillo 2009) or 'nudging' individuals towards desired behaviours (Vallgårda 2012), that cannot be explicitly coerced. As shown by McDermott (2007), one example of how individual behaviour may be shaped in relation to health is through the use of 'risk discourses' in which 'physical inactivity and obesity are understood as due to an individual's inability to make the 'right' choices to commit to a healthy lifestyle' and therefore function as 'moral technologies' that help to guide individual conduct (p. 318). The specific case of sport/PA participation represents one area of public health promotion to which these observations can also be applied.

Where sport/PA policy is concerned, recent decades have seen national governments significantly increase their interest (Green and Houlihan 2006) and investment (Grix 2015) in sport – an increase that has seen the governance of sport undergo significant changes. For Green and Houlihan (2006), a governmentality perspective offers ways of moving beyond the 'straightforward assumptions' (p. 67) upon which many policy analyses have been based and enables better analysis of processes such as autonomisation and responsibilisation in the context of national sport organisations. Similarly, Grix (2015) describes how while sport studies have been relatively slow to draw upon the 'mature debates' (p. 24) of political sciences, approaches such as the 'governance narrative' – which shifts focus from 'big government' to more indirect processes of governing through networks, partnerships and devolution – and governmentality, which encourages both 'individual and institutional conduct which is consistent with government objectives' (p. 126). Along these lines, Piggin *et al.* (2009) used a governmentality approach to establish 'how certain governing ideas within sport and recreation policy are formulated' such as encouraging PA participation and 'promoting ideas about the value of elite sporting success' (2009, p. 89). In terms of the Olympic Games specifically, Chatziefstathiou and Henry (2009) assert that Olympism 'operates as a source of governmentality' and represents 'an overt philosophy of behaviour' that provides values, principles and behaviours that holds legitimacy from micro to macro levels of society (p. 4).

These examples bear out the distinction between 'government' – the official structures which set formal policy – and 'governing'/'governmentality' – which refers to a more abstract set of 'tactics' (Foucault 1994) and 'techniques' (Dean 1999, Ferguson 2009) that may be used to shape individual conduct in relation to wider objectives. A governmentality perspective is particularly suitable for the present study as it enables a more sophisticated of government targets that concern an area of population management that is inherently uncontrollable and demands the use of more indirect forms of governance. Furthermore, the increased political use of sport by governments (Green and Houlihan 2006, Grix 2015) along with the specific values and behaviours advocated by the Olympic Games (Chatziefstathiou and Henry 2009) demonstrates how the

London 2012 sport/PA participation legacy represents an ideal site to approach with the broader complexity offered by a governmentality perspective.

Methods

This research aimed to understand more about how the proposed London 2012 pre-event sport/PA participation legacy objectives were constructed by selected policy actors between the UK's official decision to bid for the 2012 Games in 2003 and the staging of the event in 2012. The focus was therefore not upon the sport/PA legacy policy of the Games as a whole, which has continued to develop since 2012 and as a post-event Olympic legacy may require at least 15 years to be accurately measured (Gratton and Preuss 2008). Specifically, the emphasis of this study was upon policy content pertaining to the pre-event sport/PA participation targets – encompassing both the broader claims published in the bidding stage and the specific pre-event sport/PA participation legacy policies that were published following London's selection as host in 2005.

As documentary content allows access to political processes that would otherwise be inaccessible (Harrison 2001), this research analysed policy documents and media articulations of certain policy developments produced by selected organisations between 2003 and 2012. The increasing number of organisations involved in the delivery of the Games (Chappelet and Kübler-Mabbott 2008) further emphasises the practical need to limit the organisations selected for analysis, and data collection therefore focused upon policy published by four state organisations: the UK government's Department for Culture, Media and Sport (DCMS), the Department for Health (DH), Sport England and the Greater London Authority (GLA) along with the London 2012 Bid Team/ LOCOG. The emphasis upon state organisations is attributable to the fact that host governments are chiefly responsible for Olympic legacy planning. LOCOG was also selected on the basis that 'the legal form of an OCOG is increasingly becoming that of a government agency' (Chappelet and Kübler-Mabbott 2008, p. 91). The selection of documents was restricted to policy documents authored exclusively by the organisations named in this section. For example, although the official DCMS meta-evaluation of the Games features extensive work upon the sport/PA legacy of the Games, its authors acknowledge that no guarantees can be made regarding the 'accuracy' or 'completeness' (DCMS 2011) of the contributions made to this work by external organisations.

Although the selection of specific organisations may risk ignoring important policy articulations from others, the advantage of focusing upon the five listed here was that it better enabled the researchers to identify contradictions and inconsistencies in material produced by the same organisation(s) over an extended period of time. In choosing relevant organisations, emphasis was placed upon state organisations that held a national level responsibility for the design and delivery of the legacy of the Games. International bodies such as the IOC and regional organisations such as the Nations and Regions Group were therefore not considered. Focus was also restricted to policy around the Olympic Games and mass sport/PA participation – thus excluding that concerning the Paralympic Games and the legacy for disability sport, primarily owing to the scope of the study and the extra debates and issues that would be entailed. As the UK government's size demanded that only certain departments were used for analysis, departments were selected on the basis of their contribution to the published sport and activity participation legacy targets of London 2012. Despite the change of UK government in 2010, this research treats the UK government as one consistent entity as the foremost concern was its role as an Olympic host government as opposed to any comparison between different UK administrations.

The one exception to the above criteria was the Greater London Authority's (2009) *A Sporting Future for London*, as London's high population distinguishes its role in promoting sport in London from those of other local organisations. With these criteria established, specific documents were selected purposively (Silverman 2010), on the basis that they either concerned the sport and activity participation legacy specifically, or – more commonly – covered this as one of several strands of the event's legacy as a whole – either in terms of its initial proposal, planning or adjustment (such as those made following the change of government in 2010). Also included was the UK government's 2011 *Public Health Responsibility Deal*, on the basis of its content regarding responsibility for public health in the years around London 2012.

From these sources, 16 policy documents with a total combined length of 642 pages were analysed. These documents provided official accounts of the various stages of the sport/PA participation legacy's proposal, planning and delivery within the broader context of the event's legacy as a whole. Additionally, extra sources were collected that pertained to four significant events in the development of the sport/PA legacy that were not completely covered in official documents: the first official announcement of London's intention to bid for the Games in 2003, its selection as host city for the 2012 Games in 2005, the 2010 announcement of *Places People Play* and the 2011 admission that the pre-event sport/PA participation targets had been abandoned. In order to address these gaps, a further 30 pages of data were collected, which took the form of speeches and media articulations of specific policy developments. The overall dataset consisted of 22 different sources which contained a total of 672 pages of content. A full timeline of the key events in the development of the sport/PA participation legacy and the documents used for analysis is provided in Table 1.

Analysis of the selected documents followed Braun and Clarke's (2006) six phases of thematic analysis (familiarisation with data, generating initial codes, searching for themes, reviewing themes, defining and naming themes, producing the report), but with one modification. This concerned the initial reading of the documents, where one preliminary stage was added in order to establish whether content related to sport and activity participation legacy – with unrelated content being disregarded. This was particularly necessary in the analysis of documents that covered every aspect

Table 1. Timeline of key events and policy documents relating to the London 2012 sport/PA legacy.

Year	Key Events	Documents Published
2003	**Bidding phase: Potential of 2012 Games to increase sport/PA participation highlighted but no formal target published in Candidate File**	
	UK government announces London bid for 2012 Games	
2004	London 2012 Candidate File submitted to IOC	*London 2012: A Vision for the Olympic Games and Paralympic Games* (London 2012 Bid Team)
		London 2012: Response to the questionnaire for cities applying to become Candidate cities to host the Games of the XXX Olympiad and the Paralympic Games in 2012 (London 2012 Bid Team)
		London 2012 Candidate File (London 2012 Bid Team)
2005	**Planning phase: Pre-event sport/PA participation targets published in 2008 following selection of London as host**	
	London selected as Host City for 2012 Games	*Towards a One Planet Olympics* (LOCOG)
2007		*London 2012 Sustainability Policy* (LOCOG)
		Our Promise for London 2012 (DCMS)
2008	2012 Legacy plans published	*Before, During and After: making the Most of the London 2012 Games.* (DCMS)
		Sport England Strategy 2008–2011 (Sport England)
2009		*Be Active Be Healthy: A Plan for Getting the Nation Moving* (DH)
		A Sporting Future for London (Mayor of London/GLA)
		Towards a One Planet 2012 (LOCOG)
2010	**Change of government: labour administration succeeded by Conservative-led coalition government which confirms the abandonment of the 2008 pre-event participation targets in 2011**	
	UK General Election sees Labour government replaced by Coalition government	Plans for the Legacy from the 2012 Olympic and Paralympic Games (DCMS)
	Places People Play participation legacy initiative announced	
2011	Coalition government announces abandonment of official sport/PA participation legacy targets	The Public Health Responsibility Deal (DH)
2012	Coalition government announces new sport/PA participation legacy plans	Creating a Sporting Habit for Life: A New Youth Sport Strategy (DCMS)
		Beyond 2012: the London 2012 Legacy Story (DCMS)
	2012 Summer Olympic Games staged in London	The Get Set Story: How London 2012 Inspired the UK's schools (LOCOG)

of the event's legacy, which were defined by the DCMS (2008) as including 'making the UK a world-leading sporting nation', 'transforming the heart of East London', 'inspiring a new generation of young people', 'making the Olympic Park a blueprint for sustainable living' and 'demonstrating that the UK is a creative, inclusive and welcoming place to live in, visit and for business' (p. 1). Within these legacy areas, the sport/PA participation legacy was detailed underneath the first 'promise' (to make the UK a 'world-leading sporting nation'), which in turn was divided into three headline ambitions: 'inspiring young people through sport', 'getting people more active' and 'elite achievement' (DCMS, 2008, p. 6). Furthermore, it is worth clarifying that the term 'sport/PA participation legacy' as used in the present document does not refer to 'elite achievement' – as the focus of the study was upon mass participation sport and discretionary/leisure PA. Material pertaining to elite sport was therefore disregarded.

Findings and analysis

Constructions of sport/PA and their relationship with health

Across the documents examined, there was significant inconsistency in how 'sport' and 'PA' participation were constructed in terms of their intended effects upon public health and wider society. On a definitional level, some sources claimed a clear distinction between sport and PA (Sport England 2008) while others acknowledged that 'on the ground the division is far more blurred' (GLA 2009, p. 9). Beyond these terminological issues, sport's social value was articulated in varying ways. For example, the DCMS (2008) emphasised the risks of failing to use the Games to promote PA participation:

> By 2050 60% of men and 40% of women could be clinically obese, if we do nothing. The London 2012 Games are our best chance in a generation to encourage people to be more physically active and to give them the opportunities they need to do so. (DCMS 2008 p. 22)

This warning is consistent with the empirical evidence that no previous Olympic Games has been proven to have caused a permanent increase in PA participation (Bauman *et al.* 2001, Veal 2003, Tsuoros *et al.* 2007). The use of statistics to emphasise the importance of using London 2012 to succeed where its predecessors could not resonates with accounts of how 'tactics and calculations' (Foucault 1994) and 'techniques' and 'forms of knowledge' (Rose *et al.* 2006) contribute towards the process of governing and shaping individual conduct. In this case, ostensibly scientific predictions around obesity rates based on current statistics are set against the one-off nature of the Games in order to emphasise the vital effort required to increase PA. This logic also resonates with the notion of 'risk discourses' (McDermott 2007) which function in (neoliberal) societies where populations are understood in relation to 'discourses of responsibilisation, choice and self-governance' and issues such as individual health/obesity are therefore linked to the inability of individuals 'to commit to a healthy lifestyle'. A 'risk discourse' therefore acts as a 'moral technology' through which 'regulatory practices seeking to shape and guide people's conduct are deployed' (2007, p. 318). A similar logic can be seen in the present example, as the DCMS's rationale is primarily phrased in indirect terms such as 'providing opportunities' and 'encouraging' increased participation. Despite these parallels with McDermott's (2007) understanding of how 'risk discourses' may be used in the promotion of healthy lifestyles, the specific context of the London 2012 Olympic legacy features a number of additional factors that must be considered in relation to the dynamics of sport/PA and health. These include the link between these issues of individual responsibility and the one-off nature of the Games (DCMS 2008), as well as the proclaimed broader benefits of sport/PA, such as the assertion that PA participation 'boosts concentration and feeds through directly into improved academic performance' (DCMS, 2010, p. 2).

This focus upon the 'risks' or negative consequences of failing to promote sport/PA was not the only way in which the unique opportunity offered by London 2012 was articulated. Other sources approached the issue in more positive terms, emphasising the broader positive consequences of sport/PA instead:

> Sport can act as a great leveller – allowing people from all backgrounds to come together and join in positive activity. It can help our young people stay healthy, and it can help tackle issues such as obesity, academic underachievement and crime. (Johnson, cited GLA 2009, p. 5)

This paean to sport, authored by then Mayor of London Boris Johnson, echoed Sport England (2008) assertion that 'sport can and does play a major role in achieving wider social and economic benefits – notably on the health front' (p. 1). While these positive views of sport are long-established (e.g. Smith and Westerbeek 2007), this emphasis upon the rewards of sport/PA participation contrasts with the warnings of the 'risks' of failing to participate examined above. Just as a 'risk discourse' can be used as one indirect means of promoting health (via sport/PA), these articulations of the potential incentives of sport/PA participation suggest that a parallel 'reward discourse' could be argued to function similarly. These policy emphases upon 'risk' and 'reward' are comparable in how both can be understood as indirect attempts to 'steer' (Vallentin and Murillo 2009) individuals towards desired behaviours that cannot be brought about by direct coercion. Beyond this similarity, the more optimistic emphasis upon potential rewards or benefits of sport/PA participation could be linked to the unique status of sport – and indeed the Olympic Games – in relation to broader goals such as community development (Grix and Carmichael 2012) and social integration (Smith and Westerbeek 2007).

Three features of the evidence examined in this section can be seen as factors which may have facilitated the use of indirect governmental techniques such as 'risk' and 'reward' discourses. First, the inherent difficulties faced by governments in trying to promote health (Osborne 1997) – in this case via sport/PA participation – and sport/PA participation (e.g. Grix and Carmichael 2012, Weed *et al.* 2012) represent significant challenges. Second, the increased planning and social responsibilities demanded of Olympic legacy planning (e.g. Fussey *et al.* 2011, Leopkey and Parent 2012a) are consistent with how the claims examined in this section moved beyond the proclaimed benefits of sport/PA alone and extended into other areas such as education and crime. Third, the deployment of the indirect governmental techniques described here can be seen more broadly as symptomatic of sport's growth into a major public policy concern (Green and Houlihan 2006, Grix 2015). Overall, this illustration of how both the 'risks' and 'rewards' of sport/PA participation were emphasised in policy relating to London 2012's pre-event participation targets demonstrates how Olympic legacies are both long-term exercises in social responsibility (Fussey *et al.* 2011) and social constructions that can be continually reshaped and contested. In terms of sport/PA participation legacy targets and PA policy in general, the chief implication of this evidence is that appreciating the social complexity of precisely what constitutes sport or PA – and the ultimate effects of these constructs upon 'health' – is a clear requirement for Olympic legacy planners and sport/PA policy makers.

'Inspiration': the unique nature of the Olympic Games

Although certain features of UK state policy around the legacy of London 2012 can be understood in relation to longer term trends regarding sport/PA's status in contemporary politics, others were more explicitly connected to the specific context represented by the Olympic Games. The perceived special status of the event was most readily apparent in the intangible notion of 'inspiration' and became heavily linked to the proposed sport/PA participation legacy following Lord Coe's speech to the IOC before the final vote in Singapore:

> We can no longer take it for granted that young people will choose sport. Some may lack the facilities. Or the coaches and role models to teach them. Others, in an age of 24-hour entertainment and instant fame, may

> simply lack the desire. We are determined that a London Games will address that challenge. So London's vision is to reach young people all around the world. To connect them with the inspirational power of the Games. So they are inspired to choose sport. (Coe 2005, cited in London 2012, 2005, para. 36–40)

Coe's vision implies that factors in increasing participation such as coaches and role models are best provided by the Olympic Games. This assumption resonates with Chatziefstathiou and Henry (2009) account of Olympism's historical capacity to define itself as 'the reference point for what constitutes sport' (p. 24–5). Coe's emphasis upon the 'inspirational power' of the Olympics in relation to young people was soon echoed in UK government policy. In its official legacy plans, the DCMS proclaimed that the Games would 'inspire every person, young and old, to take part in a range of sporting activities and to lead healthier, more active lives' (p. 19) while in 2010 Coe himself announced *Places People Play* with the statement that it would 'harness the inspirational power of the Games to promote sport and leave a lasting legacy of facilities' (Coe, cited in Slater 2010, para. 27). These examples illustrate how early references to the unique 'inspiration' and 'power' of the Games evolved into formal statements about how the event could bring about a mass sport/PA participation legacy despite substantial evidence to the contrary (e.g. McCartney *et al.* 2010; Weed *et al.* 2009).

This inconsistency between the apparent reliance upon the 'inspiration' and 'power' of the Olympic Games in official legacy policies and the practical challenge of increasing participation points to a deeper contradiction. On the surface, 'inspiration' resonates with the broad view that hosting sport events can generate 'civic pride, self-confidence, or a festival atmosphere' (Burgan and Mules 1992, p. 709); three intangible constructs that are difficult to prove (or disprove). However, the specific use of 'inspiration' in relation to the London 2012 sport/PA participation legacy can be linked to more complex assumptions upon which the Olympics are based. Central to these assumptions is the concept of Olympism, which has been described as a 'philosophy of behaviour' or 'set of values' accepted across the global context of world sport that may also be internalised at individual level (Chatziefstathiou and Henry 2009, p. 4). This understanding of the Olympic Games both helps to explain the unique status they enjoy in contemporary sport and underpins the references to 'inspiration' in relation to sport/PA participation examined above. In terms of the broader workings of governmental tactics (Foucault 1994), this example demonstrates how the use of 'inspiration' represented a specific means for UK policy to link the global status of the Olympics to a set of established assumptions regarding individual conduct in relation to sport and physical culture.

From the bidding stage onwards, the inherent 'inspiration' and 'power' of sport and the Olympic Games were also deployed enthusiastically in relation to broader social objectives than sport and PA participation alone:

> Throughout our country there is an appreciation that the Olympic Games and Paralympic Games are a power for good. For London 2012, that power for good will be the most powerful catalyst imaginable for the regeneration of one of our most underdeveloped areas. It will accelerate the most extensive transformation seen in London for more than a century. Tens of thousands of lives will be improved by new jobs and sustainable new housing, new sports venues and other facilities. (London 2012, 2004, p. 1)

These sentiments were echoed after London had been selected as host, with the innate 'inspiration' of the Games further linked to social objectives relating to obesity, health and crime (GLA 2009). These claims are consistent with the ways in which the sport/PA participation legacy was articulated in relation to the unique status of the Games, as in both cases the underpinning assumption is that the Olympics are capable of stimulating broad social changes that could not be achieved otherwise – which echoes MacAloon's (2008) description of the 'magical properties of today's highly fetishized legacy talk in Olympic circles' (p. 2069). As much as elite sport success may be argued to increase participation and public health (Grix and Carmichael 2012), the statements examined in this section demonstrate that the Olympics have an additional moral dimension that allows policy makers to emphasise its potential for social benefits that extend beyond sport. Along with the long-established assumptions around Olympism and sport (Chatziefstathiou and Henry 2009), these statements about the event's special social status show how the repeated references to the 'inspiration' of the event in official legacy policy represented a specific governmental technique (Rose *et al.* 2006) that fitted congruently with both the stricter Olympic legacy requirements (Fussey *et al.* 2011) and the increasing importance of sport in government policy (Green and Houlihan 2006).

Abandonment of pre-event participation targets

In March 2011, the UK government admitted that the pre-event sport participation targets published by the DCMS (2008) were to be abandoned following three years of negligible progress (Gibson 2011). This acknowledgement followed reports in May 2010 that the target of one million more people participating in PA had been 'quietly dropped' (Weed 2013, p. 95). The following year, a 'new approach' to the Olympic sport/PA participation legacy was published, which emphasised 'reaching out to young people more effectively' (Hunt, cited in DCMS 2012, p. 1) instead of increasing mass participation. Given the ambitious rhetoric of both the bidding stage and the DCMS' formal announcement of its pre-event participation targets, this policy shift represents a crucial event in the development of the legacy of London 2012.

Following the 2010 UK general election, the Labour government that had overseen the first seven years of bidding and planning for the 2012 Games was replaced by a Conservative-led coalition. Against a backdrop of national and global economic instability, the coalition government sought to justify widespread reductions in public spending in relation to the preceding Labour government's perceived fiscal irresponsibility (e.g. Landale 2013). Although these debates extended well beyond sport and the Olympic Games, the justification of coalition policy in relation to mistakes made previously by Labour – as well as the coalition's broader effort to distinguish itself from its predecessor's more target-driven approach to policy (Weed 2013) – were also evident in the abandonment and replacement of the 2008 pre-event sport/PA participation targets.

For example, the issue of how 'legacy' itself should be measured was strongly disputed. The DCMS's (2008) pre-event participation targets were announced alongside the claim that legacy includes 'not just what happens after the Games, but what we do before and during them' (p. 8). Four years later, new Minister for Sport Hugh Robertson argued otherwise:

> 2012 is not the end of the story; it's the start of one. For us to think we could start all of this and get it done by 2012 was foolish. Government is to blame for allowing people to believe this was the date by which all this should be judged. Legacy is what it says on the can. In 2012 we should start the legacy. (Robertson, cited Gibson 2012, para. 7–8)

These competing views are consistent with recent accounts of how no clear consensus exists regarding precisely when legacy should be measured and that the term itself is inherently subjective (MacAloon 2008, Leopkey and Parent 2012b). For SME hosts with similar political systems to the UK, this lack of clarity regarding legacy measurement has significant implications. Most importantly, the fact that one government can design legacy plans according to a specific timescale only to leave office shortly after their publication is problematic – particularly when the succeeding administration justifies wider policy changes in relation to the perceived failures of its predecessor.

Beyond the specific policy approaches of different UK governments, rationales for the abandonment and replacement of the sport/PA participation targets also referred more broadly to the late 2000s financial crisis. For example, the central policy change around the sport/PA legacy concerned the decision to focus upon encouraging a 'habit' of sport participation in young people (DCMS 2012). This contradicted the DCMS' (2008) claim that its pre-event participation targets were intended to apply to all demographics, with specific reference made to female participation, the disabled, ethnic minorities, the elderly, and people from 'more deprived areas' (p. 23). For then Culture Secretary Jeremy Hunt, this policy shift was unavoidable:

> I do think it's reasonable to ask whether, with resources as constrained as they are, if it's an appropriate use of taxpayers' money to be focusing on adult participation when really what we want is to be getting young people into a habit for life. (Hunt, cited Gibson 2011, para. 3)

In this instance, the legacy planners responsible for the pre-event sport/PA participation targets were ultimately powerless in trying to ensure their realisation. This 'powerlessness' is consistent with observations about the difficulty of ensuring or 'guaranteeing' health (Osborne 1997, Vallgårda 2012) – which in this case, apply similarly to sport/PA participation. Despite the enthusiasm with which the pre-event sport/PA targets were announced and the discursive tactics (Foucault 1994, Rose *et al.* 2006) that were deployed in their pursuit, the attribution of their abandonment to the broader economic situation represents a clear warning for future SME hosts and legacy planners.

The ambitious nature of London's attempt to be the first Games to achieve a permanent legacy for sport/PA was also emphasised both before and after the abandonment of the initial pre-event participation targets. In 2009, the DH acknowledged that although no previous Games had brought about a 'lasting increase in physical activity', London 2012 would 'break new ground in delivering a health legacy' (DH 2009, p. 21). Three years later, then Culture Secretary Jeremy Hunt introduced the coalition government's new participation legacy plans with similar reference to the unprecedented nature of what London 2012 was attempting:

> The UK has been attempting something that no other host nation has achieved – to harness the power of the Olympics and Paralympics to create a deep and lasting legacy of sports participation in every community … Yet what we've also learnt over the last six years is that there can be no 'plug and play' sporting legacy from the Games. (Hunt, cited DCMS 2012, p. 1)

The broader significance of these statements about the ambitious nature of bringing about a sport/PA participation increase lies in how the challenge of increasing participation depends upon sport/PA policy's ability to work against long-established social structures (Girginov and Hills 2009) relating to the provision of sport/PA opportunities. Along with the links between the London 2012 legacy and the UK economy explored previously, this challenge provides a further example of how the planning of Olympic legacies must be sensitive to various external factors that may affect their attainment. In this case, the sentiments expressed by Hunt here had already been established in academic literature on SME legacies.

The evidence examined in this section demonstrates that despite the lofty rhetoric with which the DCMS' (2008) pre-event sport/PA participation targets were announced, their ultimate abandonment in 2011 can best be understood in terms of broader social and political factors. Three specific factors have been identified here. First, the change of UK government in 2010 saw the Labour government that oversaw the design of the first legacy plans replaced by a coalition that sought to justify much of its policy in relation to the alleged financial irresponsibility of its predecessor. Second, this perceived irresponsibility was argued to have mitigated the effects of the late 2000s financial crisis in the UK, enabling key policy makers to rationalise the abandonment of the participation targets on economic grounds. Third, the acknowledgements of the inherent challenge of attempting to bring about the stated participation increase further emphasise the difficulty of using SMEs to attract new people to sport/PA. For future SME hosts, these three factors must all be considered in the design of policies around potential legacies. Given the extensive use of governmental 'tactics' and 'techniques' (Foucault 1994, Rose *et al.* 2006) geared towards the promotion of the DCMS' (2008) sport/PA participation targets, their ultimate abandonment and replacement has broader implications for how processes of government can be understood. Despite characterisations of (neoliberal) governmentality as overly negative (Ferguson 2009), this particular example shows how there are circumstances where attempts to manage populations can be frustrated by uncontrollable environmental factors.

Conclusion

This research aimed to understand more about how the pre-event London 2012 sport/PA participation legacy targets were constructed and reconstructed by key policy actors between 2003 and 2012. While this aspect of the event's legacy – and broader UK policy regarding sport/PA and health – have continued to develop since 2012 (e.g. HM Government 2015), this study focused specifically upon the published intention to bring about a pre-event sport/PA participation increase, which was abandoned in 2011. For future SME hosts and policy makers, it is concluded that two sets of implications can be taken from the ultimate fate of London 2012's pre-event sport/PA participation legacy.

First, if one considers the 'tactics' (Foucault 1994) or 'forms of knowledge' (Rose *et al.* 2006) that may be used in pursuit of desired individual conduct, it can be seen that although various rhetorical strategies were deployed in policy around these legacy objectives, they were ultimately ineffective. Of these strategies, two features were most apparent. The first concerned the use of scientific – or 'expert' knowledge to cast the 2012 Games as a vital opportunity to combat the 'risk' (McDermott 2007) of obesity, alongside statements that placed more emphasis upon the various social benefits which the Games – and indeed sport more broadly – can bring. Second, the inherent 'inspiration' of the Games – premised upon these deeper assumptions around sport (e.g. Smith and Westerbeek 2007) – was enthusiastically presented as affording the event a special capacity to increase sport/PA participation in addition to addressing numerous wider social issues for the better. As has been suggested previously (e.g. Weed *et al.* 2012), host governments cannot rely on the event alone to increase or 'inspire' participation. As befits the status of the Games as a 'genuine public policy concern' (Chappelet and Kübler-Mabbott 2008, p. 91), social legacies such as sport/PA participation must therefore be pursued much more proactively.

Second, the ultimate abandonment of these pre-event targets and their accompanying policies should not be attributed exclusively to their own limitations, but also to a range of external environmental factors. The subsequent DCMS assertions that the measurement, target population and timescale of the pre-event targets were fundamentally flawed are consistent with claims that Olympic legacy is best viewed as a product of social and political processes that can be seen to evolve over time (Girginov and Hills 2008, 2009, Leopkey and Parent 2012b) as well as (ultimately vindicated) academic warnings of the difficulties of using the Games to increase sport/PA participation (e.g. Bauman *et al.* 2001, Veal 2003, Coalter 2004). Future Olympic hosts and legacy planners can learn from the fact that these empirical sources were overridden by such dominant 'styles of thought' (Rose *et al.* 2006) and popular assumptions. However, where previous analyses may have tended towards an overly negative usage of governmentality in relation to neoliberal societies (Ferguson 2009), the example of policy abandonment examined here demonstrates how the power of governing actors must be set against the competing influences of external and uncontrollable social factors.

As this research focuses specifically upon pre-event legacy policy, these conclusions do not apply to SMEs on a post-event basis. Further research will be required to evaluate the post-event success of the London 2012 sport/PA participation legacy and its implications for other SMEs. Furthermore, the UK's status as a developed country with a Western democratic model of government that fully acknowledges sport's role in public policy (Green and Houlihan 2006) should also be acknowledged. SMEs are increasingly being held in nations that differ markedly; as demonstrated by the hosting of the 2016 Summer Olympic Games by Rio de Janeiro, Brazil and the 2022 FIFA World Cup by Qatar, and future research should be both sensitive to these differences and aware of the value of examining the policy issues addressed by this research in new environments.

Disclosure statement

No potential conflict of interest was reported by the authors.

References

Agha, N., Fairley, S., and Gibson, H., 2011. Considering legacy as a multi-dimensional construct: the legacy of the Olympic games. *Sport management review*, 15 (1), 125–139. doi:10.1016/j.smr.2011.08.004

Bauman, A., Ford, I., and Armstrong, T., 2001. *Trends in population levels of reported physical activity in Australia, 1997, 1999 and 2000*. Australia: Australian Sports Commission.

Braun, V. and Clarke, V., 2006. Using thematic analysis in psychology. *Qualitative research in psychology*, 3, 77–101. doi:10.1191/1478088706qp063oa

Bullough, S.J., 2012. A new look at the latent demand for sport and its potential to deliver a positive legacy for London 2012. *International journal of sport policy and politics*, 4 (1), 39–54. doi:10.1080/19406940.2011.627357

Burgan, B. and Mules, T., 1992. Economic impact of sporting events. *Annals of tourism research*, 19 (4), 700–710. doi:10.1016/0160-7383(92)90062-T

Cashman, R., 1999. Beyond the games. *In*: R. Cashman and A. Hughes, eds. *Staging the Olympics: the event & its impact*. Netley: Griffin, 183–194.

Chappelet, J., 2012. Mega sporting event legacies: a multifaceted concept. *Papeles de Europa*, 25, 76–86.

Chappelet, J. and Kübler-Mabbott, B., 2008. *The international Olympic committee and the Olympic system: the governance of world sport*. Great Britain: Routledge.

Charlton, T., 2010. 'Grow and Sustain': the role of community sports provision in promoting a participation legacy for the 2012 Olympic games. *International journal of sport policy and politics*, 2 (3), 347–366. doi:10.1080/19406940.2010.519340

Chatziefstathiou, D. and Henry, I., 2009. Technologies of power, governmentality and Olympic discourses: a Foucauldian analysis for understanding the discursive constructions of the Olympic ideology. *Esporte e sociedade*, 4 (12), 1–28.

Coalter, F., 2004. Stuck in the blocks? A sustainable sporting legacy. *In*: A. Vigor, M. Mean, and C. Tims, eds. *After the gold rush: A sustainable Olympics for London*, 91 106. Great Britain: Institute for Public Policy Research.

Commission for a Sustainable London 2012, 2011. *Fit for purpose? A review of inclusion and healthy living across the 2012 programme*. Great Britain: Commission for a Sustainable London 2012.

Dean, M., 1999. *Governmentality: power and rule in modern society*. Great Britain: Sage Publications.

Department for Culture, Media and Sport, 2008. *Before, during and after: making the most of the London 2012 Games*. London: DCMS.

Department for Culture, Media and Sport, 2010. *Plans for the legacy from the 2012 Olympic and Paralympic Games*. London: DCMS.

Department for Culture, Media and Sport, 2011. *Report 1: Scope, research questions and data strategy: Meta-evaluation of the impacts and legacy of the London 2012 Olympic and Paralympic Games*. London: DCMS.

Department for Culture, Media and Sport, 2012. *Creating a sporting habit for life: A new youth sport strategy*. London: DCMS.

Department for Health, 2009. *Be active be healthy: A plan for getting the nation moving*. London: DH.

Devine, C., 2013. London 2012 Olympic legacy: a big sporting society? *International journal of sport policy and politics*, 5 (2), 257–279. doi:10.1080/19406940.2012.656674

Ferguson, J., 2009. The uses of neoliberalism. *Antipode*, 41, 166–184. doi:10.1111/j.1467-8330.2009.00721.x

Foucault, M., 1994. Governmentality. *In*: J.D. Faubion, ed. *Power: the essential works of Foucault 1954-1984*. England: Penguin, 201–222.

Fussey, P., *et al.*, 2011. *Securing and sustaining the Olympic city: Reconfiguring London for 2012 and beyond*. Great Britain: Ashgate.

Gibson, O., 2011. Jeremy Hunt admits London 2012 legacy targets will be scrapped. *The Guardian*. Available from: http://www.theguardian.com/sport/2011/mar/28/jeremy-hunt-london-2012-legacy

Gibson, O., 2012. Hugh Robertson admits to struggling with legacy for grassroots sport. *The Guardian*. Available from: http://www.theguardian.com/sport/2012/mar/05/hugh robertson legacy games 2012

Girginov, V. and Hills, L., 2008. A sustainable sports legacy: creating a link between the London Olympics and sports participation. *The international journal of the history of sport*, 25 (14), 20910–22116. doi:10.1080/09523360802439015

Girginov, V. and Hills, L., 2009. The political process of constructing a sustainable London Olympics sports development legacy. *International journal of sport policy and politics*, 1 (2), 161–181. doi:10.1080/19406940902950713

Gratton, C. and Preuss, H., 2008. Maximizing Olympic impacts by building up legacies. *The international journal of the history of sport*, 25, 1922–1938. doi:10.1080/09523360802439023

Greater London Authority, 2009. A Sporting Future for London? Available from: http://www.london.gov.uk/sites/default/files/a%20sporting%20legacy%20for%20Lo don.pdf

Green, M. and Houlihan, B., 2006. Governmentality, modernization, and the "disciplining" of national sporting organisations: Athletics in Australia and the United Kingdom. *Sociology of sport journal*, 23, 47–71. doi:10.1123/ssj.23.1.47

Grix, J., 2015. *Sport politics: An introduction*. Great Britain: Palgrave.

Grix, J. and Carmichael, F., 2012. Why do governments invest in elite sport? A polemic. *International journal of sport policy & politics*, 4 (1), 73–90. doi:10.1080/19406940.2011.627358

Harrison, L., 2001. *Political research: an introduction*. Great Britain: Routledge.

Heynen, N., *et al.*, 2007. *Neoliberal environments: false promises and unnatural consequences*. Great Britain: Routledge.

Hindson, A., Gidlow, B., and Peebles, C., 1994. The 'trickle down effect' of top level sport: myth or reality? A case study of the Olympics. *Australian journal of leisure and recreation*, 4 (1), 16–24.

HM Government, 2015. *Sporting future: A New strategy for an active nation*. London: UK Government

International Olympic Committee, 2013a. Olympic Charter. Available from: http://www.olympic.org/Documents/olympic_charter_en.pdf

International Olympic Committee, 2013b. *Olympic Games: Legacies and impacts*. Lausanne: IOC Library.

Kay, T., 2012. Accounting for legacy: monitoring and evaluation in sport in development relationships. *Sport in society: Cultures, commerce, media, politics*, 15 (6), 888–904. doi:10.1080/17430437.2012.708289

Kelso, P., 2011. London 2012: sport England to miss legacy target as Games fail to inspire youngsters. *The Telegraph*. Available from: http://www.telegraph.co.uk/sport/olympics/news/8944428/London 2012-Olympics- Sport England-to-miss-legacy-target-as-Games-fail-to-inspire-youngsters.html

Landale, J., 2013. David Cameron: labour's the point. *BBC News*. Retrieved from http://www.bbc.co.uk/news/uk-politics-24371521

Leopkey, B. and Parent, M.M., 2012a. Olympic Games legacy: from general benefits to sustainable long-term legacy. *The international journal of the history of sport*, 29, 924–943. doi:10.1080/09523367.2011.623006

Leopkey, B. and Parent, M.M., 2012b. The (neo) institutionalization of legacy and its sustainable governance within the Olympic movement. *European sport management quarterly*, 12 (5), 437–455. doi:10.1080/16184742.2012.693116

London 2012, 2004. *Response to the questionnaire for cities applying to become Candidate cities to host the Games of the XXX Olympiad and the Paralympic Games in 2012*. London: London 2012.

London 2012, 2005. *Singapore presentation. In: Presented at 117th International Olympic Committee Session*, 6 July 2005. London: London 2012.

MacAloon, J.J., 2008. 'Legacy' as managerial/magical discourse in contemporary Olympic affairs. *The international journal of the history of sport*, 25 (14), 2060–2071. doi:10.1080/09523360802439221

Markula, P. and Pringle, R., 2006. *Foucault, sport and exercise: Power, knowledge and transforming the self*. Great Britain: Routledge.

Mahtani, K.R., *et al.*, 2013. Can the London 2012 Olympics 'inspire a generation' to do more physical or sporting activities? An overview of systematic reviews. *British medical journal open*, 3, e002058.

McCartney, G., *et al.*, 2010. The health and socioeconomic impacts of major multi-sport events: systematic review (1978-2008). *British medical journal*, 340, c2369. doi:10.1136/bmj.c2369

McDermott, L., 2007. A governmental analysis of children "at Risk" in a world of physical inactivity and obesity epidemics. *Sociology of sport journal*, 24, 302–324. doi:10.1123/ssj.24.3.302

Murphy, N.M. and Bauman, A., 2007. Mass sporting events and physical events – are they "bread and circuses" or public health interventions to increase population levels of physical activity? *Journal of physical activity and health*, 4, 193–202. doi:10.1123/jpah.4.2.193

Osborne, T., 1997. Of health and statecraft. *In*: A. Petersen and R. Bunton, eds. *Foucault: health and medicine*. Great Britain: Routledge, 173–188.

Piggin, J., Jackson, S.J., and Lewis, M., 2009. Knowledge, power and politics. *International review for the sociology of sport*, 44, 87–101. doi:10.1177/1012690209102825

Rose, N., O'Malley, P., and Valverde, M., 2006. Governmentality. *Annual review of law and social science*, 2, 83–104. doi:10.1146/annurev.lawsocsci.2.081805.105900

Silverman, D., 2010. *Doing qualitative research*. Great Britain: Sage.

Slater, M., 2010. Lottery boost for London 2012 mass participation legacy. Available from: http://news.bbc.co.uk/sport1/hi/olympic_games/london_2012/9190546.stm

Smith, A.C.T. and Westerbeek, H.M., 2007. Sport as a vehicle for deploying corporate social responsibility. *Journal of corporate citizenship*, 25, 43–54. doi:10.9774/GLEAF.4700.2007.sp.00007

Sport England, 2008. *Sport England strategy 2008-2011*. London: Sport England.

Tsuoros, A.D., *et al.*, 2007. The Athens 2004 Olympic Games and public health: main conclusions and lessons learned. In: A.D. Tsouros and P.A. Efstathiou, eds. *Mass gatherings and public health: the experience of the Athens 2004 Olympic Games*. Denmark: World Health Organisation Regional Office for Europe, 303–310.

Vallgårda, S., 2012. Nudge—a new and better way to improve health? *Health policy*, 104, 200–203. doi:10.1016/j.healthpol.2011.10.013

Veal, A.J., 2003. Tracking change: leisure participation and policy in Australia, 1985-2002. *Annals of leisure research*, 6 (3), 245–277. doi:10.1080/11745398.2003.10600924

Vallentin, S. and Murillo, D., 2009. *CSR as governmentality*. Denmark: CBS Center for Corporate Social Responsibility.

Weed, M., 2013. London 2012 legacy strategy: ambitions, promises and implementation plans. In: V. Girginov, ed. *Handbook of the London 2012 Olympic and Paralympic Games (Volume One)*. Great Britain: Routledge, 87–98.

Weed, M., *et al.*, 2012. Developing a physical activity legacy from the London 2012 Olympic and Paralympic Games: a policy-led systematic review. *Perspective public health*, 132 (2), 75–80. doi:10.1177/1757913911435758

Weed, M., *et al.*, 2009. *A systematic review of the evidence base for developing a physical activity and health legacy from the London 2012 Olympic and Paralympic Games*. London: Department for Health.

Weiler, R. and Stamatakis, E., 2010. Physical activity in the UK: a unique crossroad? *British journal of sports medicine*, 44, 912–914. doi:10.1136/bjsm.2010.073726

Wellings, K., *et al.*, 2011. The 2012 Olympics: assessing the public health effect. *The lancet*, 378 (9797), 1193–1195. doi:10.1016/S0140-6736(11)60550-3

Group fitness instructors as local level health promoters: a Foucauldian analysis of the politics of health/fitness dynamic

Pirkko Markula and Jocelyn Chikinda

ABSTRACT

As fitness professionals, group fitness instructors play an important role in promoting recommended public health initiatives to various communities. While their practices are connected to public health policy, their certifications are often provided by commercially operated agencies in the North American context. The interrelationship of commercial and governmental control creates a complex environment where certain ways of understanding health and the fit body become dominant. In this paper, consequently, we were interested in what fitness knowledges informed Canadian group fitness instructors' practices. Approaching our topic from a Foucauldian perspective, we conducted semi-structured interviews with five instructors who had a provincially governed fitness qualification. The findings revealed that two knowledges – health as illness prevention and the aesthetics of health – strongly directed the instructors' class design despite their willingness to think, particularly about health, differently. Their certification reinforced the medical, physiological, and psychological knowledges that tend to assign health as individual responsibility, but left the social issues behind the healthy, fit body unproblematized. From a Foucauldian perspective, these dominant knowledges locked the instructors within dual control of anatomo-political and bio-political neoliberal power relations. To assist the instructors to problematize the control mechanism behind the dominant knowledge structure, we call for inclusion of broader knowledge base in their certification training through which serving the multiple needs of their various clientele can be constructively negotiated.

Canada promotes physical activity, nationwide, through such governmental public health strategies as ParticipAction supported by the Canadian Active Living Guidelines (CALG). While these strategies are not explicitly aimed at the fitness industry, it is, nevertheless, responsible for involving considerable population in healthy physical activity. As leaders of significant numbers of exercisers, certified group fitness instructors are important promoters of health. In this study, consequently, we are interested in how the governmental health policy manifests in the actual fitness instruction practices. To do this, we map what group fitness instructors learn about health in a provincially supported certification course and how governmental health policy, through these knowledges, might inform fitness industry practices. As experienced fitness instructors, we propose that the certification should provide the major foundation for quality group fitness instruction, but as feminist Foucauldian researchers we also want to problematize some of the health related knowledges endorsed by the instructor certification courses.

We locate our investigation into a broader context of neo-liberal governance of health in Canada. To do so, we draw from Michel Foucault's understanding of the operation of power/knowledge nexus within the dual influence of bio-politics of population health control and anatomo-political control of individual bodies within neo-liberal societies. We are particularly interested in the effects of power (Foucault 1977a) at the local level of fitness instruction and how power relations, through uses of certain health knowledge distributed in governmental health policy and fitness instructor certification, materially, and in-depth (Foucault 1977b), penetrate fitness practices. We then detail our method before presenting the type of knowledges that inform group fitness instructors' understandings of healthy fitness practices. We conclude by contextualizing these health and fitness practices as produced in the intersections of neo-liberal governmentality and consumerism.

Foucault, power/knowledge, and fitness

From a Foucauldian perspective, health is currently a central aspect of population control in neo-liberal societies that have undergone a broader shift from a spatial control of individual bodies to bio-political control of the entire population (Foucault 1978, 2007). According to Foucault (2007), bio-politics operates through regulatory practices assigned to a continuum of state apparatus (law, medicine, political economy, education) and is facilitated by the type of power that he called 'government.' The current purpose of the government is to improve the welfare, wealth, longevity, and health of the population (Foucault 2008). State intervention is not necessarily reduced, but is modeled based on 'the market' rationale in this neo-liberal governmentality. For instance, the state sponsored social programs are increasingly shaped according to the commercial models of industry to increase individual citizens' 'freedom' to act for themselves. As documented by several scholars (e.g. Crawford 1980, 2006, Petersen and Lupton 1996, Lupton 1997, 2013, Ayo 2012), health has turned into a personal responsibility under neo-liberalism. Within this arrangement, the governmental apparatus and a 'series of knowledges' become intertwined to support a particular rationale for governance (Foucault 2007). Governmentality, thus, can also serve as an overarching framework for situating group fitness instructor knowledge within the apparatuses of contemporary neo-liberal society.

Foucault's (2007) 'the arts of government' point to a discursive field in which exercising power is 'rationalized' by defining concepts, specifying objects of government, argumentations, and justifications. Certain types of knowledges, partly produced and proliferated by state agencies, support this reasoning. Health policy, directly a part of governmental apparatus, is inescapably intertwined with these strategies as a distributor of specific style of thought. Ayo (2012), for example, argued that in Canada, neo-liberal health promotion focuses on such individualized practices as physical activity promotion and healthy eating instead of social determinants of health (e.g. unemployment, poverty, lack of education). Relevant to our project, the Canadian Active Living Guidelines (CALG) were developed by the Canadian Society of Exercise Physiologists (CSEP) with support by the governmental Public Health Agency of Canada (PHAC) to establish healthy physical activity levels for individual citizens. From a Foucauldian perspective, these guidelines do not simply contain neutral facts, but advocate for a specific type of healthy physical activity. For example, the PHAC website emphasizes that physically active people 'live longer, healthier lives' and are 'more productive, and more likely to avoid illness and injury' (Public Health Agency of Canada 2016a). The CALG specifies the benefits of 150 minutes of moderate to vigorous intensity aerobic physical activity per week for an adult between 18–64 as reducing risk of premature death, heart disease, stroke, high blood pressure, certain types of cancer, type 2 diabetes, osteoporosis, overweight, and obesity. They link health predominantly with illness prevention while also advocating improved mental health (morale and self-esteem) as a benefit of physical activity. Physical activity, in turn, is defined based on exact time (150 minutes), intensity (moderate to vigorous), and type (aerobic). Foucault (1972) was interested in how propositions like these strategically construct knowledges that, as a part of governmentality, play a tactical role in the strategic use of power.

As health and wellbeing constitute a significant part of population control in neo-liberal society, the evidence supporting healthy physical activity is also a part of the politics of knowledge production and power relations for defining 'truth' in contemporary society. Within these conditions, Foucault (1972, p. 101–192) asserted, knowledge(s) turn into discourses, 'tactical elements or blocks operating in the field of force relations' that always manifest in material life. Through discourses, governmentality becomes a lived experience: governmental health promotion moves across a web of power networks often in unexpected and uncontrollable ways when percolating down to group fitness instructor training. In this process, phrases regarding health and fitness turn into 'knowledges' that have material effects on how exercise is practiced at fitness clubs (Markula and Kennedy 2011). Previous research has already highlighted that certain ways of knowing dominate the field of fitness and consequently, structure group fitness instructors' practices.

Healthy exercise

As regular physical activity is commonly considered a vital aspect of health in neo-liberal societies, the group fitness instructors, as exercise providers, continually engage in health discourse. While they can obtain their professional knowledge from several sources, their certification manuals and continuing education texts supply significant health information and can act as a type of policy determining their instruction practices. Some Foucauldian researchers (Markula and Pringle 2006, Smith Maguire 2007) have examined how exercise manuals and introductory university exercise texts books define health, physical activity, and exercise. These studies found that knowledge from three main scholarly disciplines – medicine, physiology, and psychology – shape the understanding of healthy physical activity in these texts.

In the exercise texts, health, based on medical and physiological information, is rather singularly defined as absence of particularly costly illnesses such as heart disease and diabetes (Markula and Pringle 2006). As noted earlier, these statements are echoed in the CALG supported by the PHAC at the governmental level in Canada. In addition, such terms as 'health benefits,' 'health behavior,' or 'healthy lifestyle' are introduced as methods of reducing the risk of illness. Specific to our study, the Fitness Leadership Certification Association (FLCA) course book, the *Exercise Theory* manual, similarly emphasizes 'healthy lifestyle' that 'refers to health behaviors aimed at reducing the risk of disease and accidents' (Hansen 2010, p. 5–1). Adopting healthy lifestyle, then, leads to 'wellness' (a combination of health and happiness) comprised of spiritual, emotional, mental, social, physical, and environmental health. Despite the broad definition of wellness, the manual focuses more narrowly on 'the relationship between healthy eating, physical activity and their relationship to healthy weights' drawing from the 'Pan-American Healthy Living Strategy' (Hansen 2010, p. 5–2). Such a proposition verifies Ayo's (2012) earlier contention that health is individualized when practices of healthy eating and exercise are privileged in neo-liberal Canadian society.

The previous research further indicates that healthy physical activity is introduced through the term 'health related physical fitness' that is comprised of four components (cardio-vascular fitness, muscle strength and endurance, flexibility, and body composition). These components, in turn, inform 'exercise prescription:' the detailed instructions on how to improve each of these four components with specific exercises (Markula and Pringle 2006). The exercise texts books in Markula and Pringle's (2006) study further introduced specific exercise prescription guidelines by the American College of Sport Medicine (ACSM). The FLCA *Exercise Theory* manual similarly details the components of health related fitness and, referring to both the ACSM and the CALG guidelines, explains that health related fitness leads to improved quality of life, decreased risk of disease, and an ability to perform everyday tasks with ease. The concept of health related fitness, thus, provides the phrases and propositions through which the broader discourse of health materializes in the everyday practice of fitness instruction. The FITT formula, in turn, defines the frequency, intensity, time, and type of training to correspond to the physiological changes resulting from regular exercise program. Therefore, it further operationalizes the components of health related fitness into the practical level physical training. By manipulating the FITT, a group fitness instructor can build in improvement of physical fitness while the body adapts to training. The components of health related fitness together with the FITT formula comprise the exercise prescription for a group exercise class that typically consists of a warm-up, cardiovascular component, muscular conditioning, and cool-down with flexibility (Kennedy-Armbruster and Yolk 2009). Consequently, the practical content of a group exercise class is more closely dictated by the ACSM guidelines for exercise prescription than the governmentally endorsed CALG policy of health built on the principles of 'active living.'

The promotion of physical fitness (the ACSM guidelines) and active living (CALG) are, nevertheless, deeply intertwined. For example, originally the Canadian federal government's physical activity policy aligned with the early version of the ACSM guidelines (published in 1980) (Bercovitz 1998) to increase overall health through exercise: intentional physical activity to improve the components of physical fitness (Garber *et al.* 2011). Similar to the US context (Dishman 1988), only a small segment of Canadians were able to adhere to these strictly defined standards (Bercovitz 1998). In 1995, the ACSM revised its guidelines to include objectives for both exercise and more moderate physical activity (Markula and Pringle 2006). This approach, labelled the 'public health' approach by the ACSM or active living by many governmental health agencies (Bercovitz 1998, Hardman and Stensel 2003), promotes moderate intensity physical activity (any bodily movement produced by skeletal muscles, Garber *et al.* 2011) as exemplified by the CALG. The ACSM, nevertheless, continues to promote exercise as the most effective way to prevent illness, but considers active living as a starting point for an exercise regime (Garber *et al.* 2011). From the Foucauldian perspective, a physical activity policy modification as a response to initial failure to engage individual citizens in healthy behavior, represents a strategic elaboration, or a continual re-adjustment to the effects of power operations (Foucault 1980a). In this process, the actual goal of the health apparatus – building an illness free nation – has not changed, but the means are re-adjusted for desired behavioral change towards exercise adoption and adherence (Garber *et al.* 2011).

In addition to physical fitness benefits, the ACSM (Garber *et al.* 2011) now emphasizes the psychological factors – choice, preference, and enjoyment – that enhance individual's exercise behavior. Smith Maguire (2007) similarly found that the exercise manuals presented themselves as motivational experts that entice individuals to participate in self-work required for sustaining a fitness program. Therefore, psychological knowledge has now emerged to complement the medical and physiological information of the exercise benefits. Following the lead of the ACSM, FLCA *Exercise Theory* manual endorses 'behavioral change' toward health introducing such concepts as self-esteem, self-efficacy, and motivation and psychological theories such as theory of planned behavior (Hansen 2010). Healthy eating, another major aspect of individualized health promotion in neo-liberal Canada (Ayo 2012), is addressed through Health Canada's (a governmental agency) Canada's Food Guide. Tactically chosen (Foucault 1977a) governmental information of proper weight management, thus, reaches the individual group fitness instructors through their certification.

Based on a Foucauldian perspective, Markula and Pringle (2006) and Smith Maguire (2007) critiqued the definitions of health as absence of illness and physical activity as illness prevention as too singular. When healthy exercise is defined narrowly to aim for an absence of illness, physical activity is translated into tightly prescribed workouts that, from a Foucauldian perspective, turn into disciplinary techniques (Markula and Pringle 2006). Through its regulated movement, timing, and repetition, exercise operates as a normalizing practice (Foucault 1979). As a result, only one way of practicing physical activity, exercise, is accepted as 'healthy,' and thus, desirable and normal. Adherence to disciplinary techniques (and thus, normalcy) requires self-discipline, clear timetabling, and continual body measurement that are then enacted through self-surveillance: the exerciser must continually survey her adherence to exercise intensity and duration and use metrics to chart progress in order to follow the proper progression of exercise prescription. McDermott (2011) added that normalizing and homogenizing bodies through adherence to health related fitness endorse the role of medical and exercise experts whose advice for self-care is accepted as truth. Smith Maguire (2007) connected exercise advice to governmental technologies that 'individualize the question of physical fitness' (p. 125) by knitting 'self-work' together with 'broader political, economic, and social agendas and goals' (p. 126). Through its emphasis on the components of the health related fitness and the FITT formula, the FLCA *Exercise Theory* manual similarly advocates the importance of disciplinary techniques. However, its focus on wellness could open the door for understanding health more broadly. Wellness, nevertheless, is harnessed to the neo-liberal agenda of individual responsibility in the manual. For example, the group fitness leaders are advised to adopt a wellness approach that involves 'working with individual participants and groups to recognize how a responsible attitude towards personal health will improve overall wellness' (Hansen 2010, p. 5–4). This translates into an instructional practice where 'special emphasis is placed on personal initiative, responsibility and control over one's own health through appropriate lifestyle choices that reduce the risk of disease or injury' (Hansen 2010, p. 5–1). Smith Maguire (2007) further alluded that healthy lifestyle in neo-liberal society encourages engagement in additional aspects of self-care beyond physical and mental health.

The aesthetics of health

In the neo-liberal consumer society the 'looks' of the body is closely intertwined with health discourse. While not captured into governmental health policies, it operates as a part of the market driven ethos of neo-liberalism to draw from the principles of individual responsibility for good citizenship. In the fitness industry, the healthy body turns into the fit body that is often judged based on its looks. Feminist researchers, from various theoretical perspectives, have found that looking good (the ideal body) and feeling good (health) become closely intertwined, particularly through popular media texts. As Markula and Kennedy (2011, p. 4) summarized, women's health in these popular enunciations 'is culturally expressed in aesthetic terms as a thin, healthy-looking body.' Smith Maguire (2007) further indicated that the ideal feminine body provides a starting point to market fitness as a part of the healthy lifestyle through which continued consumption of the fitness industry becomes possible. Dworkin and Wachs (2009, p. 172) added that the consumerist promotion of the fit looking body corresponds to a neo-liberal imperative of constructing 'the healthy self.' Following Markula and Kennedy (2011), we label this way of knowing about fitness the aesthetics of the healthy looking body. The previous research on group fitness instructors has largely focuses on the complexities of promoting the healthy looking, fit body in commercial fitness industry[1] (Markula 1995, 2001, 2004, Berman *et al.* 2005, D'Abundo 2009, Dworkin and Wachs 2009, Mansfield 2011, Petersson McIntyre 2011, Wray 2011).

These studies reveal that body aesthetics is a central aspect of being fit. Consequently, the instructors equate the ideally beautiful body with health that they tend to emphasize as each participant's personal responsibility (D'Abundo 2009, Mansfield 2011, Petersson McIntyre 2011, Wray 2011). In this context, the obese bodies are often condemned as unhealthy based on their appearance. For example, in her study of the UK fitness gyms, Mansfield (2011, p. 92) observed that the instructors and participants engaged in gossip about their bodies

> in the construction of preferred images of female physicality and the stigmatization of fat bodies. Derogatory comments about bodies that did not match up to stylized versions of (heterosexual) femininity served to consolidate and strengthen both superior images of the body beautiful and inferior images of fat bodies.

As role models for their clients, the instructors also feel a need to maintain a fit looking body. Evans *et al.* (2005), indeed, reported that women consumers preferred instructors with thin and fit bodies.[2] Even if advocating the healthy looking body, the instructors aim to provide a comfortable and supportive learning environment. For example, instructors in D'Abundo's (2009) study, exhibited 'agency' by encouraging participants to modify exercises to their own needs. Petersson McIntyre (2011) found that striptease aerobics instructors believed their classes offered a safe place for the participants with varied body shapes. Markula (2004), however, indicated that although aware of the problems associated with the ideal fit body, the mindful instructors in her study lacked knowledge on which to ground alternative practices. For example, they were reluctant to use the improved body shape as a selling point preferring to promote such exercise benefits as relaxation and improved body alignment. Yet, they defined building a fit looking body as the ultimate aim that appealed to their clientele and thus, continued to construct these types of bodies through their practices.

Following Foucault, the fitness industry in consumer society is one locale for anatomo-political power where the dominant aesthetics of the healthy looking body ensures that women obediently discipline themselves by dieting and exercising to continually strive for the impossible ideal body. Self-surveillance acts as an extension of 'an inspecting gaze' that the individuals internalize 'without physical force or material constraints [that] controls individuals' (Markula and Pringle 2006, p. 59–60). According to Foucault (1979), self-surveillance operates as a part of panoptic power, where the gaze of the unseen 'other' monitors individuals' behavior. When the participants and instructors re-produce and re-enforce the ideal feminine body aesthetic as healthy, they follow the disciplinary techniques that subjugate them to the anatomo-political power.

Unlike the manuals in Smith Maguire's (2007) study, the FLCA *Exercise Theory* manual does not openly discuss improved appearance as an exercise benefit. It only briefly addresses body image as a psychological (not a social) issue and details eating disorders as an aspect of unhealthy eating. In addition, there is a short mention of the cultural influences and instructor role modeling in regard to body image in the FLCA *Group Exercise* manual (Kennedy-Armbruster and Yolk 2009). Consequently, the feminist, socio-cultural critique of the fit feminine healthy looks is largely absent in the FLCA group instructor training. Dominated by physiology, psychology, and medicine, the manuals remain silent on one of the main problematic issues in the broader culture of fitness.

Although some group fitness instructors aim to build these bodies in a safe environment, their practices can still be anchored in the dual knowledges of health as illness prevention and feminine aesthetics. Following Foucault, these knowledges have entered into the discursive formation of fitness supported by a combination of anatomo-political power through disciplinary techniques applied on the individual body and bio-political power that controls population usually through such governmental strategies as health promotion. Together these forces produce docile, yet useful and responsible citizens for effective workforce based on individuals taking responsibility for staying healthy despite the increasing demands from the competitive, privatized Canadian society (e.g. Dallaire *et al.* 2012, Rail 2012). In this way, anatomo-political power and bio-power are exercised through discursive formation that empowers instructors and participants to believe that regular, consistent level of exercise, as prescribed in class, will greatly enhance their looks, physical health, and wellbeing.

Group fitness instructors have a vital role as health promoters in society, yet there is no in-depth study of how they know about health, physical fitness, the body and how they reproduce these knowledges in their teaching practice. In our study, we examine what knowledges shape experienced instructors' ideas of healthy fitness practices and how these knowledges emanate from different health policies such as CALG, ACSM guidelines, or the group fitness instruction certification texts. In addition, we have chosen a group of instructors certified by the program supported by a provincial government as we were further interested in how the bio-politics of governmental health promotion might diffuse into the material level of grassroots fitness practices. Our analysis, thus, aims to further investigate how the group fitness instructors' practices might align with existing neo-liberal ideals or alternatively, if there is space for critically thinking fitness leadership. In the following section, we provide details of the group fitness instructor education in Canada, and particularly in our province, to further contextualize our research.

Context

In North America, group fitness instructor certification is a commercial industry operated by a number of providers. For example, independent national organizations such as the American

Council on Exercise (ACE), Aerobics and Fitness Association of America (AFAA), or National Strength and Conditioning Association (NSCA), the American College of Sports Medicine (ACSM), as well as a plethora of smaller providers, including Canfitpro, operated by a commercial fitness center chain FitLife in Canada, offer certifications. Some of these are accredited through the National Commission of Certifying Agencies that also sets the standards of certifications for athletic training and nursing in the USA (Kennedy-Armbruster and Yolk 2009). In this environment, FLCA was established in 1984 as an attempt to provide 'some level of guidance and quality assurance in fitness leadership' (Hansen 2010, p. iii) in Canada. It is the first Canadian provincially sanctioned fitness leadership certification association. FLCA is also 'the flagship association in the National Fitness Leadership Alliance of Canada, a partnership of not-for-profit organizations dedicated to the advancement of exercise accreditation and leadership' (Provincial Fitness Unit 2016).

The FLCA operates under the governmentally funded Fitness Unit (FU) that was established in 1981.[3] The provincial government supports the FU administration by providing about 20% of its funding. The Provincial University provides infrastructure (the office space) with rest of funding obtained through grants, fees from services (e.g., workshops and certifications), resource sales (e.g., exercise manuals), and membership dues. The FLCA, thus, operates within an organization based on private-public partnership typical to many neo-liberal governmental services. While the FU aligns itself with provincial Active Policy (Provincial Fitness Unit 2016), no governmental policy directly dictates the FU or FLCA mandate. The provincial government has an ex-officio representative without voting rights in the FU board of directors. The FU, thus, is governed by its own 'agency based board' into which 'members are appointed and elected' (personal communication, executive director FU).[4]

An executive director currently leads the FU and manages its three streams: the FLCA certifications, a fitness for life initiative, and the FU projects. Two FCLA coordinators oversee the fitness leader certifications, but more than 60 'trainers' approved by the FU deliver the actual courses. The group exercise leader certification is one of the professional certifications offered under the umbrella of FLCA. About 600–1000 group exercise leaders are trained annually and since 1986 the FLCA has certified 'well over 20,000 leaders' (Hansen 2010, p. iv). The group instructor training certification costs about $500CAD and is paid by each course participant, as one of the funding streams of FU (personal communication, executive director FU). Participation in the certification course does not require any previous fitness qualification or degree, but requires a minimum age of 18 years. The certification consists of two theory courses, a practical instruction experience, and two exams. In addition to the main certification, group exercise leaders can obtain a specialization in choreography, portable equipment, step, cycle, or mind and body fitness. The content for the FLCA certification program is reviewed in approximately 3-year intervals.

As noted earlier, textbooks that 'police' the information flow to the instructors support the theory and practice of the FLCA group fitness certification program. In the previous section, we noted that the *Exercise Theory* manual is informed by both the federal CALG that enacts behavioral change towards active living and ultimately towards wellness; and the ACSM guidelines that detail exercise prescription towards improved physical fitness. Both sources endorse physical activity as a means for illness prevention. However, it must be noted again that the CALG were developed by CSEP whose exercise physiologists are expected to draw strongly from the expertise of the ACSM, their main scholarly organization in North America. Consequently, the medical and exercise knowledge of the ACSM, an authorative organization in the North American health and exercise field, has a profound impact on the fitness instructor training through both the CALG and the exercise prescription. In this sense, the ACSM, a scholarly organization, exercises significant force over both the governmental health policy and the fitness industry practice through its powerful 'position stands' on exercise related health behaviors. Its impact, thus, should percolate down to FCLA group fitness instructors' knowledges and practices through the FU edited certification manuals.

Method

To explore the instructors' ideas about healthy fitness, we conducted face-to-face semi-structured interviews (Markula and Silk 2011). The interview guide, using open-ended questions (Patton 2006), was developed based on previous literature on predominant knowledges in the fitness industry and thus, included two major sections exploring the instructors' understanding of 'healthy exercise' and the 'aesthetics of health.' We also included specific questions of the CALG and the ACSM guidelines to find out how health policy might guide the instructors' actual fitness practices. Before conducting the interviews, we obtained ethical approval from the university ethics board. The interviews were conducted in February 2013, lasted approximately one hour and were audio-recorded for transcribing. We followed Kvale and Brinkmann (2007) suggested steps for poststructuralist interview analysis: We first identified common themes aided by the interview guide. The analysis of these themes resulted in several sub-themes and we then identified intersections, discrepancies between the emerging sub-themes.[5] Finally, we connected the themes with Foucault's theory of power/knowledge nexus within neo-liberal governmentality.

Participants

The participants were chosen through purposeful sampling (Patton 2006). We further specified the sample through convenience sampling. Our university runs an extensive campus recreation program open to students, staff, and community members. As group fitness is a large part of this program, it contracts more than 50 instructors annually to provide these classes. We obtained access to these instructors through the Campus and Community Recreation. We further narrowed down our sample through criterion sampling (Patton 2006). While all the instructors employed by the university recreation services are required to have a certification, we specifically looked for participants who had completed their group fitness certification through the Fitness Unit.[6] In addition, we looked for instructors who had a minimum of two years of experience teaching fitness classes, because we believed that they were in a better position to reflect upon the knowledges guiding their teaching practice than beginner instructors.

The participants were assigned a pseudonym to ensure anonymity, but we provide further details of their background in Table 1. While the participants had a range of educational backgrounds, three had fitness instruction as their main occupation while two held other occupations in addition to leading exercise classes. Four participants had university degrees. Typical of the contemporary fitness industry, all instructors taught several different types of group fitness classes and one was also a certified personal trainer. This meant that they were, again typical to the current fitness industry, employed by several local fitness facilities in addition to the university recreation services. With their strong educational backgrounds and extensive experience (only one instructor had taught less than 10 years), we found that these instructors readily and insightfully reflected upon both their training and their current practices within the fitness industry.

Findings

Although the interview analysis revealed a plethora of themes, for the purpose of this paper we have organized our discussion to align with the two main fitness knowledges – healthy exercise and the aesthetics of health – to provide a coherent account of our findings. Under the discussion of the first theme, healthy exercise, the instructors define their understandings of health to then detail how it translates into their actual class design. In addition, we point to some of the ways that the instructors attempt to redefine healthy fitness.

Table 1. Group exercise leader demographics.

Fitness Instructor	Ethnicity	Education	Profession	Fitness Certifications	Years Teaching	Classes Taught	Hours per week
Jenny	white	Personal Fitness Trainer Diploma	Fitness Instructor, Personal Trainer	FLCA Group, Can-Fit-Pro Certified Personal Trainer	21	MSE, Strength, Cardio, HITT	3–6
Olivia	white	Bachelor of Science	University Administrator	FLCA Group	4	Step, MSE	3
Anna	white	Bachelor of Physical Education Certified Exercise Physiologist	Personal Trainer, Health Care Exercise Coordinator, Construction Foreman	FLCA Group, and Older Adult	21	Older Adult, MSE, Chronic condition	14
Kim	white	Bachelor of Physical Education Master of Arts	Certified Exercise Physiologist	FLCA Instructor Trainer: Group Exercise, Older Adult, Resistance Trainer and Aqua-Fit Can-Fit-Pro Pre/Post Natal, Certified Exercise Physiologist	14	Parent & Tot, Boot-Camp, Stroller-Fit, Cycle, Older Adult, MSE, Aqua-fit	3–4
Laura	white	Food Science Degree	Research Lab Technician	FLCA Group, and Resistance	17	MSE, Boot-camp	3–5

'It's 100% health'

All the instructors described health as an 'incredibly important' (Anna) aspect of an exercise class. Kim exclaimed: 'Oh it's paramount' and Anna expanded: '[health] is two-thirds of what I do. The other third is fun' (Anna). Although not 'fun,' the instructors viewed health 'holistically' as 'overall perception of fitness' (Laura), as 'life balance,' or as composed of several aspects such as the mental, emotional, spiritual wellness (Jenny, Kim, Olivia). Kim specified:

> I don't necessarily think it (health) is an absence of disease, that's part of it. I think to be a healthy person there is almost an alignment of physical health, mental health, social health, spiritual health, the different aspects we could say wellness. I can use wellness and health interchangeably, but I think it's more than just the physical side of things.

While these definitions went beyond illness prevention endorsed by the ACSM, the instructors' views reflected the *Exercise Theory* manual guiding their FCLA certification. Their approach to health resonated with the governmental policy for healthy physical activity. When asked about the CALG, all the instructors endorsed its importance to their participants. For example, Olivia suggested the CALG as a resource for her participants when they asked her for exercise advice. Anna felt that following the CALG would help the participants 'maintain [their] health over a long period of time.' While Jenny claimed that she did not use the guidelines, she suggested that her participants do '60 minutes every day, just move everyday,' a variation of the CALG. Kim used the CALG guidelines for exercise advice only if asked after class. Laura had introduced the guidelines to her classes in a general way to encourage her participants to include physical activity in their day: 'It's not just about getting one class in a day, it's overall getting moving... taking the stairs instead of an elevator, parking at the farthest spot at the grocery store.' Based on these views, the instructors had internalized the governmentally endorsed health promotion policy, CALG, as an integral aspect of healthy living.

This endorsement involved the fitness instructors in the public health discourse of changing individual's behavior from unhealthy sedentary lifestyle (or a lifestyle of insufficient physical activity) to one with healthy physical activity levels as determined by governmental policy. This behavioral change model, adopted from the CSEP training manual, was also included in their *Exercise Theory* manual as well as strongly endorsed by the ACSM (Garber *et al.* 2011). The fitness instructors further believed that healthy dietary and exercise practices needed to be adopted in childhood. As a dietician, Laura was very concerned with bad eating habits in childhood:

> I see these kids coming to school with chocolate bars and pop; they don't have any perception of health...we need try and put forth a positive image for all these other people around us.

Laura's concerns also echoed the public health policy assumptions that lack of knowledge is the reason for poor health and consequently, and increased education serves as the primary tool for avoiding chronic illness and obesity (e.g. McPhail 2013). In this public health context, the individual fitness instructor needs to take responsibility for modelling healthy, active lifestyle and then educate others to inspire to similar behavior (Bercovitz 1998). This type of exercise 'leadership' is also emphasized in the *Exercise Theory* manual where the instructors are advised to 'teach internally focused behaviour that emphasizes health benefits associated with Active Living' (Hansen 2010, p. 1–9). Rail (2012, p. 232), among several other Foucauldian health scholars (e.g. Crawford 1980, Fullagar 2002, Burrows 2009, Lupton 2013, and McPhail 2013) and notes that the 'lifestyle' model focused on internalized behavioral change is deeply 'entrenched with notions of individual choice: one chooses whether to pursue this lifestyle or that other one and hence one chooses whether to be fat [fit] or not.' From a Foucauldian perspective, thus, the instructors' comments reflected the neo-liberal Canadian public health promotion (Ayo 2012) as individual's care for healthy eating, regular exercise, and positive role modeling. In addition, they openly promoted the governmental policy of healthy lifestyle despite having no recollection of it being included in their certification course. For example, Anna stated that "[the course training] did nothing for my lesson planning" but that she "felt it was important to promote health through understanding what you're doing and why you're doing it." While defining health as a central aspect of their participants' lives, the instructors did not apply public health concepts to design their classes.

Fit and healthy: practicing health-related physical fitness

Although the instructors recalled receiving minimal education on health in their certification training, they did remember a strong focus on physiology. Exercise physiology emerged as the dominant scientific foundation for quality group fitness instruction and the instructors found it an important base for their teaching knowledge. For example, for Kim, 'the first step' of good instruction was knowledge on exercise physiology and she would 'think about the science of exercise physiology' (not health) when she taught her clients. Anna also felt that 'the physiology part was really good. It was basic enough that most people in the class that I saw picked it up ... without a degree.' Nevertheless, while the instructors strongly endorsed the benefits of physiology, it did not intersect with their broad understanding of wellness. As Jenny recalled: 'Training of health...has always been just health physiologically.'

Informed by exercise physiology, the instructors focused on physical fitness in their practice. Without explicitly referencing them, all of the instructors used the ACSM guidelines for exercise prescription and the FITT formula to design the content of their classes. As instructed in their course book (Kennedy-Armbruster and Yolk 2009), their classes were organized to include a warm-up, cardiovascular segment, muscular strength and endurance segment, and a cool down. Each segment contained specific exercises designed to improve the components of health related physical fitness (aerobic endurance, muscular strength, muscular endurance, and flexibility). The FITT formula then determined the frequency, intensity, time, and type of exercise. Kim followed this structure faithfully in her classes:

> So [I] always start with warm-up, at least 5 minutes and then a combination of resistance training and cardiovascular exercises. [I'll add] aerobic work...playing with my principles of cardiovascular exercise and resistance training...that lasts 30–45 minutes. Then a cool down...I always do flexibility at the end.

According to Foucault (1991, p. 161), this type of precise use of time aims at the correct use of the body that then becomes disciplined, practiced, and useful (healthy), yet docile body. This is "a body of exercise" achieved through meticulous and detailed adherence to programs "imposed from the outside" by such organizations as the ACSM. Disciplinary exercise is repetitive and gradually progressive to assume "a growth:" continuous improvement from useful training (Foucault 1991, p. 161). The FITT formula provides the practical tools for this "organic control:" it guides the appropriate 'overloading' of frequency, intensity, and duration designed for progressively and continuously improved physical fitness (Kennedy-Armbruster and Yolk 2009). Both the ACSM guidelines and the FITT formula operate within the political anatomy of detailed bodily discipline (Foucault 1991) that locked the exercisers' bodies within dominant conceptualization of health as illness prevention (see also Markula and Pringle 2006).

As we explained earlier, the exercise prescription is designed to improve the components of health related physical fitness. The ACSM guidelines (Garber *et al.* 2011) clearly stipulate that physical fitness is predicted to decrease the risk of illnesses such as chronic heart disease, diabetes, and some forms of cancer. The ACSM, thus, promotes exercise, not physical activity advocated in governmental CALG. Although both the FLCA *Exercise Theory* manual and FLCA *Methods of Group Exercise Instruction* openly revolve around the ACSM exercise prescription, the instructors did not make a connection between exercise, physical fitness, and (health as) illness prevention. As a matter of fact, they did not articulate their lesson planning with ACSM guidelines at all or mention the ACSM as an organization involved in developing the fitness industry standards.

Regardless, the instructors promoted health related physical fitness and consequently, even if unwittingly, the narrow idea of health as an absence of illness by following the discipline set by the ACSM exercise prescription. As highly qualified and experienced fitness professionals, they turned into productive and useful neo-liberal experts whose practices intertwined the dominant knowledges of medicine (health as absence of illness) and exercise physiology (health related fitness) into unproblematized acceptance of benefits of physical fitness. Foucault (1977b, p. 186) would contend, then, that in fitness instruction, 'power relations can materially penetrate the body in depth...without...having first to be interiorised in people's consciousness.' The powerful knowledge of physical fitness as healthy (due to its predicted ability to decrease risk of illness) by the ACSM penetrated the practice of group fitness without the instructors' conscious awareness and even against their explicit desire to promote a more holistic notion of wellness.

Beyond exercise prescription?

Although the instructors carefully followed the ACSM exercise prescription, they, like the participants in D'Abundo's study (2009), 'consistently provided options and modifications' to recognize 'the different levels and types of learners' in their classes (p. 314) to create a supportive environment. Kim and Olivia, for example, aimed to include modifications 'that would be easy enough for the newcomers, but challenging and interesting enough for the veterans' (Olivia). Providing modification does not, in itself, offer an escape from a disciplinary exercise regime. Foucault (1991) explained that modification of prescribed exercise movements could act 'as a minimal threshold, as an average to be respected or an optimum towards which one must move' (p. 183). In other words, modifications, while customized to each individual, still work towards the ACSM's optimum of gradual improvement of physical fitness through appropriate duration, intensity, and frequency. The ACSM guidelines (Garber *et al.* 2011) emphasize '*individualized*' (p. 1335, emphasis original) exercise prescription adjusted to varied individual responses to exercise to provide a minimum threshold to physical fitness. Providing modification within the ramifications of these guidelines, however, continues to discipline the individual bodies to unquestioningly follow the health agenda of illness prevention, but through a more 'modest' but equally 'calculated' economy of power (Foucault 1991, p. 170).

However, when talking about exercise modifications, Laura and Anna also introduced the idea of 'functionality' that moved beyond the discussion of health related fitness to use 'applied principles of functionality by explaining how exercise benefits quality of life and talking about the similarities between exercise and daily tasks' (Laura). In a similar vein, Anna added exercises designed to support seniors' every day needs, such as tasks that challenge finger dexterity, memory games, and equipment to offer variety of movements. She further emphasized posture as the most valuable aspect of fitness for her young university students. This focus on enhanced capacity to perform daily tasks can emerge as an alternative to the medical and physiological models of healthy exercise. While still somewhat marginalized and practically unmentioned in the FLCA *Theory Manual*, such understanding can potentially expand the ways of knowing about group fitness. Despite its promise, only two instructors emphasized every day functionality in some of their classes. Laura added that functionality improved 'quality of life,' a concept that was also included in the instructor manuals. Kennedy-Armbruster and Yolk (2009) offered a psychologized definition of 'enhancing quality of life' by helping "people live happier and healthier lives through exercise" (p. 6). The *Exercise Theory* manual further stated that '[P]hysical activity influences quality of life because it increases energy and promotes physical, mental, and psychological well-being in addition to benefiting physical health' (Howley and Frank, 2007 quoted in Hansen 2010, p. 5–2). Combined with medical and physiological knowledges, psychology enters the world of fitness through the notion of 'quality of life' that can now be turned to service the rhetoric of health as individual's choice and responsibility (e.g. Bercovitz 1998).

In addition to providing modifications for participants with differing fitness levels, the instructors increasingly catered to 'special groups' with medical conditions. For example, Laura described:

> I try to give options for range of motion and positioning [to clients with medical conditions]. As long as they have the options, and know that they can use lighter weights, or no weights, and that they can do something other than a push-up, it works well. For people with chronic illnesses, every day is different for how they react: some days they have a lot of strength and other days they just don't. I think people need to hear that that they have options.

This knowledge did not draw from the governmental health promotion model of the CALG or the ACSM guidelines that, while providing three separate guidelines based on age (early years 0–5 years, children and youth, and older adults over 18 years, seniors),[7] are 'normalized' for large populations. Therefore, despite their readiness to accommodate injured and chronically ill participants, all five instructors noted that the FLCA training had not prepared them to deal with these types of clients. Three of the instructors asserted that their knowledge came from personal experience after seeking the information on their own. Laura reflected:

> Experience has [taught me]... everything. When you're a fresh FLCA trained instructor, you haven't seen all of these special circumstances. I think there was a twenty-minute lecture about special populations in the course. And until you've been teaching for a while, you're just trying to figure out the cue the bicep[s] curl without thinking of the twenty different options you can give them.

They added that the FLCA certification is limited in scope and thus, felt not qualified to help clients with chronic conditions. For example, Kim was concerned about the scope of practice: 'I think that, in the importance of safety, every instructor should have more training. There also needs to be an understanding of scope of practice, about when to refer people elsewhere and to recognize our limitations.'

The ACSM position statement (Garber *et al.* 2011) clearly specifies that their exercise prescription targets primarily 'apparently healthy adults of all ages' (p. 1335). Foucault (1991, p. 184) argued that while 'power of normalization imposes homogeneity,' it also 'individualizes' by determining exercise levels for different ages and then fitting these categories 'one to another' to determine 'normal' exercise prescription. In the process of normalization, however, 'the ill' become more 'individualized' through increased surveillance, observation, and comparative measures that take the 'norm' as their reference point (p. 184). 'The ill' are also assumed to require increased surveillance in a group fitness class and a different, individualized exercise prescription from the 'normal' exercisers. Therefore, a separate set of health care experts such as physiotherapists, nurses, or dieticians are educated through governmentally endorsed university graduate programs (and require governmental licencing) to take care of the 'ill.' The fitness instructor certification trains lower level experts and consequently, an average fitness instructor liability insurance[8] does not cover teaching 'special populations.' Nevertheless, clients with medical conditions are increasingly encouraged to take care of their health by joining the commercialized fitness industry instead of having access to the governmentally provided health care. In a neo-liberal context of the Canadian fitness industry, this leaves the instructors to expand their knowledge on their own or to exclude participants with 'special needs' who are defined to be 'out of scope' for fitness instruction due to insufficient instructor insurance coverage.

In summary, the instructors were committed to promote health holistically by embracing wellness. In practice, however, they followed the principles of health related fitness and thus, even if not aware of it, endorsed physical fitness linked to illness prevention. Their understanding of physical fitness was based on the dominant scientific knowledges of physiology, nutrition, and psychology readily laid out in their *Exercise Theory* manual. The instructors actively embraced the CALG that targets the Canadian populations rather than the US based ACSM guidelines that, nevertheless, dictated their class design. Both guidelines anchored the instructors as parts of biopolitics of health control: when not problematizing the premise of their practice, they accepted physical fitness as individualized, as each exerciser's personal responsibility for her health. They were much more aware of the problems related to the aesthetics of the healthy, fit, feminine body.

The aesthetics of health

Unlike their knowledge on physical fitness that was clearly based on physiology, the instructors did not ground their discussion of the ideal fit body on any specific 'scientific' knowledge. In addition, none of the instructors recalled any discussion of ideal body from their certification courses and indeed, such discussion were absent in the FCLA *Exercise Theory* manual. However, as Foucault (1977c, p. 167) argued, 'the centre of initiative, organization and control for this [health] politics should not be located only in the apparatuses of the state,' but should also include the 'noso-politics' of informal, social, and mediated discourses of health. In this section, we discuss how the body aesthetics intertwines with the instructors' somewhat contradictory definitions of the fit body as unhealthy, but also as a sign of healthiness.

The ideal feminine body as a health problem

The instructors identified (excess) weight as the exercisers' main body problem and motivation to join their classes. In these discussions, weight was signified as both a physical (health) and social (appearance) problem without a deeper reasoning of how these might be connected to support the continued obsession with (too much) weight. Four of the instructors indicated that their female clients come to fitness classes to lose weight. Anna even declared: 'All the time, 100% of the time. That's the first question [Do you need to lose weight?] I ask people.' Olivia exclaimed that 'certainly weight still tends to be the main motivator for a lot of people' with many exercisers trying to lose weight in specific body parts. Anna added that the physically fit body improves self-confidence: 'physical fitness, it's a good sense of a positive body image.' Interestingly, several instructors connected 'positive body image' with physical fitness and then with health. These views, again, aligned with the FLCA *Theory Manual* that emphasized body image as an individual, psychological issue. None of instructors questioned the importance of weight loss and Laura, a dietician, saw weight control as a natural part of healthy lifestyle akin to the governmental health promotion strategy and the FLCA *Exercise Theory* manual.

The instructors' discussion of weight loss as an integral part of healthy lifestyle intersects with Foucauldian analyses of obesity discourses. While not directly affected by governmental population control of obesity (Markula 2008), the explicit attachment of physical fitness and healthy weight operates as a similar form of bio-power (Foucault 2008). Parallel to socio-cultural researchers of fitness, several obesity scholars (e.g. Harwood 2009, Wright and Harwood 2009, Rail 2012, McPhail 2013, Ferry and Richards 2015) demonstrate how such practices as dieting and exercise reinforce the bio-politics through which anatomo-political power of the body and the bio-power of population control unite to discipline the individual citizens. The discourse of healthy lifestyle further reproduces 'the notion that weight loss is the right prescription and that it will improve health' (Rail 2012, p. 236) and the requirement of '*action*:' a necessary participation in strict exercise and diet regimes (Murray 2008, p. 9 emphasis original). The motivation to exercise primarily for weight loss illustrates how medicine (health), exercise science (exercise prescription), and psychology (the thin body as source of self-esteem) continue to dominate the fitness industry as well the exercisers' body narratives.

Although all exercisers had a host of body problems, Olivia spoke specifically about how some overweight participants may be intimidated in class with average sized participants: 'People likely are coming into that classroom who might feel intimidated, who might be overweight and are new to exercise. Those are the ones that you don't [want to] lose because of that pressure.' Similar to Mansfield (2011), she suspected that overweight participants could be stigmatized in a group fitness class. While not openly stating why overweight people, specifically, should maintain an exercise program, they, according to Olivia, face bigger health problems than other participants. Although obesity is defined as a major public health problem that contributes to the development of many chronic illnesses in Canada (Public Health Agency of Canada 2016b), Olivia was the only instructor who specifically referred to overweight exercisers. Therefore, while the 'obesity epidemic' is constructed as a global epidemic that represents a major health risk in public health discourse (e.g. Gard and Wright 2005, Wright and Harwood 2009, Gard 2011, Rail 2012), fitness instructors' every-day-world appeared to be populated by participants who, while wanting to lose weight, were not visibly obese.

It was, nevertheless, evident that the majority of group fitness participants believed that they carried excess weight. Similar to obesity narratives, the fit body is conflated between 'health' and 'thin' bodies (Gard and Wright 2005) and individuals are expected to actively manage their lifestyles to produce such 'a look' (Wright and Harwood 2009, Rail 2012). 'As a result,' Rail (2012, p. 242) concluded, 'the self is engaged in a life-long process of assessing and improving its weight and wellbeing through monitoring and management in accordance with free market lifestyle options.'

Similar to their *Exercise Theory* manual, some instructors preferred to remain silent on issues related to women's weight problems. Kim related:

> I don't like to talk to people about their body weight, [nor when they] talk to me about my [weight]. I just stay away from it...I tend to not talk about exercise in relation to weight loss, because we know the research isn't necessarily supporting that. But it's so ingrained in the population that that's what it is, and people talk about it. I also want to give them the best evidence-based answer on things.

Kim felt more comfortable discussing 'evidence-based' research of weight loss than problematizing it as a social issue that 'people talk about.' According to Rail (2012, p. 238), scientific knowledge (of health risks of being overweight) now helps further justify the 'maintenance of oppressive feminine norms' that have been long been used by weight-loss, cosmetics, and fitness industries. This strategy, nevertheless, masks the socio-cultural support for celebrating the aesthetics of the healthy looking body (Markula and Kennedy 2011) by emphasizing the scientifically proven health benefits of weight loss and thinness.

Although unacknowledged, instructors' personal issues with weight were apparent in the interviews. Anna's comment exemplified internalized guilt associated with eating:

> I'll complain that last night I had that piece of German chocolate cake. I'm all bummed about that because I really didn't need it, but I wanted it and I gave in... Did I feel guilty? No, but during the week I let people know that's really going to hurt you if you keep doing that every single day.

Anna, thus, used her own behavior as an example of unhealthy eating to then project guilt on her participants. Analyzed from a Foucauldian perspective, Anna engaged in 'modern confessional' (Foucault 1978) where she revealed her 'sinful,' unhealthy eating practices to receive salvation. While not admitting feeling guilty, she turned into 'a convert' who actively preached against such indulgence. As an instructor, she also occupied a position of expert who could then educate her clients about the 'truth' of serious risks of eating a piece of cake. Paraphrasing Rail (2012), Anna had embodied the health discourse of risks of overweightness that then materialized through her confession and her communication to her participants.

Despite endorsing the bio-politics of the healthy body, some of the instructors echoed the feminist critique of the ideal fit feminine body (e.g. Markula 1995, 2001, Bordo 2003, Berman *et al.* 2005, Markula and Pringle 2006, Dworkin and Wachs 2009, Mansfield 2011, Petersson McIntyre 2011). They agreed that there is pressure from the media for women to conform to the ideal body weight that can lead to eating disorders. Jenny explained:

> I think we have more bulimia, food issues and body issues than we've ever had. Women in their 30s, 40s and 50s feel like they have to be super women with perfect bikini bodies.

While acknowledging the health problems associated with the strive for the ideal fit body, Laura, like the FLCA *Theory Manual*, assigned them as an individual responsibility: 'Oh I think there's lots of pressure. I think [the participants] have more education and can dismiss some of those images that you see on TV and in magazines. But I think people need to learn acceptance.' Laura's perception aligns with Markula's (2001) findings of fitness magazine's advice on body image distortion (BID). Similar to Laura, they admitted their images creating pressure that can cause BID and lead to eating disorders. In this case, however, individual women have misperceived the images and lost their sense of reality. As a solution, the magazines suggested that the readers control their minds better to ignore such images through, as Laura suggested, increased education of how to accept their bodies. As an exercise in self-acceptance, the instructors reminded the participants of their biologically based, genetically 'inherited' body types. Laura explained:

> Every one's body type is different. 'It's my muffin top, it's my flabby thighs, it's my cellulite, it's my grandma arms, it's my double chin', I mean it's because we all are built differently. So everybody has an issue with something.

Anna described such body types as unchanging and urged her participants to accept their less than perfect body shapes:

> I found this triangle thing that's got pumpkin people and pear people. I'll [ask the participants]: 'What type are you?' and they [say] 'Maybe that's me?' Well guess what? You're not going to change that. That's OK. We're all there.

Although Laura and Anna promoted some differences in body types, they also assumed that women are born with a certain body shape that is unalterable. 'A pumpkin' or 'a pear' shape is, of course, not a fit body that nevertheless, remains achievable by specific exercises. In this discussion women's body related problems turned into individual problems that are dealt with first, a personal acceptance of biological facts and second, with increased exercise participation. From a Foucauldian perspective, Markula (2001) demonstrated how health, when conceptualized as a biological and physical manifestations of the individual body, turns into a problem where the solution lies on the individual's choice. When exercising women are persuaded to look for individual solutions to such illnesses as BID or eating disorders, these problems are divorced from their social, political, or environmental circumstances. When simply adjusting 'their behavior into the parameters of healthy femininity' (Markula 2001, p. 175), women leave the societal construction of the fit femininity unchallenged. The instructors certainly felt pressure from the clients to maintain a fit looking body.

The fit body as the healthy body

The instructors strived to be healthy role models for their clients. Having their bodies on display in the fitness class, they felt pressure by both participants and other instructors to *look* fit: Muscles needed to be toned without any wiggling or loose tissue indicating extra weight needed to be lost. Jenny explained:

> A fitness instructor should look healthy. I have an issue when I see sloppy overweight instructors, when you know they're not in shape. There's a difference to being somebody who's muscular and bigger to being out of shape and soft.

As D'Abundo also observed (2009), health and appearance intersected in the instructors' comments. On the other hand, some instructors believed that instructors with lean, muscular bodies intimidate participants. As Anna lamented: 'I don't like it when the instructors come in, head to toe skin tight clothing and super fit because that intimidates people who aren't there [yet].' Kim had a similar view: 'In some respects I very much want to be like my participants. If someone [doesn't] have the so-called ideal body they might be more relatable to the participants than the person that has this ideal body.' D'Abundo (2009) agreed that an instructor with a more average body type provided a more realistic and attainable model for her clientele, but the instructors indicated that an overweight or 'flabby' instructor will be judged more harshly than a lean and toned instructor. Olivia's comments illustrated the strength of some of these judgements:

> If I [saw] an instructor [who] was overweight, it would make me wonder how effective that instructor was. I assume if you're a fitness instructor you're going to be in shape. I would say fit, toned, [with] little body fat.

Other instructors claimed that there is, indeed, much more diversity of instructor body types now. Jenny explained: 'I think there are many more diverse types of [instructor] bodies now than there's ever been. Whether or not they are being judged I don't know, but there's definitely more diversity, good and bad.' The appearance of body became intertwined with health when the instructors discussed the ultimate goal for fitness. Olivia explained:

> I think there has been a movement towards health. But I think that there's still that persistent [drive] to achieve that ideal body. It's probably more still achieving that ideal body, but health can come in different shapes and sizes.

Other instructors also noted that the perfect body does not equal perfect health. Anna explained: 'I don't agree with [the body beautiful]. You'll never see me wear [tight fitting clothes]. There's no such thing as a totally healthy person. You might look fit and athletic, but you're not healthy.' Interestingly, the instructors indicated that the 'body beautiful' is not openly acknowledged within the fitness community despite the pervasive affects felt by instructors and participants alike. Kim elaborated:

> It's like the elephant in the room: We all know about it, but no one really talks about it. At all the fitness conferences, they've got the racks of tight clothing. It's that little tank top you might feel that you have to wear and that is what you need to be and who your participants want you to be...I don't think it [is about] being skinny, it's more about looking toned and tight and tanned. It's almost secretly required.

As the object of harsh judgment and scrutiny, an exemplary teacher with an unacceptably soft body will fail in comparison to an instructor possessing the fit looking body.

Rail (2012) located the quest for healthy, thin body within the nexus of biomedical, bioeconomical, and biocultural discourses that, in the neo-liberal society, define the contours of the ideal body size. Biomedicalization refers to the justification of an acceptable body size through medical knowledge. For example, the thin feminine ideal is now joined with the fit, healthy body that is diagnosed, visually, to prevent chronic illness and obesity. This interconnection tightens bodily control and surveillance. Combined with bioeconomic discourse of neo-liberal economics, 'the individual becomes a producer-consumer in the sense that she is imagined to produce the satisfactory thinness and health that she will enjoy and "consume"' (p. 239–240). Biocultural discourse connects the other two discourses to cultural justifications, such as the feminine body aesthetics, to further validate the need for continual bodywork. Jointly, these discourses 'shift popular perceptions toward the acceptable (thin) body and the ways in which we should understand our bodies and our selves' (p. 240). These bioprocesses distance the fit feminine body from its social critique to call for individualized solutions such as adopting a healthy lifestyle to solve women's body problems. In these conditions, Rail (2012, p. 241) observed, women are captured within 'an apparatus' where they re-produce their own capture as 'female biocitizens' who remain silent about the 'elephant in the room' that denotes women's weight problems.

Conclusion

In this study, the instructors described their passion for promoting health holistically and were keen proponents of healthy, lifelong physical activity promoted through their instructor training course and the governmental health promotion of the CALG. Although they spoke about mental and emotional health, their practices drew exclusively from principles of health related physical fitness. The US based ACSM emerged as the major force behind health related fitness promotion. Its influence, while strongly felt through the instructional practices, went unacknowledged by the instructors. Analyzed from a Foucauldian perspective, in the Panopticon of the fitness industry, the ACSM acted as the invisible gaze that controlled the commercial setting of the group fitness instructor certification, but also powerfully, yet less directly, shaped the governmental active living policy in Canada. The instructors accepted both strategies by following the exercise prescription in their class design, but also encouraging healthy, active lifestyle outside of class participation.

In addition, the instructors' discussion reflected the overall intertwining of body shape and health into the healthy-looking, fit body prevalent in the fitness industry. The governmental policy and the ACSM guidelines remain silent about the aesthetics of the healthy looking body, but this silence has also led to a repression of the problems related to this discourse that, according to the instructors, still strongly motivates their participants. Such suppression, however, has supported the continuing endorsement of the ideal (feminine) body as the healthy body in the popular media including the social media. As Foucault (1978) demonstrated, the repression of a discourse can actually lead to proliferation of actions and theories related to it. By ignoring the discourse around the aesthetics of the fit looking body, the scientific community of ACSM and the governmental health promotion policy of CALG have actually enabled the problematic body practices that effective draw from the intended message of illness prevention (in itself a problematic understanding of health). As Foucault (1977b, p. 186) observed: 'There is a network or circuit of bio-power…which acts as the formative matrix of sexuality [the fit body] itself as the historical and cultural phenomenon within which we seem at once to recognize and lose ourselves.'

Read through a Foucauldian lens, the persistence of the dominant fitness knowledges, particularly the intertwining of health and the feminine body aesthetics, reflects the combined impact of anatomo-political and bio-political power relations (Foucault 1978). When the instructors (and their participants) continued to build 'the body beautiful,' they felt the force of anatomo-political power directly on their bodies. The instructors, unquestioningly, structured their classes based on the exercise prescription to follow the governmentally endorsed guidelines and thus, became parts of the bio-political power arrangement of neo-liberal governmentality. As Foucault (1978) theorized, the anatomo-politics and bio-politics effectively work together to reinforce the governmental health promotion to endorse personal responsibility for health that, within the fitness industry context, manifested in an additional requirement to look fit. This connection was strengthened by locating healthy physical activity within the individual physiological body through the exercise prescription and within the individual mind through psychology of increased self-esteem, improved body image, and mental health.

Although the instructors subscribed to the two dominant fitness knowledges quite closely, they were not entirely unthinking, docile bodies. They worked diligently to provide the types of classes that they believed benefitted their participants. Some of the instructors had started to ground their practice on every day functional benefits of exercise, a different knowledge base that potentially can challenge the dominance of physiology and psychology of healthy fitness. Despite these emerging trends, the fitness instructors generally operated in the confines of anatomo-politics of the disciplined bodies and bio-politics of governmental health promotion without effective and acknowledged tools to problematize these forces. Their practices evolved alongside the current governmentality that, by productively infiltrating neo-liberal health policy into instructor training, defined the appropriate practice for healthy physical activity.

Implications

From a Foucauldian perspective, change takes place at the micro level of practice (Foucault 1980b). To instigate it, alternative knowledges need to enter the discursive formation of fitness through instructor training if the instructors, indeed, are to act as ethical, knowledgeable leaders. Thus, revising the governmental or national policies such the ACSM or CALG guidelines, although the ultimate goal, might not be the most realistic starting point to change group fitness instruction. However, it is possible to directly influence the policy dictating group fitness certification at two levels: lobbying for a change in the governing structure of the FU and revising the content of certification manuals.

As the FU is a part of the University governance structure, we, as researchers, have direct access to the executive director and should continue to lobby for change by asking to be included in the publications such as FLCA quarterly periodical by FU and the professional conferences they sponsor. For example, the annual FLCA conference would be an opportunity to share findings from this study as well as to open up discussion regarding the most beneficial knowledges for ethical fitness instruction. The FU has already included us in a workshop for fitness professionals where we presented our findings and offered practical tools for change from the health related physical fitness and the preoccupation of the body shape in the fitness industry.

Currently, the content of the FLCA group exercise certification course is based rather vaguely on 'evidence based information' that 'expert review committees and national alliance members' assess as suitable (personal communication, executive director FU). The two course books act as a type of grounding policy that direct the certification information and the content of these texts can be rethought to clearly conceptualize the connections between health as illness prevention, physical fitness, and the exercise prescription. The instructors also need tools to problematize these terms to then develop more variety of instructional practices. Expanding the review panel to include experts from a broad range of disciplines including social sciences and feminist research can help alleviate the dominance of exercise physiology and psychology that the instructors indicated was already delivered at sufficient level in the instructor course. As our research demonstrates, the social and cultural knowledges have a strong influence on teaching practices and should, thus, reserve a much larger role in instructor training. In addition, a more systematic and regular process of upgrading the certification content in closer collaboration with scholars from the university could be implemented. Such process can lead to further research on the structures behind the practice of fitness instruction and thus, can support possible changes to the actual certification curriculum.

Our study focused on experienced group exercise instructors with a certification that, compared to many of commercial certifications, offers thorough and sustained education. It would be interesting to compare our results to knowledges held by instructors with other types of qualifications. As FLCA also certifies personal trainers, inquiring the knowledge base of these fitness professionals can also expand our findings. We will also continue to problematize our own group fitness instruction to develop practical ways to use marginalized knowledges to create teaching practices that embrace a broader knowledge base. This praxis should also result in further research on how to implement alternatives to current dominant ways of understanding fit bodies. Our findings verify that considerable work is still required if we aim to provide fitness practices for more diverse audiences with multiple goals. This project, however, has strengthened our desire to improve current fitness services and our resolve to work together with other fitness instructors, trainers, certification bodies, and policy makers towards more theory-informed, broadly based fitness practices.

Notes

1. The existing research on personal trainers, in many ways, intersects with research on group fitness instructors (e.g., Frew and McGilligvray 2005, Smith Maguire 2007, George 2008, Donaghue and Allen 2015, Wiest *et al.* 2015). We have chosen not to detail this research here because of the differences in the certification process and the instructional practices between personal trainers and group fitness instructors.
2. Despite these pressures, the instructors are generally satisfied with their bodies, but, nevertheless, prefer to be leaner and more toned (Prichard and Tiggemann 2005, D'Abundo 2009, Mansfield 2011). There are also several psychological studies that identify group exercise instructors as a risk group for eating disorders (e.g. Martin and Hausenblas 1998, Mcnelis-Kline 2000, Smolak *et al.* 2000). In addition, 35% of the instructors in Hoglund and Normen (2002) study reported eating disorder experiences. More recently, Bratland-Sanda and Sundgot-Borgen (2015) estimated that up to 40% of group fitness instructors had symptoms of disordered eating or severe eating disorders.
3. The executive director of the Fitness Unit provided the following information:
Mission: The Fitness Unit inspires our community to be physically active through advocacy, education, working in strategic partnerships and by supporting professionalism in the exercise industry.
Vision: All [individuals] have access to safe, effective active living strategies to live healthy active lifestyles.
4. Despite our inquiry, the executive director did not provide any details regarding the constitution of the FLCA board membership. However, the *Exercise Theory* manual lists five women as the FLCA past and present directors. They include the executive director, a professor of exercise physiology outside of the host university, and three FLCA trainers.

5. The main theme, health, had the following sub-themes: health enhancement and disease prevention through physical fitness; health promotion through instructor practice; health as a personal responsibility; health linked to physical fitness; and health linked to the ideal feminine body. The second main theme, the ideal feminine body, had the following sub-themes: ideal feminine body equated with health; weight loss as a primary goal in class design; obese and over-weight bodies as unacceptable; the pressure for a fitness instructor to conform to ideal feminine body.
6. While the university hosts both the FU (and the FLCA), a certifying body, and the Campus and Community Services they operate as entirely separate units. Recreation services, thus, can hire instructors with any type of certification.
7. CSEP also provides specific guidelines for three 'special populations:' multiple sclerosis, spinal cord injury, and Parkinson's disease (http://www.csep.ca/en/guidelines/physical-activity-guidelines-for-special-populations).
8. In the North American context, contract group fitness instructors are required to finance and obtain personal instructor liability insurance. This is also a requirement for teaching at the university recreation services. This practice further reflects the neo-liberal context where the responsibility for liability of practice is moved from the employer to individually contracted (part-time) employees.

Disclosure statement

No potential conflict of interest was reported by the authors.

Funding

This work was supported by the University of Alberta [EFF-SAS].

References

Ayo, N., 2012. Understanding health promotion in a neoliberal climate and the making of health conscious citizens. *Critical public health*, 22 (1), 99–105. doi:10.1080/09581596.2010.520692

Bercovitz, K.L., 1998. Canada's active living policy: a critical analysis. *Health promotion international*, 13 (4), 319–328. doi:10.1093/heapro/13.4.319

Berman, E., De Souza, M.J., and Kerr, G., 2005. A qualitative examination of weight concerns, eating and exercise behaviours in recreational exercisers. *Women in sport and physical activity journal*, 14, 24–38.

Bordo, S., 2003. *Unbearable weight. Feminism, western culture, and the body*. Berkley: University of California Press.

Bratland-Sanda, S. and Sundgot-Borgen, J., 2015. "I'm concerned—What do I do?" Recognition and management of disordered eating in fitness center settings. *International journal of eating disorders*, 48 (4), 415–423. doi:10.1002/eat.22297

Burrows, L., 2009. Pedagogizing families through obesity discourse. *In*: J. Wright and V. Harwood, ed. *Biopolitics and the 'obesity epidemic': governing bodies*. New York: Routledge, 127–140.

Crawford, R., 1980. Healthism and the medicalization of everyday life. *International journal of health services*, 10 (3), 365–388. doi:10.2190/3H2H-3XJN-3KAY-G9NY

Crawford, R., 2006. Health as a meaningful social practice. *Health*, 10 (4), 401–420.

D'Abundo, M.L., 2009. Issues of health, appearance and physical activity in aerobic classes for women. *Sport, education and society*, 14 (3), 301–319. doi:10.1080/13573320903037655

Dallaire, C., *et al.*, 2012. The gap between knowing and doing: how Canadians understand physical activity as a health risk management strategy. *Sociology of sport journal*, 29, 325–347.

Dishman, R.K., 1988. *Exercise adherence: Its impact on public health*. Champaign, IL: Human Kinetics.

Donaghue, N. and Allen, M., 2015. People don't care as much about their health as they do about their looks: personal trainers as intermediaries between aesthetic and health-based discourses of exercise participation and weight management. *International journal of sport and exercise psychology*. doi:10.1080/1612197X.2015.1016086

Dworkin, S.L. and Wachs, F.L., 2009. *Body panic: gender, health, the selling of fitness*. New York: New York University Press.

Evans, R.R., Cotter, E.M., and Roy, J.L.P., 2005. Preferred body type of fitness instructors among university students in exercise classes. *Perceptual and motor skills*, 101, 257–266.

Ferry, M.D. and Richards, D., 2015. Biopedagogy digitalized: 'Educational' relations among participants on an online weight loss surgery forum. *Critical public health*, 25, 63–77. doi:10.1080/09581596.2014.940849

Foucault, M., 1972. *The archaeology of knowledge and the discourse on language*. London, UK: Tavistock Publications.

Foucault, M., 1977a. Truth and power. *In*: C. Gordon, ed. *Power/knowledge: Selected interviews and other writings 1972–1977*. New York: Vintage Books, 109–133.

Foucault, M., 1977b. The history of sexuality. *In*: C. Gordon, ed. *Power/knowledge: selected interviews and other writings 1972–1977*. New York: Vintage Books, 183–193.

Foucault, M., 1977c. The politics of health in the eighteenth century. *In*: C. Gordon, ed. *Power/knowledge: selected interviews and other writing 1972–1977*. New York: Vintage Books, 166–182.

Foucault, M., 1978. *History of sexuality, volume 1: introduction*. London: Penguin Books.

Foucault, M., 1979. *Discipline and punish*. New York: Random House Vintage Books.

Foucault, M., 1980a. Confessions of the flesh. *In*: C. Gordon, ed. *Power/knowledge: selected interviews and other writings 1972–1977*. Harlow, UK: Harvester, 194–228.

Foucault, M., 1980b. Two lectures. *In*: C. Gordon, ed. *Power/knowledge: selected interviews and other writings 1972–1977*. Harlow, UK: Harvester, 78–108.

Foucault, M., 1991. *Discipline & punish: the birth of the prison*. London: Penguin Books.

Foucault, M., 2007. *Security, territory, population: lectures at the College de France 1977–1978*. New York: Palgrave MacMillan.

Foucault, M., 2008. *The birth of biopolitics: lectures at the Collège de France, 1978–1979*. Basingstoke: Palgrave Macmillan.

Frew, M. and McGilligvray, D., 2005. Health clubs and body politics: aesthetics and the quest for physical capital. *Leisure studies*, 24, 161–175. doi:10.1080/0261436042000300432

Fullagar, S., 2002. Governing the healthy body: discourses of leisure and lifestyle within Australian health policy. *Health*, 6 (1), 69–84.

Garber, C.E., *et al*., 2011. Quantity and quality of exercise for developing and maintaining cardiorespiratory, musculoskeletal, and neuromotor fitness in apparently healthy adults: guidance for prescribing exercise. *Medicine & science in sports & exercise*, 1334–1359. doi:10.1249/MSS.0b013e318213fefb

Gard, M., 2011. Truth, belief and the cultural politics of obesity scholarship and public health policy. *Critical public health*, 21, 37–48. doi:10.1080/09581596.2010.529421

Gard, M. and Wright, J., 2005. *The obesity epidemic: science, morality and ideology*. London: Routledge.

George, M., 2008. Interactions in expert service work: demonstrating professionalism in personal training. *Journal of contemporary ethnography*, 37, 108–131. doi:10.1177/0891241607309498

Hansen, S., ed., 2010. *Exercise theory manual*. 3rd ed. Edmonton, Alberta: Alberta Fitness Leadership Certification Association.

Hardman, A.E. and Stensel, D.J., 2003. *Physical activity and health: the evidence explained*. London: Routledge.

Harwood, V., 2009. Theorizing biopedagogues. *In*: J. Wright and V. Harwood, ed. *Biopolitics and the 'obesity epidemic'*. London: Routledge, 15–30.

Hoglund, K. and Normen, L., 2002. A high exercise load is linked to pathological weight control behaviour and eating disorders in female fitness instructors. *Scandinavian journal of medicine & science in sports*, 12, 261–275. doi:10.1034/j.1600-0838.2002.10323.x

Kennedy-Armbruster, C. and Yolk, M.M., 2009. *Methods of group exercise instruction*. 2nd ed. Champaign, IL: Human Kinetics.

Kvale, S. and Brinkmann, S., 2007. *Interviews: learning the craft of qualitative research interviewing*. London: Sage.

Lupton, D., 1997. Bodies, pleasures and practices of the self. *In*: D. Lupton, ed. *The imperative of health: public health and the regulated body*. Thousand Oaks: SAGE, 131–157.

Lupton, D., 2013. Quantifying the body: monitoring and measuring health in the age of mHealth technologies. *Critical public health*, 23 (4), 393–403. doi:10.1080/09581596.2013.794931

Mansfield, L., 2011. Fit, fat and feminine? The stigmatization of fat women in fitness gyms. *In*: E. Kennedy and P. Markula, ed. *Women and exercise: the body, health and consumerism*. New York: Routledge, 81–100.

Markula, P., 1995. Firm but shapely, fit but sexy, strong but thin: the postmodern aerobicizing female bodies. *Sociology of sport journal*, 12, 424–453.

Markula, P., 2001. Beyond the perfect body: women's body image distortion in fitness magazine discourse. *Journal of sport and social issues*, 2, 158–179. doi:10.1177/0193723501252004

Markula, P., 2004. Tuning into oneself:" Foucault's technologies of the self and mindful fitness. *Sociology of sport journal*, 21 (3), 302–321.

Markula, P., 2008. Governing obese bodies in a control society. *Junctures*, 11, 53–66.

Markula, P. and Kennedy, E., 2011. Introduction: beyond binaries: contemporary approaches to women and exercise. *In*: E. Kennedy and P. Markula, ed. *Women and exercise: the body, health and consumerism*. New York: Routledge, 1–26.

Markula, P. and Pringle, R., 2006. *Foucault, sport and exercise: power, knowledge and transforming the self*. London: Routledge.

Markula, P. and Silk, M., 2011. *Qualitative research for physical culture*. London: Palgrave Macmillan.

Martin, K.A. and Hausenblas, H.A., 1998. Psychological commitment to exercise and eating disorder symptomatology among female aerobics instructors. *Sport psychologist*, 12, 180–190.

McDermott, L., 2011. "Doing something that's good for me": exploring intersections of physical activity and health. *In*: E. Kennedy and P. Markula, ed. *Women and exercise: the body, health and consumerism*. New York: Routledge, 197–226.

Mcnelis-Kline, C.M., 2000. Body image, social physique anxiety and eating disorders in aerobic instructors. *Dissertation abstracts international section B: the sciences and engineering*, 61 (2–B), 1090.

McPhail, D., 2013. Resisting biopedagogies of obesity in a problem population: understandings of healthy eating and healthy weight in a Newfoundland and Labrador community. *Critical public health*, 23, 289–303. doi:10.1080/09581596.2013.797566

Murray, S., 2008. Pathologizing fatness: medical authority and popular culture. *Sociology of sport journal*, 25, 7–21.

Patton, M.Q., 2006. *Qualitative research and evaluation methods*. 3rd ed. Thousand Oaks, CA: Sage.

Petersen, A. and D. Lupton, D., 1996. *The new public health: Health and self in the age of risk*. London: Sage.

Petersson McIntyre, M., 2011. Keep your clothes on! Fit and sexy through striptease aerobics. *In*: E. Kennedy and P. Markula, ed. *Women and exercise: the body, health and consumerism*. New York: Routledge, 247–265.

Prichard, I. and Tiggemann, M., 2005. Objectification in fitness centers: self-objectification, body dissatisfaction, and disordered eating in aerobic instructors and aerobic participants. *Sex roles*, 53 (1–2), 19–28. doi:10.1007/s11199-005-4270-0

Provincial Fitness Unit., 2016. *National fitness leadership alliance*. Available from: http://www.provincialfitnessunit.ca/nfla/.

Public Health Agency of Canada., 2016a. *Physical activity*. Available from: http://www.phac-aspc.gc.ca/hp-ps/hl-mvs/pa-ap/index-eng.php.

Public Health Agency of Canada., 2016b. *Risk factor atlas*. Available from: http://www.phac-aspc.gc.ca/cd-mc/atlas/index-eng.php)

Rail, G., 2012. The birth of the obesity clinic: confessions of the flesh, biopedagogies and physical culture. *Sociology of sport journal*, 29, 227–253.

Smith Maguire, J., 2007. *Fit for consumption: sociology and the business of fitness*. London: Routledge.

Smolak, L., Murnen, S.K., and Ruble, A.E., 2000. Female athletes and eating problems: A meta-analysis. *International journal of eating disorders*, 27, 371–380. doi:10.1002/(ISSN)1098-108X

Wiest, A.L., Andrews, D.L., and Giardina, M.L., 2015. Training the body for healthism: reifying vitality in and through the clinical gaze of the neoliberal fitness club. *Review of education, pedagogy, and cultural studies*, 37 (1), 21–40. doi:10.1080/10714413.2015.988505

Wray, S., 2011. The significance of westerns health promotion discourse for older women from diverse ethnic backgrounds. *In*: E. Kennedy and P. Markula, ed. *Women and exercise: the body, health and consumerism*. New York: Routledge, 161–179.

Wright, J. and Harwood, V., 2009. *Biopolitics and the 'obesity epidemic.'*. London: Routledge.

Health, physical activity and the body: an inquiry into the lives of female migrant cleaners in Denmark

Verena Lenneis and Gertrud Pfister

ABSTRACT
Numerous reports identify minority ethnic women as a population group which is greatly affected by chronic illness. Health authorities tend to attribute their health problems to their lifestyle, for example refraining from participation in recreational physical activity (PA). However, little is known about the perspectives of the targets of health promotion, that is, their perceptions of and lived experiences with health recommendations. In this article we investigate minority ethnic women's attitudes and practices, in particular with regard to PA. We conducted semi-structured interviews with 33 female migrant cleaners from non-western countries which provided insights into their everyday lives. We analysed the material drawing on the literature related to minority ethnic women and recreational PA, with a focus on Foucauldian scholars who have used the concepts of governmentality and disciplinary power. The interviewees considered weight loss the main benefit of recreational PA; this did, however, not lead to participation. Constraints to participation were exhaustion and lack of time caused by the demands of the women's jobs and a 'second shift' at home. These findings confirm that the preoccupation with a healthy lifestyle is a privilege that requires socio-economic resources. Therefore, health policies must adapt to the needs of marginalised groups and take structural factors into consideration, such as the organisation of the labour market and the gendered division of work.

Introduction

> The health messages we constantly get bombarded with seldom reach a home where people are badly integrated and speak another language. That's why we have to initiate [more] health campaigns specifically targeting immigrants. (Allan Krasnik, Professor of Public Health at the University of Copenhagen, quoted in Ringgaard 2012)

Krasnik's statement refers to the well-documented poor health status of ethnic minorities in Denmark (Singhammer 2008, Holmberg *et al.* 2009), which he attributes to an unhealthy lifestyle caused by a lack of knowledge. This explanation also implies that members of ethnic minorities would make the 'right choices' if they knew more about the benefits of a healthy lifestyle. In this article we will, among other things, discuss whether health messages really do not reach the migrant population or whether there are other causes for their non-compliance with health recommendations, including participation in recreational physical activity (PA). Our informants were 33 first-generation migrants from various non-western countries who, as a rule, came to Denmark after they had been married to men of the same ethnic background. All women worked as cleaners – an occupational group reportedly exposed to considerable health risks. Many cleaners suffer from work-related injuries and strains; they are often overweight, have high blood pressure and a low fitness level, all of which increases their risk of cardiovascular diseases (see, for example, Kumar and Kumar 2008, Jørgensen *et al.* 2011). Physiologists claim that the work of cleaners is not intense enough to have any positive effects on the prevention of lifestyle-related diseases and recommend, therefore, that they engage in recreational PA to enhance their fitness levels (Korshøj *et al.* 2013, Korshøj 2015).

However, such recommendations – and, in general, medical and behavioural science approaches to health and PA – rarely take into account the socio-economic and cultural backgrounds of groups and individuals, even though these greatly determine the opportunities they have of engaging in health-enhancing practices (see, for example, Markula *et al.* 2008, Wray 2011). Moreover, while a number of scholars have (critically) analysed current policies on PA (see, for example, among many others, Fullagar 2002, Glasdam 2009, Macdonald 2011, Piggin and Bairner 2016), there has been significantly less research on the embodied effects of these policies and on the perspectives of ('at risk') groups addressed by health-promotion campaigns (see, for example, Rail 2009, Markula and Kennedy 2011). Fullagar (2009, pp. 122–123), too, emphasises that there is 'little research that explores how people, as embodied subjects, negotiate and produce meaning about healthy lifestyle practices in the complex sociocultural, economic and political conditions of advanced liberalism.' This is particularly true of members of ethnic minorities working in menial jobs: partly due to various difficulties such as getting into contact with the migrant population and obtaining insights into their lives (see, for example, Feskens *et al.* 2006, Ahlmark *et al.* 2014), there is very little information available about the ways in which ethnic minorities make sense of the recommendations on PA.

The purpose of this paper is to explore female migrant cleaners' lived experiences with health policies and recommendations as well as with recreational PA. In this article, we will firstly give background information about health policies and the health behaviour of ethnic minorities in Denmark before presenting a review of the literature related to minority ethnic women's participation in recreational PA, with a focus on the work of Foucauldian scholars who have drawn on the concepts of governmentality and disciplinary power to analyse contemporary public health policies and the sporting practices of individuals. After providing information about the research methods of the study, we will present its findings and discuss them against the backdrop of the reviewed literature. We will conclude by emphasising that life circumstances and social structures set the frame for marginalised groups' opportunities of engaging in recreational PA – issues which health policies should pay particular attention to.

Background – health policies and the health behaviour of ethnic minorities in Denmark

Although Denmark is a universal welfare state with free health care for all residents, inequalities in health do exist (see, for example, Danish Health and Medicines Authority 2011). Numerous reports and studies identify members of ethnic minorities,[1] in particular women from non-western countries, as a population group which is greatly affected by chronic illnesses and which is less likely than members of the ethnic majority to engage in health-promoting behaviour such as participation in recreational PA (see, for example, Singhammer 2008, Holmberg *et al.* 2009). A study comparing the PA participation of the Danish mainstream population and Turkish migrants in Copenhagen revealed, for example, that only one third of Danish but two thirds of Turkish women without a formal education were sedentary in their leisure (Copenhagen Municipality 2005).

In Denmark, medical expenditures are covered by public funds; therefore, not only health authorities and politicians but also the media and the general public consider the costs caused by obesity or so-called 'lifestyle diseases' such as type 2 diabetes as a threat to the Danish welfare state (see, for example, Glasdam 2009). As a consequence, numerous policies and health-promotion campaigns have been initiated by the Danish authorities, informing citizens about the negative consequences of an unhealthy lifestyle and encouraging healthy living, particularly among 'at risk groups' such as minority ethnic women (see, for example, Danish Ministry of Health 2014). To support 'healthy living' among ethnic minority groups, the Municipality of Copenhagen has, for example, initiated weekly information meetings on health issues that are run by health coaches with an ethnic minority background (http://www.kk.dk/artikel/sundhed-p%C3%A5-dit-sprog-0). In these meetings, as well as in other health-promotion initiatives and recommendations of the Danish authorities, recreational PA plays an important role as it is regarded as an effective and inexpensive weapon in the fight against the 'wrong lifestyle' (see also, for example, National Institute of Public Health 2009). In addition, research institutes (financed by both public and private funds) put a strong focus on ethnic minorities' health (and health behaviour). One of these institutes is the Danish Research Centre for Migration, Ethnicity and Health (http://mesu.ku.dk) which, among other things, provides guidance and advice for health professionals working with ethnic minorities.

Literature review – a sociocultural perspective on minority ethnic women and their participation in recreational physical activity

The low PA participation rates of minority ethnic women is an international phenomenon (see, for example, WHO 2013) and has received much attention not only from health authorities but also from epidemiologists and public health scientists who have investigated the health hazards of sedentariness and the barriers which impede participation in recreational PA. These studies have found various constraints ranging from cultural and religious beliefs to such factors as a lack of socio-economic resources, lack of time, safety issues, language barriers, lack of social networks and support, low risk perception and a lack of knowledge of the benefits of PA (see, for example, Kreps and Sparks 2008, Caperchione *et al.* 2009, Netto *et al.* 2010). As a promising strategy to overcome these constraints and engage sedentary groups in recreational PA, scholars emphasise in particular the importance of 'culturally sensitive' health communication and PA programmes which are directed to the needs of a specific target group (see, for example, Lawton *et al.* 2006, Kreps and Sparks 2008, Caperchione *et al.* 2009, Netto *et al.* 2010). Muslim women, for example, may prefer to exercise in a single-sex environment. However, Wray (2011, p. 171) and other scholars draw attention to the fact that such approaches to health promotion are problematic as they are based on the assumption that the members of a 'high-risk group', for example, minority ethnic women, (should and) will 'change their "health behaviours" if the health promotion interventions they are targeted with are culturally sensitive.' This assumption ignores 'the wider socio-cultural and economic circumstances that influence the choices available to women, and importantly their right not to conform to health promotion rhetoric' (Wray 2011, p. 171).

Many of the scholars criticising current public health policy have drawn on Foucault's (1991, 2007) concept of governmentality to analyse the specific techniques that authorities employ to govern a population's health and guide their practices of body management. Studies in Denmark (see, for example, Vallgårda 2011) and in other western countries have revealed that health authorities use strategies which put a strong focus on the individual's responsibility for health: individuals are encouraged and expected to self-regulate their health in their own best interest (see, for example, among many others, Lupton 1995, Fusco 2006, Smith Maguire 2008, Fullagar 2009, Harrington and Fullagar 2013). Self-regulation includes avoidance of health risks; therefore, the threat of (potential) risks has been identified as a powerful strategy to foster individual responsibility for health and well-being. Ayo (2012, p. 103), for example, explains that the 'particular strength and effectiveness of deploying risks as a neoliberal tool [...] is the impending harm that it implies, thus stimulating a sense of panic, a sense of urgency, and a sense that action must be taken now.' Sociologists such as Rose (1999) emphasise, moreover, the key role that experts play in spreading information about health risks and the 'correct' lifestyle (see, for example, Crawford

2006, Fullagar and Harrington 2009). Expert advice, for example, about exercise as the 'ideal panacea' promising long life, health and happiness (Smith Maguire 2008, p. 127), derives from a broad range of organisations, institutions and authorities such as scientists and health professionals, as well as the mass media that govern 'at a distance' (Rose and Miller 1992, p. 181). However, as stressed by Foucauldian scholars, placing the responsibility to make the healthy 'choices' on the individual stigmatises those who do not comply and fails to acknowledge social structures, in particular structural disadvantages. Korp (2010, p. 801), for example, argues that the moral obligation to 'act in a healthy manner simply adds to the burden' of socially and economically disadvantaged groups such as ethnic minorities (see also, for example, Wheatley 2005, Brown *et al.* 2013).

The dominant messages of exercise as a means of achieving good health and the ideal body (see, for example, Markula and Kennedy 2011) are likely to affect the attitudes, desires, practices and experiences of minority ethnic women living in a western society. In addition, ethnic and cultural beliefs and values might have an impact on the importance and the meanings minority ethnic women ascribe to health, the possibilities they have and the choices they make. Wray (2007), for example, emphasises that cultural background, socialisation and life circumstances strongly influence perceptions and understandings of health and PA. Moreover, Wray (2007, 2011) argues that 'western-centric' knowledge about exercise and diet would devalue alternative, non-western ways of thinking and living. In her study of the perceptions of health messages among women from diverse ethnic backgrounds in the UK, Wray (2011, p. 164) found that some of her interviewees actively resisted 'dominant ideas about health, fitness and beauty and chose to ignore the hegemonic messages emanating from them.' They chose, for example, to eat traditional food which had cultural or religious meaning, although it may have been regarded as 'unhealthy' according to western standards.

Research conducted by scholars focusing on PA and sport also points to the influence of multiple, often competing discourses in ethnic communities and host societies: Walseth (2006) observed that participation in sport (but not in fitness exercises) challenged young Muslim women's ethnic identities as (competitive) sport was regarded as a men's activity and as inappropriate for young women. Jiwani and Rail's (2010) study of the meanings young Muslim Canadian women attached to PA, too, showed how women navigated between different discourses related to PA, gender and religion. Even though most of Jiwani and Rail's (2010) interviewees linked PA to staying in shape or losing weight – thus clearly articulating a desire to comply with the western ideal of the body (see also George and Rail 2006) – they supported traditional values and gave religion a higher priority than recreational PA. These findings differ from the results of Abou-Rizk and Rail's (2014) study exploring young (Christian) Lebanese-Canadian women's practices of body management. Adopting a Foucauldian perspective, and in particular drawing on Foucault's (1977) concept of disciplinary power (see also Markula and Pringle 2006), Abou-Rizk and Rail found that their interviewees had internalised the dominant discourses of individual responsibility for health and lifestyle. They were very concerned about their physical appearance, beauty and weight, and carefully monitored their body shape and their behaviour; they turned the 'gaze' upon themselves (see also Duncan 1994) and engaged in disciplinary bodily practices such as dieting and exercising to obtain the ideal slim body (in some cases they even practised extreme forms such as diet pills, starvation and compulsive exercise). Thus, these women turned their bodies into 'docile bodies' (Foucault 1977, p. 135) and became 'good citizens' who did not challenge the current ideas of beauty and health (see also, for example, Duncan 1994, Markula 2001, Bordo 2003). Abou-Rizk and Rail (2014, p. 161) suggest that their interviewees' great focus on physical appearance and thinness might be a consequence of Christian Lebanese-Canadian women's desire 'to adopt Western ideals of heteronormative femininity and whiteness so as to distance themselves from Muslim Lebanese and, more generally, from Arab women, whom they perceive as less "modern".' Although improving health and appearance seems to be an important incentive for migrants to exercise, they may also experience the joy of being physically active. The results of an interview study in Denmark showed that female migrants had adopted western body ideals and fitness discourses (Hacısoftaoğlu and Pfister 2012). However, the interviewees in this study also experienced that recreational PAs such as swimming and cycling provided a new sense of freedom and thus added to their quality of life.

Moreover, there are several studies on Muslim girls and adolescents' experiences of sport and PA, in particular of physical education in mixed-gender environments (see, for example, Benn *et al.* 2011, Dagkas *et al.* 2011, Barker-Ruchti *et al.* 2013). It must be emphasised, though, that most studies on the PAs of minority ethnic women have focused on the experiences of *young* women. Hence, it remains widely unexplored how middle-aged minority ethnic women with low levels of education working in marginal jobs position themselves in the discourses of exercise, beauty and health dominant in western societies (see, for example, Markula and Kennedy 2011).

Research questions

Inspired by the approaches and findings of the reviewed literature, the study explores female migrant cleaners' perceptions of health polices and, in particular, their lived experiences with recommendations on PA. We focused on the following questions: Do messages on health and recreational PA reach minority ethnic women with low levels of education living in Denmark? Which importance and meanings do they attach to health and to PA? Why do some of the interviewees engage in recreational PA and others do not?

The interviewees and the methods employed

This article presents some of the results of a PhD project about the everyday lives and recreational PA of female migrant cleaners. This paper focuses on the research questions stated above that we addressed using semi-structured interviews.

Recruitment of the interviewees

The interviewees were employed at four different workplaces (two hospitals and two universities in Copenhagen), but had in common that they had signed up for different worksite fitness programmes which were initiated and conducted by the Danish National Research Centre for the Working Environment and the Copenhagen Centre for Team Sport and Health, respectively. As it had turned out to be a major challenge to come into contact with migrant cleaners, both authors took part in the exercise programmes[2] and managed to form positive relationships with the participants. This made it possible to recruit them for interviews about their bodies, health, work and participation in recreational PA. The interviews took place after the programmes had ended, and we interviewed all cleaners who were willing to participate in the study. All in all we talked with 42 participants. Given the topic of this paper, however, we have only used the interviews with the 33 women who had a migrant background. It must be emphasised that this article is not about the women's experiences with the different exercise programmes but about their general attitudes towards health and recreational PA as well as their reasons for (non-)participation in recreational PA before and after attending the programmes.[3]

The interviewees

Twenty-nine of the interviewees worked as cleaners while four were former cleaners who had been promoted to the rank of supervisor. They worked 37 hours per week, starting work at either 5 or 6am and finishing at 1 or 2pm. The women were between 27 and 62 years of age (the majority were in their forties) and were all migrants from non-western countries. Eighteen women came from Turkey, around half of them with a Turkish, the other half with a Kurdish background. Three women were from Pakistan; two women each were from China, India and Macedonia; one woman each came from Kosovo, Morocco, Palestine, the Philippines, Serbia and Tanzania. Twenty-six interviewees were Muslims. The great majority of the interviewees had migrated to Denmark as young adults after being married, as a rule, to a man of the same country of origin who had either grown up in Denmark or had lived in the country for many years. Exceptions to this were two women who had married a Dane. One woman was a widow and four women were divorced; all the others lived together with their spouses. Except for one woman, all the interviewees had children; 14 of them had children aged ten or younger. The overwhelming majority of the interviewees were unskilled workers who had only attended primary school in their countries of origin (most women from Turkey had only gone to school for 5 years); one woman had never gone to school and was illiterate. As a rule, their husbands also had low levels of education and worked in low-paid jobs.

Methods and analysis

We gathered information about the women's everyday lives and recreational PA using semi-structured interviews (see, for example, Kvale 2007). In addition, we engaged in participant observation (see, for example, Creswell 2013) during the fitness programmes. In this way we got to know the participants and could engage in informal conversations about their lives. We took field notes about these conversations, as well as about our observations and reflections (see, for example, Patton 2002, Creswell 2013). The informal conversations provided important background information about the daily routines of cleaners and inspired the design of the interview guide.

Five women did not feel at ease talking in Danish and were therefore interviewed by a student in Turkish; the other interviews were all conducted by the first author. The interviews lasted 1 hour on average and took place in locations which guaranteed privacy. The main topics of the interviews were their work; their everyday lives and families; their previous experience with sport and recreational PA; their reasons for and against participating in PA; and, finally, their health-related attitudes and practices. These issues evolved from the participant observation, informal conversations and the reviewed literature presented above. Although we used an interview guide, we also encouraged the cleaners to talk about issues which they themselves found important (see, for example, Patton 2002, Kvale 2007). The interviews were recorded, transcribed and then thematically coded with the help of the software programme Atlas.ti (see, for example, Patton 2002, Bryman 2012). The themes for coding arose, on the one hand, deductively from the research questions and the conceptual framework and, on the other, inductively by including new themes in the analysis which emerged during the process of coding (see, for example, Miles *et al.* 2014).

During the whole research process we were concerned with power relations – in particular with the impact of our (in many ways) privileged position (see, for example, Aléx and Hammarström 2008, Markula and Silk 2011, Hesse-Biber 2014). Even though both of us were also migrants (from Austria and Germany), our backgrounds differed greatly from those of the interviewees: we were highly educated, had desk jobs and were now trying to understand and represent the voices of minority ethnic women from non-western countries with low levels of education working in menial jobs. As emphasised by Khawaja and Morck (2009, p. 28), 'studying the other calls for close reflections on one's own position, theoretically, personally, and politically, taking into account one's complicity in either overcoming or reproducing processes of othering and marginalisation.' Accordingly, we used self-reflexivity (see, for example, Lincoln *et al.* 2011, Markula and Silk 2011, Hesse-Biber 2014) as a strategy to consider how our 'situatedness' and biographies influenced knowledge production and power relations – in particular hierarchies created by the interview situation. We therefore paid great attention to showing respect and empathy for the participants and emphasised that not we but they were experts on their own lives. Moreover, the youth, casual dress and friendly behaviour of the first author and interviewer helped to reduce (potential) anxieties and power hierarchies during the interviews (see, for example, Hesse-Biber 2014).

To protect the interviewees' anonymity we removed all identifying information and replaced their names by pseudonyms. As the interviews were conducted in Danish or Turkish, all quotes in this article are translations.

Knowledge, attitudes and practices with regard to health and recreational physical activity – findings and discussion

The first part of this section focuses on the women's knowledge and opinions about recreational PA as part of a healthy lifestyle. We will then explore whether and, if so, how their knowledge and opinions influence their practices and subsequently discuss their reasons for participation – and, in particular, for non-participation – in recreational PA. We will pay specific attention to the question of the extent to which their physically exhausting jobs as cleaners affected their attitudes and practices.

Knowledge and opinions about health and recreational physical activity

All cleaners knew about health recommendations and considered recreational PA to be 'good for the body.' Most of them stated, for example, that recreational PA could increase their fitness, that is, their endurance and strength. A few women also referred to the role of exercise in the prevention of diabetes or high blood pressure; moreover, a number of cleaners mentioned that recreational PA could relieve stress and provide energy. In contrast, only three interviewees considered recreational PA to be a source of pleasure and enjoyment.

Even though all women agreed that cleaning was hard physical work, the majority of them believed that their job did not convey the same benefits as recreational PA. Comparisons between working and exercising were even a topic of discussion among some cleaners. Sevgi, for example, referred to the 'use of the whole body' as the benefit of recreational PA: 'The others [other cleaners], they say we also exercise at work. But I don't think so. You don't run at work. You clean and do a lot of things, but you don't sweat. I think exercise is really important for us. It's good for our bodies.' Rashida, too, ascribed great importance to sweat as proof of the hard work connected with exercise: 'When you work, you aren't out of breath. You don't sweat. But when you exercise, your heart beats and you sweat a lot.' Danica shared the opinion that work did not convey the same benefits as recreational PA and used slimness as an indicator: 'Exercise is something else. If cleaning was like exercise, all my colleagues would be skinny [laughs].'

These and other statements leave no doubt that the cleaners regarded the possibility of losing weight as by far the most important benefit of recreational PA, and this was closely linked to their discontent with their bodies. Like many other interviewees, Pinar talked about her desire to be slim. For her slimness was more than a feature of attractiveness – losing weight also seemed to promise well-being, youth and happiness: 'Every day I look in the mirror, I look at my stomach and think, oh, no, there's too much fat. I used to be beautiful … when I came to Denmark; I only weighed 52, even 50 kg. […] Now I wear size 42. […] When you are skinny, you get young and have a lot of energy. […] If I was thin, I would be really happy.' However, the women did not only monitor their own body shape – thus clearly exercising disciplinary practices of self-surveillance – they also directed their 'gaze' at others (Foucault 1977, see also, for example, Duncan 1994). The body – its looks and its weight – was a major issue in their conversations, for example, when Aysel and Ebru chatted about their colleague Danica, envying her slim and trained body: 'She is so tall and fit … we said, "Wow, look at her beautiful body!" […] Aysel and I – and you know Aysel is a bit fat – we said, "We should also get into shape"' (Ebru).

The interviewees' strong focus on the slimming effect of exercise shows that the majority regarded recreational PA only as a means to an end. Their narratives also revealed that most of them could not even imagine that exercise could be rewarding or fun. Thus, Rashida could not understand why her slim neighbour exercised. In line with their aim to lose weight, the interviewees had a very narrow definition of recreational PA: they seemed to regard exercising in a fitness centre solely as 'real training' whereas, for example, they looked upon folk dancing as being fun and perhaps as exhausting but not as an effective exercise. It might have been the fun element of dancing that precluded this activity from being classified as strenuous and thus beneficial for health and losing weight. Moreover, the major role that weight loss played in the interviews indicates that the women have internalised the cultural ideology of 'slim is beautiful' that is prevalent in western societies (see, for example, Bordo 2003). They practised self-surveillance by monitoring and judging themselves according to this ideal and confessed deviations – for example during the interviews (Foucault 1977). This reveals that the participants in our study share with many other women in western societies dissatisfaction with their body's shape and size (see, for example, Markula 2001). Our findings are consistent with the results of numerous studies, in particular those of feminist scholars who have pointed to the oppressive nature of a body ideal which is out of reach for the great majority of women who nevertheless strive for slimness and subject their bodies to obsessive control (see, for example, Bordo 2003, Riley *et al.* 2008, Markula and Kennedy 2011).

However, this ideal is influenced by culture, as the statements of some of the interviewees' (older) family members reveal: although Duygu and Meryem may be considered overweight in Danish society, older relatives were worried about their diets and subsequent weight loss: 'My family got a shock when they saw my face. They told me I'd lost way too much weight' (Duygu). Meryem had similar experiences: 'My mother-in-law, she told everybody: "Try to bring my daughter-in-law to reason ... she doesn't understand that what she's doing is not healthy."' These evaluations point to alternative, non-western body ideals and also reject the western consensus of a close connection between slimness and health (see, for example, Markula *et al.* 2008). However, the concerns of their relatives did not alter the interviewees' intentions to lose weight, which can be explained by an internalisation of the dominant discourses on the ideal body and a healthy lifestyle in Denmark. Other studies, too, found that minority ethnic women's striving for a slender physique was a consequence of their long exposure to western habits and tastes (see also, for example, Hacısoftaoğlu and Pfister 2012). Therefore, it is not surprising that our interviewees adhered to this ideal as well and regarded losing weight as an important benefit of recreational PA.

Especially the women's ideals and their strategies for losing weight indicate a certain measure of body expertise. Whereas Krasnik, as indicated in the statement quoted in the introduction (Ringgaard 2012), represents the opinions of many Danish politicians and health professionals in assuming that ethnic minorities do not possess (enough) health-related knowledge, the narratives of the interviewees show that health messages regarding recreational PA do indeed reach this group of the population. Their knowledge about and attitudes towards recreational PA are strongly shaped by the two main discourses which produce and propagate 'truths' about recreational PA. In these discourses recreational PA is addressed not only as a strategy to achieve the 'body beautiful' but also as a means of preventing illness and improving health (see, for example, Markula and Kennedy 2011). However, even though the statements of our interviewees point to 'overlapping concerns with health and appearance' (Smith Maguire 2008, see also, for example, McDermott 2011), the promise of weight loss seemed to be much more important to them than the potential health benefits of recreational PA (see also Abou-Rizk and Rail 2014). The emphasis our interviewees put on weight loss may – at least partially – be explained by the fact that slimness is visible and an aim attained relatively quickly whereas good health is a long-term goal which cannot even be traced back to any specific behaviour. The interviewees' strong focus on weight loss differs from the results of Wray (2011), who found that a group of minority ethnic women in the UK were more likely to associate participation in recreational PA with socialising and staying healthy rather than with weight loss and appearance. Wray explains these women's attitudes by pointing to their efforts to maintain their ethnic identity, which seemed to have a higher priority for them than their body shape.

Practices – participation in recreational physical activity

At the time of the interviews only nine out of thirty-three interviewees engaged in recreational PA. There is an obvious discrepancy between, on the one hand, the women's desire to lose weight as well as their knowledge about the positive effects of exercise on health and weight loss and, on the other hand, their overweight bodies (by western social norms) and their lack of participation or even intention to engage in recreational PA. This raises the question as to why the interviewees did not comply with the health recommendations, that is, did not engage in body maintenance practices and turn their bodies into 'docile bodies' (Foucault 1977). Were they not fully convinced of the (health) benefits of recreational PA? Were the prospects of health and a slim body not a strong enough incentive? Or were there other reasons which impeded or prevented participation?

We discussed the issue of engaging in recreational PA in the interviews, and the women's statements provided insights into the incentives as well as the constraints influencing their reactions to society's health policies and slimness messages.

Reasons and motives for participating in recreational physical activity

Despite their physically exhausting job, there were nevertheless nine women who exercised regularly. However, only three of them participated in recreational PA because they enjoyed it. Two of these women had participated in different types of PA over their life courses. One was Danica, who grew up in Serbia and had 'loved sports all her life.' The other was Kameljeet, who practised yoga – an activity she had already been engaged in for many years in her country of origin, India. Karima, however, had first started to participate in recreational PA 2 years previously. She had been persuaded by the nurses at her workplace to exercise in the hospital's fitness centre and was enthralled immediately. Shortly afterwards she explored PA programmes for minority ethnic women and participated in belly dancing and swimming classes. Despite family obligations and a full-time job these interviewees found the time and energy to exercise because they found it enjoyable and rewarding. Their narratives suggest that participation in recreational PA depends to a high degree on one's sporting background as well as previous and current experience and also imply that time and energy are not objective quantities but rather subjective experiences and therefore negotiable.

However, in contrast to these three women who emphasised the 'fun factor' of recreational PA, six interviewees exercised in recreational PA as a means of achieving specific goals. Four interviewees, Basima, Grace, Rashida and Xing, had joined a fitness centre with the aim of losing weight. Two women had taken up recreational PA following the advice of their general practitioners. One of these was Josephine, who had recently been diagnosed with diabetes and had started to cycle every Saturday by the beach: 'I'm taking care of my health. Because of diabetes I have to take pills. I also have to lose some weight. I have to exercise. That's what my doctor told me.' The other was Sevgi, who had undergone surgery on her abdomen and was advised by her doctor to strengthen her muscles. Sevgi and Josephine had learned that physical inactivity was a risk for their health and were determined to follow their doctors' orders. The women's compliance with advice from health professionals is consistent with the results of other studies such as a Dutch study (Schmidt *et al.* 2008) about the exercise participation of women in deprived neighbourhoods: a key motive for taking up PA was a prescription from their doctors, which they perceived as an order. The potential influence of doctors on individuals' health behaviour can be explained by the trust of lay people in experts and their expertise. Lupton (1995, p. 10) argues that governmental strategies intending to regulate a population's health heavily rely on medical experts who 'play an important role in mediating between authorities and individuals, "shaping conduct not through compulsion but through the power of truth […] (Miller and Rose 1993, p. 93)."' Although the cleaners' narratives left no doubt that they considered overweight undesirable, their stories indicate that most of them linked overweight and a sedentary lifestyle in their leisure only to a limited extent to the development of disease. While the threat of (potential) risks has been described as a powerful strategy of neo-liberal health governance to stimulate health-promoting behaviour and individual responsibility for health and well-being (see among many others, for example, Lupton 1995, Fusco 2006, McDermott 2011), it seems that the women in our study needed the authority of a doctor to feel a sense of 'urgency, and a sense that action must be taken now' (Ayo 2012, p. 103).

Reasons for not participating in recreational physical activity

The interviewees named different reasons for not engaging in recreational PA. The two most common constraints were exhaustion and lack of time. By contrast, none of the women referred to religious precepts, for example, a lack of a gender-segregated sporting environment, as a reason for refraining from recreational PA. This is surprising given the strong emphasis that public health scholars place on 'cultural sensitivity' as a strategy to increase PA participation rates among minority ethnic women (see, for example, Kreps and Sparks 2008, Caperchione *et al.* 2009). Nor were lack of motivation, interest or sporting skills stated as reasons for being physically inactive in their leisure; and only a few women referred to traits of their personality. One of these was Aisha, who brought up the above-mentioned discrepancy between exercise-related knowledge and practice: 'It's true … you should of course exercise. You get stronger. But sometimes you don't feel like it. You are just lazy. That's it.' Grace – one of two women married to a Dane – had recently changed her lifestyle by eating 'healthier' food and incorporating recreational PA into her everyday life. She described her 'transformation' from a 'couch potato' (in her leisure) into a health-conscious , responsible citizen with an internalised 'will to health' (Rose 2001) who was ready to exercise self-care (see, for example, McDermott 2011): 'I was really lazy … My husband always asked me, "Should we go for a walk?" But I always had excuses … But in the end I realised that I was on the very wrong path. I told myself I have to do something.' Josephine, too, used the term 'excuses' when talking about her previous way of life, thus implying that she did not have any 'legitimate' reasons for not participating in recreational PA. Another interviewee, Kameljeet, also turned the '(panoptic) gaze' upon herself (Foucault 1977) and 'confessed' that some aspects of her lifestyle had flaws – meaning, among other things, that she did not exercise. These explanations for non-participation in recreational PA are in line with strategies of unemployed adults in Finland who referred, for instance, to a 'weak character repertoire' to explain their unhealthy lifestyle (Pajari *et al.* 2006, p. 2606). Like our interviewees quoted above, they regarded good health as an individual responsibility or even a duty, which shows that they, too, are clearly affected by neo-liberal health discourses which emphasise and demand self-discipline and self-regulation (see, for example, Vallgårda 2011).

However, a number of interviewees rejected the notion of individual responsibility and referred instead to their ethnic identity. They used, for example, the pronoun 'we' when talking about their (sedentary leisure) habits, indicating that they regarded their way of living as an expression of a collective lifestyle rooted in the culture of their home countries. Burcu, for example, depicted Turkish people as 'passive' and 'lazy.' Hamide was convinced that Turks tired more easily than Danes – and thus were not attracted to sport and exercise. Religious Makbule emphasised that recreational PA was important, but that it was 'Allah who eventually had the power to decide' about good health and a long life. These statements show how religious ways of thinking, as well as ethnic and cultural beliefs, are embedded in individuals' mentalities, influencing their perceptions, decisions and actions (see also, for example, Wray 2007, 2011). The importance of cultural background for ways of thinking, habits and tastes is corroborated by the results of numerous studies, particularly in the field of public health, for example a qualitative study exploring Pakistani and Indian patients' engagement in recreational PA as part of their diabetes care in the UK (Lawton *et al.* 2006). Many of Lawton *et al.*'s informants did not comply with the advice of their doctors, not least because they attributed their illness to factors outside their control. Lawton *et al.* (2006, p. 49) interpreted the respondents' reflections upon their futures as 'fatalistic and surrounded by a strong sense of inevitability.'

The great majority of our interviewees, however, referred neither to personal traits nor cultural habits as reasons for not participating in PA in their leisure. Instead, they argued that their physically exhausting job and their family responsibilities made it impossible for them to exercise. All interviewees described cleaning as a strenuous and physically demanding job: they suffered from pain and work-related injuries, and having got up as early as 3:30am, they were so exhausted after 8 hours of cleaning that they could not imagine being also physically active in their free time. These findings are consistent with the results of a US-American study about Latina women's engagement in recreational PA which revealed that hard factory work led to great fatigue and no energy or desire to exercise (Skowron *et al.* 2008).

Several women had joined fitness centres for a short period of time, but terminated their membership when they started to work as cleaners. Aysel, for example, explained: 'Cleaning is really tough. When you come home, your body's dead. [...] I can't get up. I sit on the couch and can't even talk because I'm so tired.' Therefore, instead of working out, the interviewees preferred to spend their time off from work resting and relaxing – if they had the time to do so. However, after their paid work most women returned to a 'second shift' at home, that is, to housework and childcare, receiving very little support from their husbands or other family members. Hadiya's account of her daily routine at home is typical of the statements given by the interviewees: 'After work, I buy groceries on my way home. Then I tidy up my home. [...] It's me who works hard at home. In the evenings I'm in the kitchen cooking dinner for everybody and doing the dishes. [...] The next morning, I get up earlier just to make lunch boxes for my husband and the [three] children. [...] I've got a very long workday. I don't have free time at home.'

These narratives reveal that the interviewees' everyday lives – in particular their exhausting job characterised by early shifts, a high workload, fatigue after work and a low wage, combined with a strenuous 'second shift' (Hochschild 1989) at home – are the result of the intersections of social class, ethnicity and gender. As minority ethnic women with little education or proficiency in Danish, they have few options on the (gender-segregated) labour market other than to work as cleaners and accept the precarious conditions of the cleaning industry (see, for example, Aguiar and Herod 2006, Rubin *et al.* 2008). Moreover, the large number of family obligations at home point to a gender-stereotypical allocation of domestic responsibilities which seems to prevail in migrant working-class families in western countries. This assumption is consistent with the findings of a literature review on the work and family life of ethnic minorities in Scandinavian countries (Dahl and Jakobsen 2005) as well as an interview study with Turkish working-class families in Denmark (Liversage 2009). Driven by a strong ethic of care (see, for example, Miller and Brown 2005), our interviewees devoted almost all their time off from paid work to the well-being of their families, without claiming time for themselves. Their everyday struggles as minority ethnic women working in menial jobs show that life circumstances set the frame for actively pursuing a healthy lifestyle. This interpretation is corroborated by scholars such as Lupton (2013, p. 397), who stress that preoccupation with health is a 'discourse embraced by the socio-economically privileged, who are able to position "health" as a priority in their lives and have the economic and educational resources to do so' (see also Lupton 1995, Crawford 2006). Our interviewees, by contrast, not only lacked these resources; they also had to deal with the high demands of their work that often caused health problems, sometimes even serious injuries and chronic pain which posed a threat to both their working capacity and their employment (see, also Jørgensen *et al.* 2011). Cleaners (have to) use their body as a tool and not (only) as an object of self-work and a basis for identity construction (see, for example, Smith Maguire 2008). Therefore, they may be more occupied with the troubles of the present, that is, the challenges of their job and their family responsibilities, than with long-term health prospects and 'body projects' (Shilling 2012) which might 'pay off' in the future (see also, for example, Lawton *et al.* 2006).

In general, strategies for dealing with (potential) health challenges are interrelated with attitudes towards the notion of 'delayed gratification' commonly attributed to members of the middle class (see, for example, Guthrie *et al.* 2009). In this case it refers to the willingness to invest in the body and wait for a later reward, for example with regard to slimness or health. Recreational PA, too, can be considered an investment in the future that does not provide immediate benefits, either with regard to losing weight or to preventing disease. Therefore, our interviewees might associate exercise first and foremost with additional work which does not seem to provide any reward – at least not in the 'here and now.' Whereas members of the Danish mainstream population may have learned in numerous socialisation processes that playing sports can provide pleasure and social contacts (see, for example, Pfister 2011), most interviewees lacked any previous sporting experience and – as a consequence – the physical competences needed in the various sports. Therefore, they may never have had the opportunity of experiencing sport and recreational PA as something enjoyable and rewarding (see, for example, Jallinoja *et al.* 2010).

Conclusion and prospective

This article gives unique insights into female migrant cleaners' lived experiences with health recommendations and with recreational PA. It provides new knowledge about the perspectives of individuals who are considered to be at great risk of developing various lifestyle-related diseases and who are therefore the target of specific health-promotion campaigns and interventions.

In this paper we have explored and discussed whether messages about health and the benefits of PA reach minority ethnic women with low levels of education and the factors that might impede their engagement in recreational PA. We found that the interviewees knew about the health benefits of recreational PA, although maintaining or improving health was not one of their major concerns. The large majority regarded recreational PA neither as a (potential) source of pleasure, fun and relaxation nor as a means of socialising but first and foremost as a way of losing weight. Their desire to be slim indicates an internalisation of western beauty ideals with the consequence that almost all interviewees were unhappy with their (over)weight and judged their bodies (and those of others) according to how they conformed to the prevailing social norms. In spite of their knowledge about the health benefits of recreational PA and their generally positive attitudes towards it, only a few cleaners exercised regularly. The others gave different reasons for not participating in recreational PA which were embedded in multiple, often competing, discourses – that is, western discourses on individual responsibility for health on the one hand and cultural and ethnic beliefs and values on the other. Whereas some cleaners blamed themselves for not living up to the demands of 'healthy living', others referred to a collective lifestyle, in particular to a widespread disinterest in recreational PA in their countries of origin. However, by far the most important reasons for not participating in recreational PA were linked to their life circumstances. Most interviewees found it simply impossible to engage in recreational PA: on account of their physically exhausting job and their 'second shift' at home, they lacked the time and energy to exercise. These findings confirm that 'health enthusiasm', the preoccupation with a healthy lifestyle and the development of 'docile bodies' (Foucault 1977) is a form of investment in health and appearance that requires a variety of resources such as time, money and energy, that is, resources that are scarce among minority ethnic women working in menial jobs (Lupton 1995, 2013, Crawford 2006).

These results differ decisively from the findings of previous sociocultural research which mainly explored *young* minority ethnic women's practices of body management in various, often sport-related, contexts that revealed negotiations of western, ethnic and religious identities (see, for example, Walseth 2006, Jiwani and Rail 2010, Abou-Rizk and Rail 2014). The insights gained in our study emphasise that not only the intersections of gender and ethnicity play a decisive role in the lives of minority ethnic women but also those of age, family status and social class. The intersections of these categories in particular determined the life circumstances of our interviewees and, consequently, the opportunities they had of engaging in recreational PA. As minority ethnic women with neither an education nor Danish language skills, they had few options on the Danish labour market and therefore had to accept the difficult working conditions in the cleaning industry. Additionally, the manifold domestic chores they were faced with appeared to be closely connected to traditional gender norms which still seemed to prevail in their families.

These findings also make clear that even 'culturally sensitive' health communication and specific PA programmes for minority ethnic women will not necessarily lead to participation. Health promotion will only be effective if it takes the lived realities of specific population groups into consideration. Moreover, the underlying social structures and institutions such as the labour market and the gendered division of work in the nuclear family must be taken into account since they determine an individual's opportunities of engaging in a 'healthy lifestyle' and integrating recreational PA into daily routines. Providing such opportunities for minority ethnic women is important, however, not only because of the positive influences of recreational PA on health and well-being but also because of additional benefits such as relaxation, social interaction and enjoyment. It must be emphasised, though, that as exercises require time, energy and perhaps also financial resources, they could become an additional stress factor or burden for minority ethnic women who already face numerous challenges in their everyday lives. Therefore, exercise programmes must take the specific situation of migrant women working in menial jobs into consideration, in particular their exhaustion after long working hours. Due to their time constraints, one solution might be to offer recreational PA at the workplace during working hours. Moreover, programmes should pay heed to the participants' wishes and cater for their needs. They could include, for example, elements of relaxation and should try to foster enjoyment through dance or games, emphasising that PA can be more than just a means of losing weight or complying with the prevailing ideals of beauty and the body.

Notes

1. According to Statistics Denmark (2014, p. 11) 8.5% of the Danish population are members of ethnic minorities; 58% of these come from non-western countries.
2. We followed the different worksite fitness programmes to varying degrees. At two workplaces the authors observed several training sessions; at the two other workplaces the authors followed the programmes more closely and joined the cleaners' training twice a week for a period of 3 months.
3. Approximately half of our interviewees prematurely dropped out of the programmes, which in general did not seem to have an impact on participation in recreational PA after the programme had ended. However, we cannot rule out that the fact that the interviewees signed up for a worksite fitness project might have (positively) influenced their opinions about and attitudes towards recreational PA.

Acknowledgement

The authors would like to thank Pirkko Markula for her feedback and many helpful comments.

Disclosure statement

No potential conflict of interest was reported by the authors.

Funding

This work was supported by the Nordea-fonden.

References

Abou-Rizk, Z. and Rail, G., 2014. 'Judging a body by its cover': young lebanese-canadian women's discursive constructions of the 'healthy' body and 'health' practices. *Journal of immigrant and minority health*, 16 (1), 150–164. doi:10.1007/s10903-012-9757-5

Aguiar, L.L. and Herod, A., 2006. *The dirty work of neoliberalism: cleaners in the global economy*. Malden, MA: Blackwell.

Ahlmark, N., *et al.*, 2014. Survey nonresponse among ethnic minorities in a national health survey – a mixed-method study of participation, barriers, and potentials. *Ethnicity and health*, 4, 1–22.

Aléx, L. and Hammarström, A., 2008. Shift in power during an interview situation: methodological reflections inspired by Foucault and Bourdieu. *Nursing inquiry*, 15 (2), 169–176. doi:10.1111/j.1440-1800.2008.00398.x

Ayo, N., 2012. Understanding health promotion in a neoliberal climate and the making of health-conscious citizens. *Critical public health*, 22 (1), 99–105. doi:10.1080/09581596.2010.520692

Barker-Ruchti, N., *et al.*, 2013. Sport—'it's just healthy': locating healthism within discourses of social integration. *Journal of ethnic and migration studies*, 39 (5), 759–772. doi:10.1080/1369183X.2013.756674

Benn, T., Dagkas, S., and Jawad, H., 2011. Embodied faith: Islam, religious freedom and educational practices in physical education. *Sport, education and society*, 16 (1), 17–34.

Bordo, S., 2003. *Unbearable weight: feminism, Western culture, and the body*. Berkeley: University of California Press.

Brown, S., *et al.*, 2013. Risk, resistance and the neoliberal agenda: young people, health and well-being in the UK, Canada and Australia. *Health, risk & society*, 15 (4), 333–346. doi:10.1080/13698575.2013.796346

Bryman, A., 2012. *Social research methods*. Oxford: Oxford University Press.

Caperchione, C.M., Kolt, G.S., and Mummery, W.K., 2009. Physical activity in culturally and linguistically diverse migrant groups to Western society: a review of barriers, enablers and experiences. *Sports medicine*, 39 (3), 167–177. doi:10.2165/00007256-200939030-00001

Copenhagen Municipality, 2005. *Social ulighed i sundhed i Københavns Kommune* [Social inequality in health in Copenhagen Municipality] [online]. Copenhagen. Available from: http://www.kk.dk/sites/default/files/edoc_old_format/Sundheds-%20og%20Omsorgsudvalget/19-01-2006%2014.00.00/Dagsorden/13-01-2006%2013.18.44/Social%20ulighed%20i%20sundhed%20i%20K%C3%B8benhavns%20Kommune.PDF [Accessed 9 February 2016].

Crawford, R., 2006. Health as a meaningful social practice. *Health: an interdisciplinary journal for the social study of health, illness and medicine*, 10 (4), 401–420.

Creswell, J.W., 2013. *Qualitative inquiry and research design: choosing among five approaches*. Los Angeles, CA: SAGE Publications.

Dagkas, S., Benn, T., and Jawad, H., 2011. Multiple voices: improving participation of muslim girls in physical education and school sport. *Sport, education and society*, 16 (2), 223–239. doi:10.1080/13573322.2011.540427

Dahl, K. and Jakobsen, V., 2005. *Køn, etnicitet og barrierer for integration* [Gender, ethncity and barriers for integration] [online]. Copenhagen: The Danish National Centre for Social Research. Available from: http://www.sfi.dk/Files/Filer/SFI/Pdf/Rapporter/2005/0501_Kon_etnicitet_og_barrierer.pdf [Accessed 9 February 2016].

Danish Health and Medicines Authority, 2011. *Ulighed i sundhed* [Inequalities in health] [online]. Available from: http://sundhedsstyrelsen.dk/~/media/F674C77308FB4B0CA00EB038F17E239B.ashx [Accessed 9 February 2016].

Danish Ministry of Health, 2014. *Sundere liv for alle* [A healthier life for everybody] [online]. Copenhagen. Available from: http://www.sum.dk/~/media/Filer%20-%20Publikationer_i_pdf/2014/Nationale-maal/Nationale-Maal.ashx [Accessed 9 February 2016].

Duncan, M.C., 1994. The politics of women's body images and practices: Foucault, the Panopticon, and Shape magazine. *Journal of sport & social issues*, 18, 48–65. doi:10.1177/019372394018001004

Feskens, R., *et al.*, 2006. Collecting data among ethnic minorities in an international perspective. *Field methods*, 18 (3), 284–304. doi:10.1177/1525822X06288756

Foucault, M., 1977. *Discipline and punish. The birth of the prison*. London: Penguin.

Foucault, M., 1991. Governmentality. *In*: G. Burchell, C. Gordon, and P. Miller, eds. *The Foucault effect: studies in governmentality*. Chicago, IL: University of Chicago Press, 87–104.

Foucault, M., 2007. *Security, territory, population: lectures at the Collège de France, 1977-78*. Basingstoke: Palgrave Macmillan.

Fullagar, S., 2002. Governing the healthy body: discourses of leisure and lifestyle within Australian health policy. *Health*, 6 (1), 69–84.

Fullagar, S., 2009. Governing healthy family lifestyles. *In*: J. Wright and V. Harwood, eds. *Biopolitcis and the 'obesity epidemic'*. New York, NY: Routledge, 108–127.

Fullagar, S. and Harrington, M., 2009. Negotiating the policy imperative to be healthy: Australian family repertoires of risk, leisure, and healthy lifestyles. *Annals of leisure research*, 12 (2), 195–215.

Fusco, C., 2006. Inscribing healthification: governance, risk, surveillance and the subjects and spaces of fitness and health. *Health and place*, 12 (1), 65–78. doi:10.1016/j.healthplace.2004.10.003

George, T. and Rail, G., 2006. Barbie meets the Bindi: constructions of health among second-generation South Asian Canadian women. *Journal women's health urban life*, 4 (2), 45–67.

Glasdam, S., 2009. *Folkesundhed: I et kritisk perspektiv* [Public health in a critical perspective]. Copenhagen: Nyt nordisk forlag Arnold Busck.

Guthrie, L.C., Butler, S.C., and Ward, M.M., 2009. Time perspective and socioeconomic status: a link to socioeconomic disparities in health? *Social science & medicine*, 68 (12), 2145–2151. doi:10.1016/j.socscimed.2009.04.004

Hacısoftaoğlu, I. and Pfister, G., 2012. Transitions: life stories and physical activities of Turkish migrants in Denmark. *Sport in society*, 15 (3), 385–398.

Harrington, M. and Fullagar, S., 2013. Challenges for active living provision in an era of healthism. *Journal of policy research in tourism, leisure and events*, 5 (2), 139–157. doi:10.1080/19407963.2013.793519

Hesse-Biber, S.N., ed. 2014. *Feminist research practice: a primer*. Thousand Oaks, CA: Sage Publications.

Hochschild, A., 1989. *The second shift*. New York, NY: Avon Books.

Holmberg, T., Ahlmark, N., and Curtis, T., 2009. *'State of the art report' - Etniske minoriteters sundhed i Danmark* [Ethnic minorities' health in Denmark]. Copenhagen: National Institute of Public Health, University of Southern Denmark.

Jallinoja, P., Pajari, P., and Absetz, P., 2010. Negotiated pleasures in health-seeking lifestyles of participants of a health promoting intervention. *Health*, 14 (2), 115–130.

Jiwani, N. and Rail, G., 2010. Islam, hijab and young Shia Muslim Canadian women's discursive constructions of physical activity. *Sociology of sport journal*, 27 (3), 250–267.

Jørgensen, M.B., *et al.*, 2011. Health disparities between immigrant and Danish cleaners. *International archives of occupational and environmental health*, 84 (6), 665–674. doi:10.1007/s00420-010-0607-2

Khawaja, I. and Morck, L.L., 2009. Researcher positioning: muslim 'otherness' and beyond. *Qualitative research in psychology*, 6, 28–45. doi:10.1080/14780880902900713

Korp, P., 2010. Problems of the healthy lifestyle discourse. *Sociology compass*, 4 (9), 800–810. doi:10.1111/soco.2010.4.issue-9

Korshøj, M., *et al.*, 2013. A 24-h assessment of physical activity and cardio-respiratory fitness among female hospital cleaners: a pilot study. *Ergonomics*, 56 (6), 935–943. doi:10.1080/00140139.2013.782427

Korshøj, M., 2015. *Physical work demands and fitness – Effects on risk factors for cardiovascular disease from a randomized controlled trial among cleaners*. Thesis (PhD). University of Copenhagen.

Kreps, G.L. and Sparks, L., 2008. Meeting the health literacy needs of immigrant populations. *Patient education and counseling*, 71 (3), 328–332. doi:10.1016/j.pec.2008.03.001

Kumar, R. and Kumar, S., 2008. Musculoskeletal risk factors in cleaning occupation – a literature review. *International journal of industrial ergonomics*, 38 (2), 158–170. doi:10.1016/j.ergon.2006.04.004

Kvale, S., 2007. *Doing interviews*. London: SAGE Publications.

Lawton, J., *et al.*, 2006. 'I can't do any serious exercise': barriers to physical activity amongst people of Pakistani and Indian origin with Type 2 diabetes. *Health education research*, 21 (1), 43–54. doi:10.1093/her/cyh042

Lincoln, Y.S., Lynham, S., and Guba, E., 2011. Paradigmatic controversies, contradictions, and emerging confluences, revisited. *In*: N.K. Denzin and Y.S. Lincoln, eds. *The SAGE handbook of qualitative research*. Thousand Oaks, CA: Sage, 97–129.

Liversage, A., 2009. Life below a 'language threshold'? *European journal of women's studies*, 16 (3), 229–247. doi:10.1177/1350506809105307

Lupton, D., 1995. *The imperative of health. Public health and the regulated body*. London: Sage Publications.

Lupton, D., 2013. Quantifying the body: monitoring and measuring health in the age of mHealth technologies. *Critical public health*, 23 (4), 393–403. doi:10.1080/09581596.2013.794931

Macdonald, D., 2011. Like a fish in water: physical education policy and practice in the era of neoliberal globalization. *Quest*, 63 (1), 36–45. doi:10.1080/00336297.2011.10483661

Markula, P., 2001. Beyond the perfect body: women's body image distortion in fitness magazine discourse. *Journal of sport & social issues*, 25 (2), 158–179. doi:10.1177/0193723501252004

Markula, P., Burns, M., and Riley, S. 2008. Introducing critical bodies. *In*: S. Riley, *et al.*, eds. *Critical bodies – representations, identities and practices of weight and body management*. New York, NY: Palgrave Macmillan, 1–23.

Markula, P. and Kennedy, E., 2011. Introduction: beyond binaries: contemporary approaches to women and exercise. *In*: E. Kennedy and P. Markula, eds. *Women and exercise – the body, health and consumerism*. New York, NY: Routledge, 1–25.

Markula, P. and Pringle, R., 2006. *Foucault, sport and exercise: power, knowledge and transforming the self*. London: Routledge.

Markula, P. and Silk, M.L., 2011. *Qualitative research for physical culture*. Basingstoke: Palgrave Macmillan.

McDermott, L., 2011. 'Doing something that's good for me': exploring intersections of physical activity and health. *In*: E. Kennedy and P. Markula, eds. *Women and exercise – the body, health and consumerism*. New York, NY: Routledge, 197–227.

Miles, M.B., Huberman, A.M., and Saldaña, J., 2014. *Qualitative data analysis: a methods sourcebook*. Thousand Oaks, CA: Sage Publications.

Miller, Y. and Brown, W., 2005. Determinants of active leisure for women with young children – an ethic of care prevails. *Leisure sciences*, 27 (5), 405–420. doi:10.1080/01490400500227308

Miller, P. and Rose, N., 1993. Governing economic life. *In*: M. Gane and T. Johnson, eds. *Foucault's new domains*. London: Routledge, 75–106.

National Institute of Public Health, 2009. *KRAM-undersøgelsen i tal og billeder* [The KRAM study in numbers and pictures] [online]. Odense: University of Southern Denmark. Available from: https://sundhedsstyrelsen.dk/da/sundhed/~/media/D31E9AF3077A420099E6D5228BCAEC85.ashx [Accessed 9 February 2016].

Netto, G., *et al*., 2010. How can health promotion interventions be adapted for minority ethnic communities? Five principles for guiding the development of behavioural interventions. *Health promotion international*, 25 (2), 248–257. doi:10.1093/heapro/daq012

Pajari, P.M., Jallinoja, P., and Absetz, P., 2006. Negotiation over self-control and activity: an analysis of balancing in the repertoires of Finnish healthy lifestyles. *Social science & medicine*, 62 (10), 2601–2611. doi:10.1016/j.socscimed.2005.11.005

Patton, M.Q., 2002. *Qualitative research and evaluation methods*. Thousand Oaks, CA: Sage Publications.

Pfister, G., 2011. Muslim women and sport in diasporas: theories, discourses and practices - analysing the case of Denmark. *In*: T. Benn, G. Pfister, and H.A. Jawad, eds. *Muslim women and sport*. London: Routledge, 41–76.

Piggin, J. and Bairner, A., 2016. The global physical inactivity pandemic: an analysis of knowledge production. *Sport, education and society*, 21 (2), 131–147.

Rail, G., 2009. Canadian youth's discursive constructions of health in the context of obesity discourse. *In*: J. Wright and V. Harwood, eds. *Biopolitics and the 'obesity epidemic'*. New York, NY: Routledge, 141–157.

Riley, S., *et al*., 2008. *Critical bodies: representations, identities and practices of weight and body management*. Basingstoke: Palgrave Macmillan.

Ringgaard, A., 2012. Ingen gider forske i indvandreres sundhed [Nobody cares to do research about immigrants' health]. *Videnskab.dk*, 26 September. Available from: http://videnskab.dk/krop-sundhed/ingen-gider-forske-i-indvandreres-sundhed [Accessed 26 October 2015].

Rose, N., 1999. *Powers of freedom: reframing political thought*. Cambridge, UK: Cambridge University Press.

Rose, N., 2001. *Inventing our selves: psychology, power, and personhood*. Cambridge: Cambridge University Press.

Rose, N. and Miller, P., 1992. Political power beyond the state: problematics of government [online]. *The british journal of sociology*, 43 (2), 173–205. doi:10.2307/591464. Available from: http://www.jstor.org/stable/591464?seq=1#page_scan_tab_contents

Rubin, J. *et al*., 2008. *Migrant women in the European labour force* [online]. European Commission. Available from: http://ec.europa.eu/social/BlobServlet?docId=2098&langId=en [Accessed 16 May 2016].

Schmidt, M., *et al*., 2008. Which factors engage women in deprived neighbourhoods to participate in exercise referral schemes? *BMC public health*, 8, 371. doi:10.1186/1471-2458-8-371

Shilling, C., 2012. *The body and social theory*. London: Sage Publications.

Singhammer, J., 2008. *Etniske minoriteters sundhed* [The health of ethnic minorities] [online]. Central Denmark Region: Centre for Public Health. Available from: https://www.regionsyddanmark.dk/dwn510078

Skowron, M.A., Stodolska, M., and Shinew, K.J., 2008. Determinants of leisure time physical activity participation among Latina women. *Leisure sciences*, 30 (5), 429–447. doi:10.1080/01490400802353174

Smith Maguire, J., 2008. *Fit for consumption: sociology and the business of fitness*. London: Routledge.

Statistics Denmark, 2014. *Indvandrere i Danmark 2014* [Immigrants in Denmark 2014] [online]. Copenhagen. Available from: http://www.dst.dk/pukora/epub/upload/19004/indv.pdf [Accessed 9 February 2016].

Vallgårda, S., 2011. Addressing individual behaviours and living conditions: four Nordic public health policies. *Scandinavian journal of public health*, 39 (6), 6–10. doi:10.1177/1403494810378922

Walseth, K., 2006. Young muslim women and sport: the impact of identity work. *Leisure Studies*, 25 (1), 75–94. doi:10.1080/02614360500200722

Wheatley, E.E., 2005. Disciplining bodies at risk: cardiac rehabilitation and the medicalization of fitness. *Journal of sport and social issues*, 29 (2), 198–221. doi:10.1177/0193723504270870

WHO, 2013. *Physical activity promotion in socially disadvantaged groups: principles for action* [online]. Copenhagen: WHO Regional Office for Europe. Available from: http://www.euro.who.int/__data/assets/pdf_file/0005/185954/E96817eng.pdf

Wray, S., 2007. Health, exercise, and well-being: the experiences of midlife women from diverse ethnic backgrounds. *Social theory and health*, 5 (2), 126–144. doi:10.1057/palgrave.sth.8700100

Wray, S., 2011. The significance of western health promotion discourse for older women from diverse ethnic backgrounds. *In*: E. Kennedy and P. Markula, eds. *Women and exercise – the body, health and consumerism*. New York, NY: Routledge, 161–180.

Are they 'worth their weight in gold'? Sport for older adults: benefits and barriers of their participation for sporting organisations

Claire R. Jenkin, Rochelle M. Eime, Hans Westerbeek, Grant O'Sullivan and Jannique G. Z. van Uffelen

ABSTRACT

The ageing global population has led to an increased focus on health for older adults. However, older adults have not been a specific priority for some sporting organisations (SOs). Thus, there is an emerging opportunity for this age group to be considered within international sport policy. The aim of this study was to understand the benefits and barriers that SOs encounter when engaging older adults. Eight focus group interviews (n = 49) were held with representatives of Australian national sporting organisations (NSOs), and older adults who were either sport club or non-sport club members. The socioecological model domains, interpersonal, organisational and policy, were used as a framework for thematic analysis, and organisational capacity building concepts were utilised to explain the findings. Common perceived benefits included interpersonal benefits (intergenerational opportunities and role models) and organisational benefits (volunteering, financial contributions and maximised facility usage) for engaging older adults. Common perceived barriers included interpersonal barriers (competing priorities and perceived societal expectations), organisational barriers (lack of appropriate playing opportunities, lack of facility access and lack of club capacity) and policy barriers (strategic organisational focus on children and elite sport and risk management). Whilst participation in sport is not common for older adults, their involvement can be invaluable for sport clubs. It is not anticipated that any policy focus on older adults will significantly increase active participation for this age group. However, any increase in older adults' sport participation either through actively playing, supporting family and friends and/or volunteering will contribute to the positive health of individuals, sport clubs and the community.

Introduction

The populations of developed countries such as Australia are ageing, and the proportion of people aged 50 years and over in Australia is projected to increase to 39% by 2061 (Australian Bureau of Statistics 2015). This is a public health issue as ageing is typically associated with a decline in physical (Paterson *et al.* 2007), mental (Bishop *et al.* 2010) and social health (Sirven and Debrand 2008).

Research on older adults has linked participation in physical activity to improved physical (Haskell *et al.* 2007, Rydwik *et al.* 2013), mental (Chodzko-Zajko *et al.* 2009) and social health

(Toepoel 2013). Furthermore, regular physical activity can also prevent or delay the onset of many chronic conditions, such as cardiovascular disease or diabetes (Haskell *et al.* 2007). However, participation in physical activity tends to decline with age (Australian Bureau of Statistics 2013–2014).

An ageing population, therefore, has a number of policy implications relating to chronic diseases and associated health care resources. As participation in physical activity is a modifiable behaviour that can result in health benefits at the population level, the role that physical activity can play to prevent or delay the onset of age-related diseases is a national government health priority (Australian Institute of Health and Welfare 2014).

Australian national preventative health policy

In Australia, there have been a number of previous preventative health initiatives that promoted healthy lifestyles, such as the 'Life, be in it!' campaign launched in 1975 (Fullagar 2002). The establishment of the Australian National Preventative Health Agency (ANPHA) in 2009 resulted in a more structured federal approach, with specific funding for preventative health management. The 2009 'Australia: the healthiest nation by 2020', and the 2010 'Taking Preventative Action' strategies were also developed (Australian Department of Health and Ageing 2010). However, the ANPHA was abolished in 2014. Despite the lack of a current specific preventative health department, the Department of Health does provide physical activity guidelines, indicating the minimum amount of physical activity that is needed for health benefits, with specific guidelines for older adults (Australian Department of Health 2014).

The decline in physical activity amongst older adults and the implications this has on their health and the national health system is clearly a priority for the national health policy agenda. In Australia, the State and National governments have identified connections between health and sport specifically. In State Government, sport and recreation is within the health portfolio, and in the Commonwealth Government, there is an appointed Minister for Health, Aged Care and Sport. Also, sport clubs have been identified as a potential setting for health promotion activities internationally (Kokko *et al.* 2009, Eime *et al.* 2010). Therefore, the nexus between sport, older adults and health are connected in principle.

Australian national sport policy

Sport is a form of leisure-time physical activity which, similar to physical activity more broadly, sees a decrease in participation with age (Breuer and Wicker 2009, Eime *et al.* 2009, Palacios-Cena *et al.* 2012). Sport participation rates for older adults in Australia are very low. A recent Australian study of 520,102 sport participants reported that fewer than 10% were over the age of 50 years (Eime *et al.* 2016). This low participation rate may in part be an effect of national sport policy which typically has a stronger focus on youth sport participation.

In Australia, the Australian Sports Commission (ASC) is the principal government agency that is responsible for sport. It allocates both elite and community-based federal funding for sport. The ASC also provides structure and funding to the NSOs, the national governing bodies of sport and their respective state/territory sporting organisations (SSOs). Most sport in Australia is participated within community-based sport clubs that are registered with their respective SSO.

A main focus of Australian sport policy is elite sport and international sporting success, which is an integral part of Australia's national identity (Stewart *et al.* 2004). This is identifiable through the allocation of federal funding. The 2015–16 Australian federal government's budget for sport is $134 m, with 84% of this funding allocated to elite sport, and only 16% to community-based sport (Australian Sports Commission 2015a). This focus is also identifiable through the ASC 2015–19 Corporate Plan, which has four focus areas: 'Win' (international success); 'Play' (increase participation); 'Thrive' (develop sustainable NSOs) and 'Perform' (ensure the ASC achieves organisational excellence)

(Australian Sports Commission 2015b). As 'Win' is the first focus area, this suggests that elite sport is the priority participation group. For community-based sport, the main focus in the 'Play' area is children through the Sporting Schools programme. Thus, older adults are not a main priority group in the national sport policy agenda and are therefore unlikely to be prioritised by NSOs.

As has been identified in Australian and other national sport systems (Green 2007, Phillips and Newland 2014), Australian national sport policies promote two contesting policies for sporting organisations (SOs) to consider when consolidating their own implementation priorities. As funding is often specifically linked to success in achieving policy objectives, engaging under-represented population groups such as older adults may be intentionally not prioritised, as organisations strive to achieve outcomes in line with state and national policy.

There are many reasons why older adults are less likely to participate in sport. The socio-ecological model can be used to understand sport participation behaviour from various perspectives. The model states that there are four interrelated domains that can influence behaviour: intrapersonal, interpersonal, organisational and policy (Sallis *et al.* 2008), and that these domains often include themes that can link and influence each other. With respect to the policy domain of the model, there are clear agendas towards elite sport and younger sport participants and not older adults specifically in Australia.

There has been extensive research in regard to the participation determinants of physical activity and some research on the determinants of sport participation, but mainly from the perspective of children and young adults (Kalakanis *et al.* 2001, Dwyer *et al.* 2006, Casey *et al.* 2009a). Of the current research on the determinants of older adults participating in sport, these predominantly focus on specific sports that are recognised as traditional for older adults, such as bowls (Heuser 2005) or golf (Siegenthaler and O'dell 2003, Cann *et al.* 2005) rather than sports in general. Further research has investigated mainly the intrapersonal determinants and partially interpersonal determinants of older adult sport participation (Dionigi 2002, Kolt *et al.* 2004, Litchfield and Dionigi 2012, Heo *et al.* 2013). Whilst the intrapersonal determinants are an important consideration, to our knowledge, there is no known research that investigates the determinants of participation in sport for older adults from an organisational and policy perspective and only limited research from the interpersonal perspective. Therefore, these domains are the focus of investigation in this study. To fully understand the reasons why older adults either do or do not participate in sport, and to develop sport policy accordingly, the perspective of SOs must be taken into consideration.

Studies on organisational determinants of sport and physical activity participation have mainly focused on sports' organisational capacity building through resources, volunteer capacity (Shibli *et al.* 1999, Cuskelly 2004) and in health promotion initiatives (Joffres *et al.* 2004, Cairns *et al.* 2005, Casey *et al.* 2009b). Capacity building of SOs is stated as a priority of national sport policy (Australian Sports Commission 2015b). However, there is limited knowledge of how factors at the organisational level, including policies that drive strategic direction, may affect participation in sport for older adults. Therefore, this study investigated the potential benefits and barriers of trying to engage older adults for SOs, from the perspective of both older adults and representatives from NSOs. The findings will be interpreted through the lens of the interpersonal, organisational and policy domains of the socioecological model and implications will be related to concepts of organisational capacity building.

Methods

This study utilised qualitative research methods and collected data via eight focus group interviews with 49 participants.

These interviews were used to gain the perspectives of representatives of NSOs, older adults who were involved in a sport club and older adults who were not involved in a sport club. Due to a lack of research within this specific area, focus group interviews were used to provide breadth of data, as the inclusion of diverse points of view were deemed important to understand organisational context more broadly. Focus group interviews enable participants to discuss and challenge their own, and their peers' views, in a social situation (Patton 2002). We also wanted to explore potential differences in gender, different sports, and with those involved or not involved in sport clubs. As such, two of these focus group interviews were with representatives of NSOs (Tennis Australia and Cricket Australia), four with sport club members (female tennis club members, male tennis club members, female cricket club members and male cricket club members) and two with non-sport club members (female non-sport club members and male non-sport club members). For this study, sport has been defined as 'a human activity capable of achieving a result requiring physical exertion and/or physical skill which, by its nature and organisation, is competitive and is generally accepted as being a sport' (Australian Sports Commission 2009).

Sport selection

To gain a broader understanding of how SOs can engage with older adults, representatives of one sport with a high proportion of older adults' participation, and another sport with a low proportion of older adults' participation, were interviewed for this study. These sports were identified using the Australian national Exercise, Recreation and Sport Survey (ERASS) 2010 data. ERASS was a joint initiative between the ASC and state and territory departments of sport and recreation in Australia, to determine the proportion of adults aged 15 years and older who participated in sport (Australian Sports Commission 2010). This survey was used to identify participation of people aged 50+ years in a range of sports in Australia.

The 10 most frequently played sports and the 10 least frequently played sports for older adults (defined for this study as adults aged 50 years and older) were ranked according to participation rates in this age group. The sports were also considered in the context of existing relations with NSOs, and each sport's appropriateness for older adults. The research team defined a sport's appropriateness as one that could be realistically played by older adults with a range of physical abilities. From this analysis, tennis was selected from the 10 most frequently played sports, and cricket was selected from the 10 least frequently played sports for both genders.

Participant recruitment

NSOs were recruited with the support of the ASC. The ASC was consulted for appropriate contacts within the two NSOs, who then recruited colleagues for the NSO focus group interviews. Paid employees of Tennis Australia and Cricket Australia with an interest in community-based sport participation were eligible to participate. Sport club members were recruited with the support of the two NSOs, who recommended sport clubs to contact for focus group interview participation. Additional sport clubs were also contacted independently by the research team for participation. Sport club Presidents or Secretaries were initially contacted, and they recruited eligible participants from their respective clubs. Eligible participants were aged 50 years or over, and either actively played the sport in the club or were involved in the coaching or administrative aspect of the club. Two interviews were held with tennis club members and two interviews with cricket club members. Each sport club member interview was stratified for gender. For the remaining two interviews, non-sport club members were invited to participate. These participants were recruited through public advertisements or community groups. Eligible participants for the non-sport club member interviews were aged 50 years or over and did not belong to a sport club. These two interviews were also stratified for gender.

Procedures

The focus group interviews were semi-structured interviews, and the socioecological model was used as a framework to develop the interview schedule. The socioecological model (Sallis *et al.*

2008) can be used to understand sport participation behaviour from various perspectives. As previously stated, current research on older adults and sport has mainly focused on the intrapersonal domains of participation, with some research on the interpersonal domains. Thus, this study focused on the interpersonal, organisational and policy domains of the model, and how themes within these domains may influence each other. The socioecological model is increasingly being used within the area of sport participation, including with adolescents (Casey *et al.* 2009a, Toftegaard-Støckel *et al.* 2011, Eime *et al.* 2013) and people living in socio-economically deprived neighbourhoods (Cleland *et al.* 2010). It has also been used in ageing literature for understanding health behaviours (Marquez *et al.* 2009) and mobility limitation (Yeom *et al.* 2008).

The NSOs' focus group interviews were the first interviews held. As the focus of this study was on the organisational perspective of older adults' participation, themes arising from their discussions were used to inform the subsequent focus group discussions for the sport club and non-sport club members.

Potential participants received an information sheet, an informed consent form and a demographic questionnaire before their respective interviews. The interviews were held in a variety of settings, including the respective NSO offices, sport clubs and in a university setting. Two academic facilitators attended each interview, with one leading the discussions and the other taking notes of any non-verbal communication. Discussions about benefits and barriers for SOs lasted for 20–30 minutes, and the interviews were recorded using voice recorders. Ethics approval was obtained from the Victoria University Human Ethics Committee, and all participants signed informed consent forms.

Analysis

After each focus group interview, the two facilitators undertook a debriefing meeting to discuss the issues that arose in each interview. These discussions influenced the initial coding of the data. The interview recordings were transcribed by a professional transcription service. The transcriptions were then reviewed by the lead author/focus group facilitator for accuracy of the transcription and this process provided initial emersion in the data. The authors decided to analyse the data using a mixture of realist and constructionist epistemological approaches, with a greater emphasis on the realist approach. A realist approach suggests treating participants' responses as 'potentially "true" pictures of "reality"' (Silverman 2010) and a constructionist approach involves 'accessing various stories or narratives through which people describe their world' (Silverman 2010).

The transcripts were analysed using a hybrid approach of content and thematic analyses (Patton 2002) by the lead author. Content analysis utilised the socioecological model as the analysis framework to determine the main themes within each of the socioecological domains (Sallis *et al.* 2008) that were deemed appropriate for this study (interpersonal, organisational and policy). The transcripts were coded using NVIVO 10, and thematic analysis with a mix of latent and semantic coding was then used to develop emerging themes within the socioecological domains.

Semantic coding involved analysis of what the participant had said, whereas latent coding involved analysis of the reasoning why a statement was made (Braun and Clarke 2006). Semantic coding was mostly used, but where body language and group dynamics or tensions impacted verbal responses, latent coding was used. Data for the latent coding were derived from non-verbal communication, such as group agreement or raised eyebrows, noted by the secondary academic facilitator during the interviews. The themes and subthemes of the coding tree were discussed throughout the coding process by the wider research team as a form of peer debriefing and this contributed to analytical rigour (Lincoln and Guba 1985).

Findings

There were 49 participants in the eight focus group interviews. Average group size was 6 participants and group size ranged from four to nine participants. Although the recommended optimal interview includes 6–12 participants (Morgan 1996), it has been suggested that smaller interview size of three to four participants can also provide useful results (Morgan 1995, Peek and Fothergill 2009). Participants in the NSO focus group interviews were mainly male (85%) and their mean age was 41 years (range of 23–67 years). Their positions within their respective organisations ranged from Community Sport Officers to Senior Development Managers. Both the tennis and the cricket sport club member interviews had an equal spread of male and female participants, and the mean age was 62 years (range of 50–85 years). There was also an equal spread of male and female participants in the non-sport club member interviews. The mean age of these participants was 57 years (range of 51–65 years).

Data from each interview was analysed separately, but as common themes emerged across groups, and agreed upon by authors, it was decided to group the findings from the focus group interviews according to the relevant domains of the socioecological model (interpersonal, organisational and policy) (Sallis *et al.* 2008). Themes that were most commonly discussed are presented under each domain heading, and themes that influenced other themes are discussed in a separate section. The findings of the study are presented through the lens of the perceptions of the study and are representatives of the participants within this study. Therefore, the opinions and quotes presented may not be reflective of all older adults (Anderson 2010).

Organisational benefits for SOs

Interpersonal benefits

The main perceived interpersonal benefit described was *intergenerational opportunities*. Minor benefits such as role modelling, mentoring and member diversity were also discussed.

Participants discussed various social *intergenerational opportunities* that SOs could derive from engaging older adults. It was felt that parents or grandparents who were engaged with a sport often introduced their child or children to that sport, thus increasing youth participation and club membership. Furthermore, older adults who had children or grandchildren playing in a sport club can have a vested interest in the club, to ensure it provided a safe environment for their families: 'We do it for the kids … it's like a big family' (51-year-old female cricket club member). Thus, the sport club could be strengthened by the social relationships and the influence of family members.

Participants felt that older adults were often *role models* for younger club members, as older adults who played sport were often seen as local heroes in the community: 'I think that they're worth their weight in gold those guys. And they have great stories, and they should be celebrated. I'd love to have a beer with them' (39-year-old male NSO participant). It was further suggested by participants that older adults could provide *mentoring*, in addition to teaching sport etiquette and sport-specific knowledge, to younger players. Also, participants believed that if sport clubs encouraged older adults to become club members, it can provide the club with greater *member diversity* and would therefore be more representative of the wider community.

Organisational benefits

The main organisational benefit discussed was *volunteering*. Other common benefits mentioned were financial contributions and maximised facility usage. Minor themes included increased volunteer capacity to run a sport club and maintaining a sporting fan base.

All of the groups felt that older adults contributed to sport clubs through *volunteering*, and therefore club capacity, mainly through being involved on the club committee. In particular, it was believed that older adults often undertook more volunteering roles than younger adults, and were also more likely to do this over a longer time period than younger people: 'They're home and hosed if you get people our age because we slot into all the volunteer roles' (51-year-old female cricket club member). This links to an increased volunteer capacity to run a sport club. One group mentioned that older adults sometimes undertook the maintenance of club facilities for free, to reduce club expenditure. This enabled club income to be used elsewhere to benefit the club.

Numerous participants believed that older adults were often more *financially stable* than some younger adults. They discussed the perception that older adults would be more disposed to support club functions, and to socialise in club facilities after a match than younger players: 'With the sporting clubs, financially they need members, so if you're involved with it, you tend to put your hand in your pocket more as well' (54-year-old non-sport club member). Also discussed was the assertion that older adults could provide an additional revenue stream through membership fees.

Another organisational benefit identified was *maximised facility usage*. Participants believed that if sport clubs engaged retired older adults, they could utilise club facilities during off-peak periods, such as during the school day: 'In most states there are [facilities] everywhere, they are underutilised' (67-year-old male NSO participant). This could benefit SOs by providing additional income for the sport club.

Maintaining a *sporting fan base* was another organisational benefit discussed. One NSO identified the importance of older adults to SOs: 'They love the game. So they pay for subscriptions on TV. They pay, you know, as members of clubs. They pay as fans to attend games. So both in a development sense and a commercial sense, they are important' (49-year-old male NSO participant). This NSO felt that older adults were an age group that were already engaged as fans and so were eager to explore new avenues to enhance this engagement through providing opportunities to play sport.

Organisational barriers for sporting organisations

Interpersonal barriers

The two main interpersonal barriers were *competing priorities* and *perceived societal expectations*.

Participants felt that their life schedules had changed and many felt older adults faced *competing priorities* that left less time for participation in sport. For example, they discussed how the retirement age had risen in recent times; meaning adults were working to a later age. Even when older adults were retired, it was discussed how these adults were often responsible for caring for their children, grandchildren or elderly parents, and so may not have time to participate in sport themselves: 'People are so committed now and so many older people mind their grandchildren' (70-year-old female tennis club member). Groups also discussed how working patterns had changed, which resulted in increased weekend and evening work, when sporting activities were often scheduled. Another competing priority discussed was the prioritisation of spectatorship over active participation for some non-sport club members. SOs are in competition with these other priorities, and as some of these, such as work and caring, are often non-negotiable, older adults may be less likely to spend their time in a sport club or playing sport.

One of the NSOs felt that the media and the general public influenced their organisational priorities:

> I think the media and the general population make that decision [which participants to prioritise] for us and unless we are successful [at elite sport], we're not viewed as being serious about our sport. So we have to create our champions in order to maintain some sort of … level of importance out within the community. (58-year-old male NSO participant).

Perceived societal expectations of older adults who played sport were also discussed as a barrier for SOs to engage older adults: 'I'll say I'm going to tennis. "Oh do you still play tennis?" Like hell, once you get over fifty, you shouldn't be playing' (70-year-old female tennis club member). Another participant agreed with this statement: 'Some people also perceive it as culturally, or as not really appropriate, to play competitive [sport] any longer once you're getting older, especially on the female side' (43-year-old female NSO participant). If older adults playing sport is not common within society, SOs may be persuaded to focus on age groups that are more likely to play sport, thus be reluctant to specifically focus on this older age group.

Organisational barriers

The main organisational barriers were a *lack of appropriate playing opportunities*, a *lack of access to playing facilities* for older adults and a *lack of volunteer capacity within sport clubs*. Other less discussed barriers included competitiveness and marketing.

A *lack of appropriate playing opportunities* was widely discussed. Numerous participants felt that there was a lack of age-appropriate teams for older adults to play sport with or compete against: 'At some point the realisation came "I can't compete with those kids anymore" and there's really nowhere else to go' (62-year-old male cricket club member), and 'If … they're just playing Sat comp or something, they quite often could play against a 12-year-old, which I think puts off a lot of our 50+ people' (27-year-old male NSO participant).

Similarly, it was felt that there was a *lack of access* to playing facilities. There was also sometimes a lack of facility capacity for all to participate. Consequently, where senior sport teams did exist, there was often a struggle to access community sport facilities. Inappropriate sport facilities were also discussed by both male and female tennis club members: 'Flexi-paved courts are absolutely detrimental to knees, any joints, they are not good for older people to play on.… I can't play on a flexi-paved court anymore, because my knees hurt' (64-year-old female tennis club member).

Another common barrier discussed was a *lack of volunteer capacity*. Participants felt that most sport clubs were run by voluntary committees. Therefore, there was often a lack of capacity to engage an additional age group or to run beginner sessions for older adults, as the clubs' priorities were often participation for children and youth: 'If you're bringing in players on a level where there's a club [that] doesn't have enough volunteers to spend the time with them and teach someone those skills, it becomes a little hard' (29-year-old female NSO participant).

Numerous older adult participants discussed that whilst competition was often still important to them, a *drive to participate in competition tended to decline with age*, as older adults tended to prefer more social forms of participation. These participants felt that sport clubs were inherently traditionally competitive, and therefore often unattractive to older adults, as competitive sport was perceived to increase the likelihood of injury: 'If you play competitive sports, you're still going to compete. You're not going to say, "Oh no, you can get it". It doesn't work that way, because it just naturally happens' (51-year-old male non-sport club member). It was also felt that sport clubs may not want older adults who cannot adhere to high playing standards.

Marketing was also discussed by participants. Participants felt that player representation on marketing materials needed to be diversified to show that sport was for all ages: 'It would be really good if they showed a range of women who are playing, not just the young uns [sic], perhaps a few older women?' (69-year-old female cricket club member). Other participants discussed that there was a lack of awareness or misconceptions of current participation opportunities for older adults: 'I think there has to be a lot of older men and women out there that would like to play. But they don't know how to go about it' (85-year-old female tennis club member).

Conversely, one older adult participant felt that there were no disadvantages for sport clubs to engage older adults: 'I don't see any disadvantages at all, and I think there are many advantages to the clubs [to attract older adults]' (51-year-old female cricket club member).

Policy barriers

The main policy barriers identified were a *strategic organisational focus on younger age groups* and *elite level sport*, in addition to *risk management* specifically for older adults. A minor barrier was potential difficulties of working with organisations outside of the traditional NSO structure.

The main barrier discussed was the *strategic organisational focus of SOs*. One focus was elite sport, and the other focus was on younger age groups in community-based sport. Participants felt that organisations tended to focus on children and younger age groups for numerous reasons. One reason given was that younger people were a larger age group than older adults, and thus more economically viable to target. A second reason was that organisations often focused on the maintenance of fan bases, and as older adults were usually already fans of a sport, there were limited incentives for further engagement: 'We tend to focus on the players that we currently have and then recruiting new players and fans, so that's very much pitched at younger age groups' (49-year-old male NSO participant). The final discussed reason was that children who engaged in sport at a young age would become 'hooked for life': 'I think all our research says that you have to engage them early... and they're likely to play for a club or play for longer' (31-year-old male NSO participant). However, a number of sport club participants in this study started playing that sport in their adult years. This was often influenced by their family or friends: 'My daughter roped me into doing a bit of cricket and I thought, "Oh that looks like fun!"' (69-year-old female cricket club member), and 'A friend of mine played tennis, so I joined in [as an adult] and actually from then we played every week' (68-year-old male tennis club member).

Another commonly discussed barrier was *risk management*. This consisted of insurance concerns and additional resources that may be needed for older adults. There were perceived concerns about the cost and additional paperwork involved in insuring older adults to play sport: 'It's [insurance] a lot of money ... and that would have an age factor in it, so if you're over a certain age I'm guaranteeing that insurance wouldn't cover you' (54-year-old male non-sport club member). Another concern was that older adult competitions would require additional resources, such as extra first-aid facilities. Participants felt that these risks could deter sport clubs from engaging with older adults.

Working and communicating with external SOs was also discussed as a policy barrier by the NSOs. Participants felt that there can be a lack of structure or communication with some external organisations, and thus it may be difficult to fully maximise the engagement opportunities available.

Linked themes of the socioecological model

In line with the socioecological model, there were links between the different domains and key themes (see Figures 1 and 2). This occurred both within the individual domains and also across different domains.

Organisational benefits of sport participation

Four linked themes (represented by arrows) emerged for the benefits SOs could receive when engaging older adults. One linkage was within the interpersonal domain, one within the organisational domain and two between interpersonal and organisational domains (see Figure 1). For example, volunteering was associated with intergenerational opportunities and this association could go in both directions. If an older adult was volunteering in a sport club, and thus engaged with the club, their children or grandchildren were often introduced to that sport. Also, if an older adults' family were involved within a sport, older adults were likely to have a vested interest in that club, and thus may help to run the club. Volunteering was also linked with the organisational domain of an increased capacity to run a sport club.

The findings of role modelling and enabling a greater member diversity (to include older adults) were linked. As older adults were often seen as role models for younger players, the higher number of older adults in a club may result in more role models. Greater member diversity was also linked with maximised facility usage. If sport clubs diversified their membership to include older adults, there would be an opportunity for the club to encourage retired older adults to use the facilities during off-peak periods.

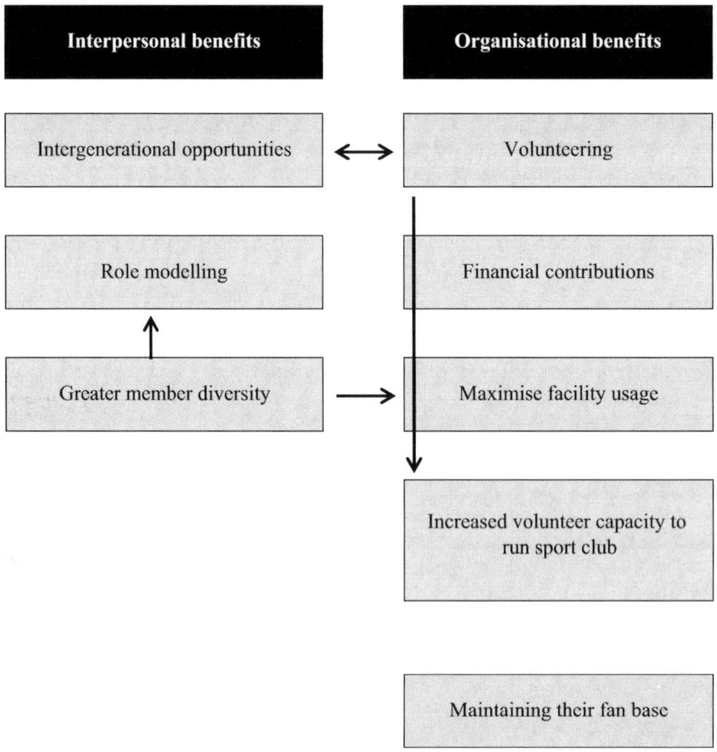

Figure 1. Linked themes of the socioecological model: benefits for sporting organisations of engaging older adults.

Organisational barriers of sport participation

Ten linked themes (represented by arrows) emerged for barriers that SOs may encounter when engaging older adults across the three domains. Seven were mutually linked, and the main theme was a focus on children and youth, and the subsequent focus on strategic organisational priorities (see Figure 2), as this was most influential on other themes. The focus on children and youth can result in a lack of appropriate playing opportunities or lack of club volunteer capacity for older adults. As the findings suggest, there was a lack of age-appropriate teams for older adults to play sport with, or compete against, their peers. Sport is most popular for younger age groups, as they have the highest participation rates in sport (Eime *et al.* 2014). Consequently, sporting opportunities are usually directed towards children. Children and young people's sport participation is often prioritised by sport clubs, as they are the priority age group for SOs and national sport policy. Therefore, older adults may not be able to access playing facilities to play sport during peak hours. Sport clubs are run by volunteers, and as such will have finite resources to engage with participants and also finite playing/facility capacity, as they may be 'full' with younger participants. SOs may prioritise engaging with younger people and may not always have the capacity to also engage a new group, such as older adults.

Another linked theme to the organisational focus on children and youth was perceived societal expectations. As sport was most commonly played by children and young people, it could be unusual for older adults to be seen actively playing sport. Therefore, older adults' sport participation may go against perceived societal expectations. This can be negatively linked to competing priorities in two different ways. Older adults prioritise their children's sport participation over their own, as national sport policy, SOs and the media heavily promote the health and social benefits of sport participation for children. From a SO perspective, if the priorities of NSOs are influenced by the media and the general public (and vice versa), then older adults may experience a lack of

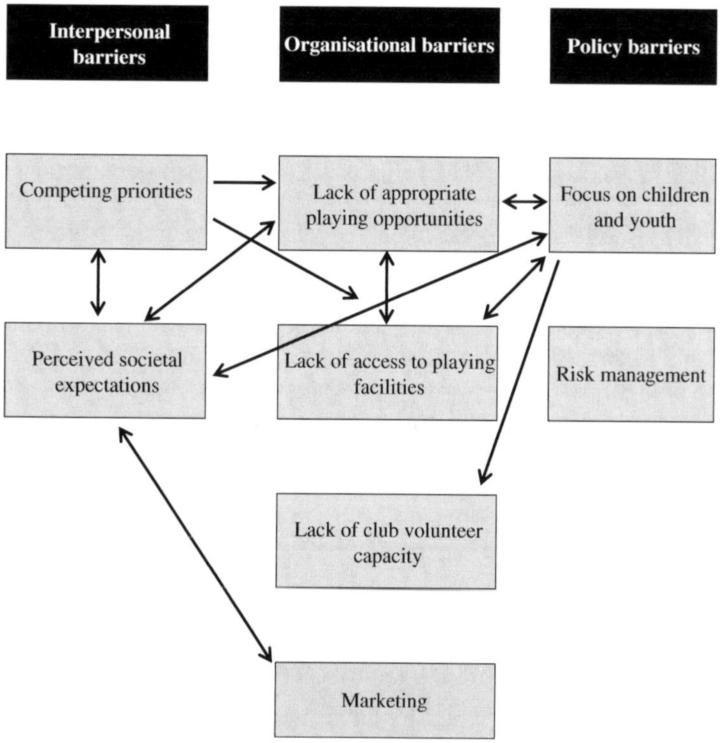

Figure 2. Linked themes of the socioecological model: barriers to sporting organisations of engaging older adults.

appropriate playing opportunities, as SOs may focus on children's playing opportunities instead. Older adults could also lack access to playing facilities, as youth sport is deemed to be more important and therefore given priority to the limited community sport facilities.

Marketing was another barrier that was linked to other themes. Sport marketing materials often reflect organisational priorities or what the general public expect to see, so usually depicts children or young people playing sport, or elite sport people. As such, these materials can perpetuate societal norms and imply that it is unusual for older adults to play sport.

Discussion

The study explores the benefits and barriers that SOs encounter when engaging older adults in sport from the perspective of SOs, older sport club members and older non-sport club members. These findings can provide guidance to SOs on how to better engage more older adults in sport participation. There were a number of key interpersonal and organisational benefits, in addition to interpersonal, organisational and policy barriers identified and discussed. Furthermore, links were discovered between these three domains of the socioecological model. Whilst this study focused on the Australian context, the findings can be relevant internationally. For example, the findings could be applicable in countries that have similar socio-demographic characteristics and for similar sports used in this study.

The majority of the themes were common across the diverse groups interviewed. This suggests that the organisational benefits and barriers discussed may be relevant for both high and low participation sports, for both SOs and sport clubs, in addition to men and women. Consequently, if national sport policy was amended to also prioritise older adult participation, the findings from this study may benefit other similar sports.

Benefits of sport participation for SOs

The main benefits that emerged from this study for SOs engaging older adults were the organisational domain of volunteering and the interpersonal domain of intergenerational opportunities.

Previous research has shown the importance of volunteers to the continued survival of community sport, and sport clubs in particular (Cuskelly *et al.* 2006, Hoye *et al.* 2008, Breuer *et al.* 2012). Most of the research has shown that parents of children who play within sport clubs are the primary club volunteers (Doherty 2006, Whittaker and Holland-Smith 2016). The findings of this study suggest there is further scope for older adults to contribute to the capacity of sport clubs through volunteering. Furthermore, the findings suggest that older adults may be stimulated to undertake this role for a longer period than younger people. The role of older adults in the management of sport clubs has been recognised in some literature (Adamson and Parker 2006), and the findings from this study reinforce this. Whilst volunteering by older adults may occur without their active participation in a sport club, opportunities for them to participate in sport can make them feel valued. This further development of already engaged people (Chaskin 2001) is likely to ensure a vested interest to continue supporting that sport club. Adults are a critical human capital resource for sport clubs and reductions in club membership by adults may have medium- to long-term impact on sport clubs' capacity to support junior participants (Eime *et al.* 2009).

Intergenerational opportunities were also identified as a key benefit for sport clubs, and can be linked to volunteering. The influence of interpersonal factors on the sports children play, such as family members, and parents in particular, has been previously documented (Greendorfer and Lewko 1978, Ullrich-French and Smith 2006). The findings of this current study suggest that engagement of older adults in sport clubs may influence the participation in sport by their children and grandchildren. The role of older adults in sport clubs should be promoted by providing active participation opportunities to further engage this age group in age-appropriate social play or competitive teams. Engaging older adults will help sport clubs to remain sustainable and could increase their capacity. However, there are barriers that may hinder this engagement.

Barriers to sport participation for SOs

The main identified barrier to participation in sport for older adults was a policy focus on children and young people in community-based sport.

The two NSOs in this study stated that their strategic organisational focus for community-based sport was on children and youth. This can result in a lack of organisational capacity to engage other age groups, such as older adults. Due to the national sport policy priorities, it is likely that this focus is reflected in most other NSOs in Australia, so is not unique to the organisations who participated in this study. Targeting organisational capacity could offer an opportunity for intervention through engaging concepts of capacity building. For example, engagement with relevant external, non-sporting community organisations could offer a possible solution (van Uffelen *et al.* 2015). Relevant non-SOs, such as community organisations for the aged, have experience with engaging this population group, and could be used as an additional resource. An example of this would be the Rusty Rackets programme that Tennis South Australia ran in conjunction with Active Ageing Australia (van Uffelen *et al.* 2015). Whilst research has suggested that engaging with non-sporting community organisations may require SOs to devote more time to engage and consolidate these relationships (Casey *et al.* 2012), developing these relationships could prove beneficial in the long term. However, organisational capacity building strategies specific to the population group of older adults are unlikely to be widely adopted, when the current sport policy landscape prioritises younger age groups.

The focus on children and youth contributes to both interpersonal and organisational barriers to engage older adults. The current research suggested that there was a lack of appropriate playing opportunities for older adults within sport clubs, for example, they wanted to play against their peers rather than younger players. Thus, older adults may be less inclined to play sport if there is a lack of appropriate opportunities to do so. This concept supports previous literature (Alexandris and Carroll, 1999, Scheerder *et al.* 2005), indicating that appropriate playing opportunities need to be developed if older adults' sport participation is to increase.

A lack of appropriate playing opportunities was also linked to a lack of access to playing facilities. It has been previously discussed that there are limited community sport facilities for all people who play sport (Estabrooks *et al.* 2003). Some sport club facilities will lack the capacity to cater for more participants. High priority age groups for sport clubs, such as children, are likely to be given priority access to these limited facilities. However, this barrier could be partially overcome by encouraging sport clubs to offer their facilities to retired older adults during off-peak periods.

This lack of access and appropriate playing opportunities can also be linked to perceived societal expectations. There is evidence that older adults wishing to play sport can experience some resistance from society (Grant 2001). Sport is often seen as the realm of young people within society, and for older adults to participate, they may have to overcome the barrier of societal expectations. However, as populations are ageing (World Health Organisation 2015), societal expectations of older adults have the potential to change. If appropriate playing opportunities were developed in partnership with non-sporting external community organisations, this could create the opportunity to challenge current societal expectations. This awareness and societal acceptance could then provide support for a change in focus of national policy.

Another engagement barrier identified within this organisational focus was marketing. Sport marketing for increasing participation is often in line with strategic organisational priorities, showing sports that are most often played by younger people (Hunt *et al.* 2001), which means imagery or reference to (offerings for) other age groups may be absent. This can discourage other age groups from participating in sport, and being active members of sport clubs, as they may feel that there is not a place for them within sport. If marketing was diversified to reflect all age groups, then older adults may see sport as being a viable physical activity option, and could also help to change societal perceptions about adults playing sport throughout their lifespan.

The final interpersonal domain barrier linked with a focus on children and youth was that of competing priorities. Older adults often experience competing priorities, such as caring for their children, grandchildren and/or elderly parents, as well as working responsibilities. In sport, parents often prioritise their children's participation over their own. This can be due to the idea that sport provides vital developmental benefits for children, which is widely promoted by national sport policy, SOs and the media (Alexander *et al.* 2011). Sport clubs could perhaps navigate around the issue of competing priorities by developing intergenerational opportunities. They could, for example, run concurrent sessions, where older adults can play sport with their peers, whilst their children or grandchildren are also playing sport at the same venue. This example could complement the capacity building suggestions to further provide opportunities for older adults to play sport.

National identity and the long-standing federal sport policies have a powerful influence on sports' organisational strategies and focus. With projections indicating a dramatic increase in the proportion of older adults worldwide (World Health Organisation 2015), a shift in national policies from prioritising elite sport might start occurring, with an obvious move towards favouring the targeted inclusion of older adults in sport. Studies such as this may well be the early drivers of such policy change. However, the SO's and club's capacity to strategically focus on older adults requires consideration.

In this study, a number of participants had started playing sport during their adult years, and this was influenced by their children's sport participation, and also related to motivation to maintain their own physical health. Therefore, there is scope to engage older adults in active sport participation, even if they had not previously participated. In addition to this, sport clubs, and consequently SOs, can also benefit from engaging older adults. These opportunities are in volunteering, maximised facility usage and the use of older adults to attract and retain young people. SOs and clubs can start to engage older adults by providing appropriate playing opportunities, such as age-specific competitions or social play sessions, and modify the way sport is advertised to show a breadth of participants.

Despite these suggestions, some of the barriers to engage older adults in sport may be difficult to practically overcome for numerous reasons. Although beyond the scope of this paper, it is acknowledged and noted that contemporary sport and its club structures is often anchored in a performance (elite sport) driven framework. This socialises club participants (positively or negatively) into sport participation experiences for life. Future research into the participation of older adults in sport could further investigate how much a sport performance focus earlier in life detracts from (re)engaging with sport and its structures later in life. Also, as previously discussed, research confirms that sport clubs are largely run by volunteers, and thus often lack the capacity to develop participation opportunities for a new age group (Jurbala 2006). Furthermore, within certain sport clubs, there may be insufficient facility playing space or time to accommodate more people or programmes. The present study's findings support this previous research. To mitigate this lack of capacity, SOs could support sport clubs to develop their capacity using the suggested partnerships with external non-sporting community organisations to implement age-appropriate participation programmes for older adults.

All of the socioecological domains play a role in influencing behaviour. This paper focuses on the under-researched areas of interpersonal, organisational and policy domains, but acknowledges that the intrapersonal domain is also an influence that can contribute to older adult behaviour change. The influence of this domain on older adults has been widely researched, including elements of social gerontology such as the development of social identity (Heo *et al.* 2013) or ageing identity (Dionigi 2006) through sport, in addition to intrapersonal benefits and barriers that may influence older adults' sport participation, such as their physical health (Kolt *et al.* 2004) or to have fun (Heo *et al.* 2013). Thus, any practical implementations must consider the determinants broadly and include all domains of the socioecological model, to ensure a holistic and multilayered approach to engaging older adults in sport is undertaken.

The intrapersonal health benefits, identified in previous research, on how sport has contributed towards a positive ageing process (Dionigi 2002, Kolt *et al.* 2004), suggests that this area provides a great opportunity to develop a collaborative relationship between sport and health organisations. Older adults are not always considered specifically in sport policy, and health policy does not specifically promote sport as a preventative health measure. Thus, health policy should consider giving sport a stronger role in preventative health for older adults, to diversify the physical activity options available to this age group.

A strength of this study was that the perspectives of older adults who played sport, and those who did not play sport, were sought, in addition to perspectives of NSOs' representatives. This provided a more holistic approach to understanding the organisational benefits and barriers of engaging older adults from the contexts of these various groups. As this was a qualitative study, there was limited scope to engage a wide variety of NSOs and sport clubs. Two NSOs, and members of eight sport clubs, participated in this study. Therefore, the opinions expressed by these organisations may not always be reflected in other sports or other sport clubs. However, the findings were often common across the different focus group interviews, thus suggesting that the findings could be related to other sports with similar attributes to tennis and cricket for both male and female participants. Future research should engage other NSOs and sport clubs in different geographical areas and with different socio-demographic populations to investigate if similar themes emerge. There are also opportunities to conduct and evaluate implementation strategies such as a trial programme in a sport club, in partnership with one or a number of NSOs and external non-sporting community organisations, to determine if these strategies increased the sport participation of older adults.

Conclusion

This research illustrates that there are wide ranging potential benefits for SOs to engage older adults, but that there were also barriers to this engagement. Whilst the participation rate of older adults in sport is unlikely to increase dramatically, the findings of this study suggest that they are 'worth their weight' in terms of participating in sport clubs, through sheer engagement and volunteering. Currently, the national sport policy priorities of children/youth participation and the focus on elite sport is likely to be a contributing factor to low sport engagement for older adults. This may be further facilitated by a lack of organisational capacity and resources that specifically prioritise strategies for SOs to engage older adults. It is not anticipated that any policy and/or strategic focus on older adults will significantly increase active participation in sport for this age group. However, any increase in older adults' sport participation, either through actively playing, supporting family and friends and/or volunteering, will contribute to the positive health of individuals, sport clubs and the community.

Acknowledgements

Claire Jenkin is supported by an Australian Sports Commission–ISEAL Victoria University PhD scholarship. Jannique van Uffelen was supported by an Australian Sports Commission–ISEAL Victoria University Senior Research Fellowship. We thank the Australian Sports Commission for their help with recruiting the National Sporting Organisations and also thank these National Sporting Organisations and the older adults who participated in this study.

Disclosure statement

No potential conflict of interest was reported by the authors.

Funding

Claire Jenkin is supported by an Australian Sports Commission–ISEAL Victoria University PhD scholarship. Jannique van Uffelen was supported by an Australian Sports Commission–ISEAL Victoria University Senior Research Fellowship.

References

Adamson, L. and Parker, G., 2006. There's more to life than just walking": older women's ways of staying healthy and happy. *Journal of aging and physical activity*, 14, 380.

Alexander, K., Stafford, A., and Lewis, R., 2011. *The experiences of children participating in organised sport in the UK.* London: NSPCC.

Alexandris, K. and Carroll, B., 1999. Constraints on recreational sport participation in adults in Greece: implications for providing and managing sport services. *Journal of sport management*, 13, 317.

Anderson, C., 2010. Presenting and evaluating qualitative research. *American journal of pharmaceutical education*, 74, 141. doi:10.5688/aj7408141

Australian Bureau of Statistics, 2013–2014. *Participation in sport and physical recreation* [online]. Available from: http://www.abs.gov.au/ausstats/abs@.nsf/mf/4177.0 [Accessed 8 June 2015].

Australian Bureau of Statistics, 2015. *Animated population pyramids* [online] Available from: http://www.abs.gov.au/websitedbs/d3310114.nsf/home/Population%20Pyramid%20-%20Australia [Accessed 10 July 2015].

Australian Department of Health, 2014. *Australia's physical activity and sedendary behaviour guidelines* [online]. Available from: http://www.health.gov.au/internet/main/publishing.nsf/Content/health-pubhlth-strateg-phys-act-guidelines#chba [Accessed 8 October 2015].

Australian Department of Health and Ageing, 2010. *Taking preventative action - a response to Australia: the healthiest country by 2020.* The report of the National Preventative Health Taskforce. Canberra: Australia.

Australian Institute of Health and Welfare, 2014. *Preventing and treating ill health* [online]. Available from: http://www.aihw.gov.au/australias-health/2014/preventing-ill-health/ [Accessed May 2014].

Australian Sports Commission, 2009. *ASC recognition. What is defined as a sport?* [online] Available from: http://www.ausport.gov.au/supporting/nso/asc_recognition [Accessed 10 August 2015].

Australian Sports Commission, 2010. *Exercise, recreation and sport survey* [online]. Available from: http://www.ausport.gov.au/information/casro/ERASS [Accessed 20 September 2015].

Australian Sports Commission, 2015a. *Australian sport policy* [online]. Available from: https://secure.ausport.gov.au/clearinghouse/knowledge_base/organised_sport/sport_and_government_policy_objectives/australian_sport_policy_documents [Accessed 31 August 2015].

Australian Sports Commission, 2015b. *2015-19 corporate plan* [online]. Available from: http://www.ausport.gov.au/__data/assets/pdf_file/0004/643207/Corp_plan_web.pdf [Accessed 28 October 2015].

Bishop, N.A., Lu, T., and Yankner, B.A., 2010. Neural mechanisms of ageing and cognitive decline. *Nature*, 464, 529–535. doi:10.1038/nature08983

Braun, V. and Clarke, V., 2006. Using thematic analysis in psychology. *Qualitative research in psychology*, 3, 77–101. doi:10.1191/1478088706qp063oa

Breuer, C. and Wicker, P., 2009. Decreasing sports activity with increasing age? Findings from a 20-year longitudinal and cohort sequence analysis. *Research quarterly for exercise and sport*, 80, 22–31. doi:10.1080/02701367.2009.10599526

Breuer, C., Wicker, P., and Von Hanau, T., 2012. Consequences of the decrease in volunteers among German sports clubs: is there a substitute for voluntary work? *International journal of sport policy and politics*, 4, 173–186. doi:10.1080/19406940.2012.656681

Cairns, B., Harris, M., and Young, P., 2005. Building the capacity of the voluntary nonprofit sector: challenges of theory and practice. *International journal of public administration*, 28, 869–885. doi:10.1081/PAD-200067377

Cann, A.P., Vandervoort, A.A., and Lindsay, D.M., 2005. Optimizing the benefits versus risks of golf participation by older people. *Journal of geriatric physical therapy (2001)*, 28, 85–92. doi:10.1519/00139143-200512000-00004

Casey, M.M., *et al.*, 2009a. Using a socioecological approach to examine participation in sport and physical activity among rural adolescent girls. *Qualitative health research*, 19, 881–893. doi:10.1177/1049732309338198

Casey, M.M., Payne, W.R., and Eime, R.M., 2009b. Building the health promotion capacity of sport and recreation organisations: a case study of Regional Sports Assemblies. *Managing leisure*, 14, 112–124. doi:10.1080/13606710902752588

Casey, M.M., Payne, W.R., and Eime, R.M., 2012. Organisational readiness and capacity building strategies of sporting organisations to promote health. *Sport management review*, 15, 109–124. doi:10.1016/j.smr.2011.01.001

Chaskin, R.J., 2001. Building community capacity: a definitional framework and case studies from a comprehensive community initiative. *Urban affairs review*, 36, 291–323. doi:10.1177/10780870122184876

Chodzko-Zajko, W.J., *et al.*, 2009. Exercise and physical activity for older adults. *Medicine & science in sports & exercise*, 41, 1510–1530. doi:10.1249/MSS.0b013e3181a0c95c

Cleland, V., *et al.*, 2010. Individual, social and environmental correlates of physical activity among women living in socioeconomically disadvantaged neighbourhoods. *Social science & medicine*, 70, 2011–2018. doi:10.1016/j.socscimed.2010.02.028

Cuskelly, G., 2004. Volunteer retention in community sport organisations. *European sport management quarterly*, 4, 59–76. doi:10.1080/16184740408737469

Cuskelly, G., Auld, C.J., and Hoye, R., 2006. *Working with volunteers in sport theory and practice*. 1st ed. New York, NY: Routledge.

Dionigi, R., 2006. Competitive sport as leisure in later life: negotiations, discourse, and aging. *Leisure sciences*, 28, 181–196. doi:10.1080/01490400500484081

Dionigi, R.A., 2002. Resistance and empowerment through leisure: the meaning of competitive sport participation to older adults. *Loisir et societe*, 25, 303–328+245. doi:10.1080/07053436.2002.10707591

Doherty, A., 2006. Sport volunteerism: an introduction to the special issue. *Sport management review (Sport Management Association of Australia & New Zealand)*, 9, 105–109.

Dwyer, J.J., *et al.*, 2006. Adolescent girls' perceived barriers to participation in physical activity. *Adolescence*, 41, 75.

Eime, R., *et al.*, 2014. *Sport participation in Victoria and the contribution of sport to physical activity levels*. Ballarat: Federation University, Victoria University.

Eime, R., Payne, W., and Harvey, J., 2009. Trends in organised sport membership: impact on sustainability. *Journal of science and medicine in sport*, 12, 123–129. doi:10.1016/j.jsams.2007.09.001

Eime, R.M., *et al.*, 2016. Age profiles of sport participants. *BMC sports science, medicine and rehabilitation*, 8, 1. doi:10.1186/s13102-016-0031-3

Eime, R.M., *et al.*, 2010. Does sports club participation contribute to health-related quality of life. *Medicine and science in sports and exercise*, 42 (5), 1022–1028.

Eime, R.M., *et al.*, 2013. A systematic review of the psychological and social benefits of participation in sport for children and adolescents: informing development of a conceptual model of health through sport. *The international journal of behavioral nutrition and physical activity*, 10, 98. doi:10.1186/1479-5868-10-98

Estabrooks, P.A., Lee, R.E., and Gyurcsik, N.C., 2003. Resources for physical activity participation: does availability and accessibility differ by neighborhood socioeconomic status? *Annals of behavioral medicine*, 25, 100–104. doi:10.1207/S15324796ABM2502_05

Fullagar, S., 2002. Governing the healthy body: discourses of leisure and lifestyle within Australian health policy. *Health*, 6, 69–84.

Grant, B.C., 2001. 'You're never too old': beliefs about physical activity and playing sport in later life. *Ageing and society*, 21, 777–798. doi:10.1017/S0144686X01008492

Green, M., 2007. Olympic glory or grassroots development? Sport policy priorities in Australia, Canada and the United Kingdom, 1960–2006. *The international journal of the history of sport*, 24, 921–953. doi:10.1080/09523360701311810

Greendorfer, S.L. and Lewko, J.H., 1978. Role of family members in sport socialization of children. *Research quarterly. American alliance for health, physical education and recreation*, 49, 146–152.

Haskell, W.L., *et al.*, 2007. Physical activity and public health: updated recommendation for adults from the American College of Sports Medicine and the American Heart Association. *Medicine & science in sports & exercise*, 39, 1423–1434. doi:10.1249/mss.0b013e3180616b27

Heo, J., *et al.*, 2013. Promoting successful aging through competitive sports participation: insights from older adults. *Qualitative health research*, 23, 105–113. doi:10.1177/1049732312457247

Heuser, L., 2005. We're not too old to play sports: the career of women lawn bowlers. *Leisure studies*, 24, 45–60. doi:10.1080/0201436042000250131

Hoye, R., *et al.*, 2008. Volunteer motives and retention in community sport: a study of Australian rugby clubs. *Australian journal on volunteering*, 13, 40.

Hunt, K., Ford, G., and Mutrie, N., 2001. Is sport for all? Exercise and physical activity patterns in early and late middle age in the West of Scotland. *Health education*, 101, 151–158. doi:10.1108/09654280110398725

Joffres, C., *et al.*, 2004. Facilitators and challenges to organizational capacity building in heart health promotion. *Qualitative health research*, 14, 39–60. doi:10.1177/1049732303259802

Jurbala, P. 2006. Sport, the voluntary sector, and Canadian identity. [Accessed 20 September 2007].

Kalakanis, L.E., *et al.*, 2001. Parental activity as a determinant of activity level and patterns of activity in obese children. *Research quarterly for exercise and sport*, 72, 202–209. doi:10.1080/02701367.2001.10608953

Kolt, G.S., Driver, R.P., and Giles, L.C., 2004. Why older Australians participate in exercise and sport. *Journal of aging and physical activity*, 12, 185–198.

Kokko, S., Kannas, L., and Villberg, J., 2009. Health promotion profile of youth sports clubs in Finland: club officials' and coaches' perceptions. *Health promotion international*, 24 (1), 26–35.

Lincoln, Y.S. and Guba, E.G., 1985. *Naturalistic inquiry*. Beverly Hills, CA: Sage Publications.

Litchfield, C. and Dionigi, R.A., 2012. The meaning of sports participation in the lives of middle-aged and older women. *The international journal of interdisciplinary social sciences: annual review*, 6, 21–36. doi:10.18848/1833-1882/CGP

Marquez, D.X., *et al.*, 2009. Health promotion for successful aging. *American journal of lifestyle medicine*, 3, 12–19. doi:10.1177/1559827608325200

Morgan, D.L., 1995. Why things (sometimes) go wrong in focus groups. *Qualitative health research*, 5, 516–523. doi:10.1177/104973239500500411

Morgan, D.L., 1996. *Focus groups as qualitative research*. Newbury Park, CA: Sage publications.

Palacios-Cena, D., *et al.*, 2012. Sports participation increased in Spain: a population-based time trend study of 21 381 adults in the years 2000, 2005 and 2010. *British journal of sports medicine*, 46, 1137–1139. doi:10.1136/bjsports-2012-091076

Paterson, D.H., Jones, G.R., and Rice, C.L., 2007. Ageing and physical activity: evidence to develop exercise recommendations for older adults. This article is part of a supplement entitled Advancing physical activity measurement and guidelines in Canada: a scientific review and evidence-based foundation for the future of Canadian physical activity guidelines co-published by Applied Physiology, Nutrition, and Metabolism and the Canadian Journal of Public Health. It may be cited as Appl. Physiol. Nutr. Metab. 32 (Suppl. 2E) or as Can. J. Public Health 98 (Suppl. 2). *Applied physiology, nutrition, and metabolism*, 32, S69–S108.

Patton, M.Q., 2002. *Qualitative research & evaluation methods*. Thousand Oaks, CA: SAGE Publications.

Peek, L. and Fothergill, A., 2009. Using focus groups: lessons from studying daycare centers, 9/11, and Hurricane Katrina. *Qualitative research*, 9, 31–59. doi:10.1177/1468794108098029

Phillips, P. and Newland, B., 2014. Emergent models of sport development and delivery: the case of triathlon in Australia and the US. *Sport management review*, 17, 107–120. doi:10.1016/j.smr.2013.07.001

Rydwik, E., *et al.*, 2013. Adherence to physical exercise recommendations in people over 65–the SNAC-Kungsholmen study. *The European journal of public health*, 23, 799–804. doi:10.1093/eurpub/cks150

Sallis, J.F., Owen, N., and Fisher, E.B., 2008. Ecological models of health behavior. *Health behavior and health education: theory, research, and practice*, 4, 465–486.

Scheerder, J., Vanreusel, B., and Taks, M., 2005. Stratification patterns of active sport involvement among adults social change and persistence. [Stratification de la participation sportive chez les adultes: changement social et persistance]. *International review for the sociology of sport*, 40, 139–162;273;375;277–278. doi:10.1177/1012690205057191

Shibli, S.T., *et al.*, 1999. The characteristics of volunteers in UK sports clubs. *European journal for sport management*, 6, 10–27.

Siegenthaler, K.L. and O'dell, I., 2003. Older golfers: serious leisure and successful aging. *World leisure journal*, 45, 45–52. doi:10.1080/04419057.2003.9674304

Silverman, D., 2010. *Doing qualitative research: a practical handbook*. 3rd ed. London: Sage.
Sirven, N. and Debrand, T., 2008. Social participation and healthy ageing: an international comparison using SHARE data. *Social science & medicine*, 67, 2017–2026. doi:10.1016/j.socscimed.2008.09.056
Stewart, B., *et al.*, 2004. *Australian sport - better by design: the evolution of Australian sport policy*. London: Routledge.
Toepoel, V., 2013. Ageing, leisure, and social connectedness: how could leisure help reduce social isolation of older people? *Social indicators research*, 113, 355–372. doi:10.1007/s11205-012-0097-6
Toftegaard-Støckel, J., *et al.*, 2011. Parental, socio and cultural factors associated with adolescents' sports participation in four Danish municipalities. *Scandinavian journal of medicine & science in sports*, 21, 606–611. doi:10.1111/sms.2011.21.issue-4
Ullrich-French, S. and Smith, A.L., 2006. Perceptions of relationships with parents and peers in youth sport: independent and combined prediction of motivational outcomes. *Psychology of sport and exercise*, 7, 193–214. doi:10.1016/j.psychsport.2005.08.006
van Uffelen, J.G.Z., *et al.*, 2015. *Active and healthy ageing through sport*. Report prepared for the Australian Sports Commission. Melbourne: Victoria University, Institute of Sport, Exercise and Active Living (ISEAL).
Whittaker, C.G. and Holland-Smith, D., 2016. Exposing the dark side, an exploration of the influence social capital has upon parental sports volunteers. *Sport, education and society*, 21 (3), 356–373.
World Health Organisation, 2015. *World report on ageing and health* [online]. Available from: http://apps.who.int/iris/bitstream/10665/186468/1/WHO_FWC_ALC_15.01_eng.pdf?ua=1 [Accessed 16 June 2016].
Yeom, H.A., Fleury, J., and Keller, C., 2008. Risk factors for mobility limitation in community-dwelling older adults: a social ecological perspective. *Geriatric nursing*, 29, 133–140. doi:10.1016/j.gerinurse.2007.07.002

What difference does dance make? Critical conversations across dance, physical activity and public health

Beccy Watson, Brett Lashua and Pip Trevorrow

ABSTRACT

Critical conversations concerning if and how dance 'fits' within current (dominant) discourse across physical activity (PA), public health (PH) and sport policy are presented here in the form of commentaries from a 'collective' research base and individual 'worldviews' that includes the director of an established community-based dance organisation, a local authority PH commissioner and three academic researchers (a sociologist, cultural geographer and technologist). Dynamic dialogue between all parties has been encouraged throughout the research process (January–December 2015). From our viewpoints, discursive differences and occasional disciplinary dilemmas are regarded as potentially knowledge producing. We share transcribed parts of our critical conversations to illustrate how evaluating dance as PA represents opportunities for challenging if not disrupting some discursive terrain, whilst concurrently being somewhat constrained by that terrain. Our broader research remit contributes to ongoing debates surrounding 'what works' in relation to PA. Our dynamic interactions are thus constitutive of and productive within wider circuits or discourses of policy and provision. Paradigmatic rivalry or epistemological 'tensions' may well be hindering attempts to demonstrate that dance does have positive impacts on health. Acknowledgement and engagement with these tensions can arguably inform policy and practice in effective and meaningful ways and contribute further to debates regarding an evidence base seeking to 'prove' the benefits of activity-based programmes and interventions as we look across PA, PH and sport.

Introduction

This paper is based upon critical conversations focused on dance: dance as a form of physical activity (PA), dance as linked to but distinct from sport and dance in the context of public health (PH). Our conversations stem from research (with an evaluative element) carried out by a group of academics in conjunction with an established community-based dance programme Dance Action Zone Leeds (DAZL), run for young people in a major city in the North of England that is commissioned via PH. We (academic researchers) were commissioned by DAZL to undertake pilot research to contribute to an evidence base on their work with young people. Details of DAZL's programmes and an indication of their success in attracting and retaining young people in dance activities can be found at www.dazl.org.uk. Our aim in the research has been to gather rich and meaningful data that illustrate 'real-life' impacts at a local level for young people engaging in dance programmes provided by DAZL. We have gathered data via a 'mapping and monitoring' approach to dance provision that links areas of 'health inequalities' (as identified by local authority/NHS-recognised IMD) with DAZL's participant demographics to highlight the significance of delivery in specific areas, captured in an online GIS map. We have so far explored the range and intensity of PA occurring in two specific dance programmes for girls (aged 12–16 years) including the use of monitoring technology and incorporated the use of local, qualitative mapping with participants to complement focus groups and semi-structured interviews. This initial research approach was deemed appropriate (by key stakeholders and academic researchers) as an effective means of exploring the community development model that DAZL operates. We draw on cultural geography, sociology, and information technology to analyse DAZL's effectiveness locally and, where possible, to inform a national agenda focused on dance engagement as a significant contributor to health, to which the 'DAZL model' is a key contributor.

In this paper, we seek to contribute to ongoing debates surrounding the question of 'what works' in relation to PA impacts using community dance as our focus – the 'what works' conundrum is evidently a recurring theme in our conversations. We do not claim to offer definitive answers to the problem, rather we draw on our interactions as a feature of wider 'circuits' of policy, provision and programme delivery. These wider circuits are arguably significant yet receive relatively little attention in dominant discourse where specific forms of evidence and evaluation procedures inform an articulation of ideas around, in this instance, dance, PA, PH, sport, which in reality is multifaceted and 'messy'. Dancing to the 'choreography' of dominant discourses present across sport, PA and PH policy agendas is challenging for a community-based organisation such as DAZL, not least in relation to austerity. Broader policy contexts reflect reduced central government support and devolved spending to local authorities across arts and health (Arts Council England, 2016, Harvey 2016; Local Government Association 2016). Meanwhile, 'Sporting Future: A new strategy for an active nation' (Sporting Future 2015) and the subsequent Sport England 'Towards an Active England' Strategy 2016–20 (Sport England 2016) reflect a rhetoric of doing more in relation to tackling inactivity and investing in children and young people, both of which are fundamental to the work that DAZL does. This is also the case in the context of Public Health England's policy on 'everybody active' (PHE 2014). On the face of it, the recent Sport England strategy reads very positively for DAZL as it explicitly states that it will fund and support dance as a named activity. How and which forms of dance will come to be invested in will be intriguing to observe. Value for money and return on investment are explicit elements of key performance indicators, as is the emphasis on behaviour change models to get people more active with an implicit tone of individual responsibility for health despite some passing references to community involvement. Emergent neoliberal 'healthiest' discourses of self-regulation and self-surveillance are apparent undercurrents (LeBesco 2011). Sport England states that they will look anew at evaluation, stating, 'We will also develop new ways of evaluating the broader outcomes of sport, especially mental wellbeing, individual development and social and community development' as a means of demonstrating commitment to their policy priorities (Sport England 2016, p. 7). Discourses embedded and evident across these policy areas demand attention in their own right and might usefully be examined in further, future analysis of the conversations we shared as researchers and stake holders. Such discourse analysis is beyond the scope of this present paper.

Critiques of the value and significance of evaluative research inform our engagement with a 'what works' agenda. Calls for specific programme evaluations to be subject to more scrutiny have been established for some time in PH (Baum 1995), sport (Coalter 2010) and in social science research more broadly (Pawson 2003). There is evidence of growing recognition of the role of qualitative research in evidence-based evaluation (Rossi *et al.* 2004, Lub 2015), critiques of standard evidence-based approaches in health and challenges to the hierarchical position of quantitative findings (Freshwater *et al.* 2010), taking a more holistic approach to health (Roe and Lysaker 2012), mixed methods in PH more generally (Kaur 2016), mixed methods in dance and PA evaluations (Sebire *et al.* 2016) and stake holder–researcher relations in PH (Oliver *et al.* 2013, Dagenais *et al.* 2015). We cannot attend to these debates in detail here but draw on them at times in our extrapolation of implications for dance in relation to PA, PH and sport.

Central to our manuscript are the voices and commentaries of our collective involvement and our individual 'worldviews' and that is what we want to give 'space' to. We seek here to address 'what works' from a position of 'listening in' to general, yet nonetheless telling, voices and opinions of the Director of the dance organisation (D), a local authority PH commissioner (C) and three academic researchers comprising (in a disciplinary sense) a sociologist (S), a cultural geographer (G) and a technologist (T). We openly share and examine some discursive differences and dilemmas that occur when attempting to carry out 'meaningful' research. We suggest that these challenges can also be potentially knowledge producing, and capturing and commenting on the dialogue between the five voices as interested parties and key stakeholders is illuminating (Dagenais *et al.* 2015). Whilst we do not address the value or impact of the dance programme directly, we suggest that it allows opportunities to consider critically the unique position dance represents when we start to unpack ongoing tensions surrounding the effective 'measurement' of health-related programmes, including evidence-based and value-based research (Freshwater *et al.* 2010). We are also cognisant of discourses within discourses, thus some terms and expressions may well require analysis in their own right beyond our musings here, such as 'health inequalities', 'wellbeing' and others that are referenced in our conversations. What we hope to convey is the range of issues facing dance (as health) providers as they work through wider circuits of policy context. Milton *et al.* (2014) provide a useful reminder that academic work is more 'messy' in real life than published papers suggest and equally that non-academics often display a greater understanding of rationales and associated research designs than perhaps they are given credit for.

Present positions: setting the scene and our worldviews

In terms of crafting the paper, we use researchers'/authors' licence to present selected features of our conversation (Gildersleeve and Kuntz 2011, Cake *et al.* 2015). These conversational narratives offer 'analysis of critical reflective practice in action and demonstrate how narrative can function as a powerful tool for reflection' (Cake *et al.* 2015, p. 472) across our diverse disciplinary worldviews. We have labelled individual comments with the letters indicated above and the use of 'we' in the general text represents a joint position expressed by the authors. In many ways, the core of the critical conversation included here was touched upon at various research planning meetings; however, it was only when the research was well under way that we decided to record and analyse this in a more formal manner (audio recording and transcription). 'We' – academics and practitioners alike – have a commitment to engaging with, and demonstrating how the dance programme makes a positive difference to the lives of its participants. This might seem glaringly obvious but it is important to state in relation to the ever-expanding domain of evidence-based policy. In many ways, the material presented speaks for itself in terms of outlining priorities and tensions. What is fascinating is how little time we all have available to really question why we are gathering certain data and offering up particular conclusions. And of course, this is dramatically influenced by our disciplinary 'homes' and our vested interests in any evaluation-based work, as Lub (2015, pp. 6–7) states '...practitioners and policy makers will continue to make use of different types of qualitative evaluations – emphasizing different purposes and starting from different paradigms'.

The sociologist (S) began by revisiting the reasons we had agreed to meet and summarising the questions that, in preparation, we had been asked to address beforehand.

S: The key topic for discussion today is what we see as being links and related tensions between dance, physical activity (PA) and public health (PH). And where dance does or doesn't fit in relation to sport and PA? Thanks to C for the idea of 'worldviews' in response to my guiding questions in preparation for this meeting on (1) an outline of our individual professional/disciplinary position, (2) perceived tensions surrounding task of gathering evidence on 'what works' and (3) perceived links between dance, physical activity, (sport) and public health. (...) A key starting point appears to be that for all of us involved in this research – practitioner, commissioner and researchers alike – we share an aspiration that dance be given equitable status to sport and that dance be given equal recognition – that dance, in relation to PA and PH, is not somehow subsumed into sport. I often use the term 'discourse' to describe our everyday sets of ideas about things and I'm intrigued by the prevailing discourses of dance, sport, PA and PH. C and D have shared their view of the five main parts of the DAZL model and what it is trying to achieve around participation, around community involvement, around dance development, around celebration and around artistic development and vocation. It is very much about community development in that sense. So it is a challenge (for researchers) to examine that and to 'monitor' physical activity intensity.

C: There's a strong consensus that the DAZL dance programme is a very successful public health programme and (...) after 15 years it seems really timely to do some research and also there's national interest in the model. So building an evidence base is now fairly critical if the model is something that might be considered to be rolled out.

This is significant because it highlights the longevity of DAZL and indicates that the programme is well established and by implication it 'works' because it has kept going and growing (as is evident in their annual reports, see: www.dazl.org). Pawson (2003) argues that the historical context of programmes is poignant; DAZL is not a new or one-off type intervention and that links to C's point above about the DAZL model being 'rolled out' or as Pawson describes, the 'transferability' of programmes (2003, p. 479).

C: [What] I'm really interested in is in increasing PA levels and seeing whether DAZL does contribute to increased levels, accepting those are quite difficult and challenging things to measure. I'm also interested in DAZL's effectiveness in improving mental well-being amongst children. That's in the broadest possible sense. But also evidence around its wider benefits as a community based programme so about empowering local communities to have ownership and I mean that side of it is really coming up the public health agenda again. You know, there's a real focus on that and I think DAZL is an absolute phenomenal model of that. So those are the areas with my aerial view that I'm interested in though I suppose really PA is at the top of that list.

We can see here how, from a PH agenda, the DAZL dance programme is targeting many policy issues through its ambitious aspirations. And, we can see how measuring PA levels is a priority. C's passion and enthusiasm for the programme clearly matters and arguably 'counts' in assessing the effectiveness of the DAZL model in question. C is involved in the dance sector beyond the role of PH commissioner having worked directly on establishing DAZL as a dance practitioner (and having been a dance performer and choreographer). One of the things requiring further attention in evaluative research is the values led enthusiasm of key individuals in projects like DAZL. A wide range of actors and agents inform this including, in this instance, long-serving dance instructors, key local authority figures and also significant community members including parents. We might consider this as a feature of transformative potential (Watson *et al.* 2013) as articulated in relation to some active recreation and sport programmes, that is considering if and how engagement in activity programmes can have impacts beyond interventions. From a qualitative, social science perspective, this can include assessing the instrumental effectiveness of provision; it may involve examining the 'meaning' of programmes and sometimes policy and may have emancipatory outcomes in terms of participants' engagement in the research process (Lub 2015).

D: I started as a young person through DAZL. So I suppose I'm an example of how the model can work. (...) They've changed throughout the years. You know, when we started, it was really just about engaging young people. Like DAZL programmes were just about getting them to like engage with school and any form of PE.

From the outset, we can see how involvement and engagement is of primary concern to the Director of DAZL. One reading is that if we engage people first, then PA and 'health' will follow assuming the 'right' programmes are in place. As a commissioner, C faces the demands of policy makers and funding bodies and therefore gathering evidence has a particular sense of urgency. Health, as D implies, is not an end in itself, yet 'engagement' is a potential means to that end. In this, we see a compelling illustration that practitioners have a good idea themselves of what works and they are also aware of shifting policy goal posts. We might say they have a realist view on knowing that they have to be responsive to policy priorities.

D: […] obviously as the organisation evolves then also public health and funding, a lot of things are driven by funding and different governments. (…) Then (previously) it was more about trying to get more young people to do 5 hours a week. But it's not just about getting inactive young people active it's about, it's more, it's how we, how we now show (what works) in our practice because in another four more years or five more years, what else are we going to have to show?

In response to D's comments, each of us offered our disciplinary worldview:

G: I like very much the idea of 'worldview' and it has been useful to hear more about these. I feel that cultural geography and the mapping (of dance provision that we have done as part of the research) in particular is a really interesting way to think about where dance takes place and, maybe not just DAZL, but it does have resonance with a question you asked, D, about why the girls come to it and whether it's place-specific or whether it's a model that might be replicable.

D: Yes, I'm interested in looking at the context they come from first rather than going straight into like a randomised control trial (RCT) and saying 'oh, if the young person gets involved in DAZl they do this many hours a week' and we show that they're physically active. (…) I feel like we really have to look at the communities and where they come from and then I suppose it's like that whole person centred approach and like looking at the whole person and like understanding their backgrounds and I don't always think that you can demonstrate that in a medical way. So for me I guess it's how we get the balance between both.

S: Balance is significant, yes. I am interested in the kind of dialogue that emerges when people come together with different specialisms and different agendas. (…) as a sociologist/social scientist, for me, understanding is always in or from a social and cultural context.

T: Being more from the sort of technology side of things, I have been looking at behaviour change and PA as part of the research that I do. So for instance, looking at whether wearable technologies do impact on and change people's exercise behaviours.

In the above discussion, our preliminary worldviews, or paradigmatic starting points, stand in some contrast. In *The Paradigm Dialog* (1990), Egon Guba described paradigms as 'options for inquiry' and also as 'basic belief systems' (p. 9). For Kuhn (1996, p. 23), 'paradigms gain their status because they are more successful than their competitors in solving a few problems that the group of practitioners has come to recognise as acute'. This continues to inform debates concerning how we address 'what works' via evaluation (Lub 2015). It is unsurprising that each of us turns to the tools that are most familiar and successful in trying to puzzle out an understanding of dance. Each option for inquiry – e.g. health, sociology, geography or technology, and how it can be applied to dance – is clearly limited in that each view shapes not just what we are looking for in the research, but also inflects the kinds of questions that each of us was able to ask while also contouring how the results can be interpreted. It followed that tensions between our worldviews were discussed next.

Tensions around what works and researching what works

C: I think there's a tension around a medical model of research that public health will always be interested in because it's come from that background.

Scrutinising the discursive terrain of different research projects helps to illustrate real tensions and issues that practitioners face. For example, there is an ongoing tension of how programmes and/or interventions arguably have to negotiate between 'buttering up' in the sense of courting favour and yet at times 'butting up' against (current) dominant policy and decision-making contexts which seek evidence of a particular (positivist) kind (Freshwater *et al.* 2010). PH's underpinning of epidemiology informs a research agenda informed by (hard) 'evidence' and (medical) 'science' (Oliver *et al.* 2013, Roe and Lysaker 2012). This is not only a qualitative/quantitative issue in research terms although dichotomies that favour the latter (and are implicitly dismissive of the former) tend to persist and prevail (Rossi *et al.* 2004, Lub 2015, Kaur 2016). Baum (1995) pointed out some 20 years ago that as PH had begun to take on sociocultural and environmental approaches, 'so the questions asked by PH researchers have become more complex, more embedded in social, political and economic factors' (1995, p. 459). It is therefore worth considering whether evidence-based policy demands are engaging with complexity (Pawson 2002, Dagenais *et al.* 2015, Kaur 2016) in ways that go beyond policy-driven 'measures' of success (e.g. Nesta assessment in 'Identifying what works for local physical inactivity interventions' PHE 2014). There are evidently policy-based questions relating to objectives that aim to increase activity levels. This tension is evident from policy-maker and practitioner perspectives in our critical conversation when outlining the challenges associated with evaluating the DAZL model.

> C: How do we measure the whole complex, rich nature of something like DAZL and the asset based community development side? At one end there's definite pressure for an RCT and you know that whole sort of gold standard research approaches and at the other end we just don't want to lose sight of the fact that it's more complex than an RCT will ever capture. So that mixed methods side is important. (...) I guess, the national interest in our dance model and how to build an evidence base for that versus the local needs which is sort of more like evaluating our practice locally, on the ground. (...) And I suppose the other tension is me as a commissioner versus you as researchers and your individual interests.

This latter point is picked up in some ways in recent attempts to bridge the academic policy divide (Fieldhouse *et al.* 2014, Milton *et al.* 2014, Dagenais *et al.* 2015)

> D: How do we track [PA]? How do we know is it making them more physically active? Or are they doing it just because, it's like, it's kind of hard because I guess I'm saying are they coming to more sessions because they love to dance or are they coming to more sessions because of their friends?

This shows practitioner impassioned engagement and alongside this, practitioner's questions that asked why participants attend DAZL programmes, the university researchers added more world-view-specific lines of questioning.

> G: It is something about 'well, where does dance take place and who's involved' and that's where I tried to get to in terms of places and people; we can ask questions of how those two interrelate and to understand something about people by looking at the places and we can understand something about places by looking and by talking to and observing the people. So they work together dialectically. And I think maps are lovely and wonderful things and in the wider sense, the online map is already, has already opened up some really interesting questions about where dance takes place and I'm really curious to find out where the more qualitative maps, as part of telling the story of these young girls' lives, where that leads us. For me as a researcher they [maps] are kind of stories, like mysteries or detective stories that allow us to try and puzzle things out and I find that really exciting. And I think the tension is, it's not an answer and I think, part of the commission was 'here's DAZL, here's the work that's being done' and instead of neat answers all of it (research) is going to generate more questions.

Comments indicate that stakeholders are often aware of tensions associated with research and building an evidence base in relation to securing resource allocation (Milton *et al.* 2014). They also demonstrate 'real-world' tensions when, as outlined earlier, there is an interest in 'rolling out' the DAZL programme in other (geographical) areas. Pawson (2003) states how the potential for 'transferability' of programmes is a *raison d'etre* of much evaluation-based research; however, against the ideal of transferability, dialogue such as ours also illustrates degrees of incommensurability in cross-paradigmatic communication (Wight 1996). It indicates that qualitative research is still seeking to establish 'rigour' in evidence-based research (Freshwater *et al.* 2010). To address these challenges, we return to our discussions of how we considered dance as a central organising concept.

Dance: it's just not sport, but so what?

> D: And with the sport thing, I think dance and sport need to be separate because I think to a lot of our young people sport is very off-putting.

In addition to entering into a five-way conversation from different worldviews, we had different views when defining dance: is dance a sport, or like sport? Or is it an art? In what ways does dance align, or not, with PA and health? What about the social and cultural significance of dance as a leisure activity? This next section centres on our discussion of the horizons and limits of dance.

T: There does tend to be a clash between what's seen as sport and PA. From the research I've done sport and PA is very much generated around a particular activity, like hockey, netball, things at school. Whereas public health to me is more about active lifestyles and because you could be walking or cycling to somewhere you're being physically active but it's not classed as sport and physical activity.

D: Is it to do with the people and us coming through (...) to really embed those people from the community to deliver into the community, so is it that the model? And is it about dance? Is it because people just love to dance? Or is it that they have these personal connections with these individuals that make people want to come and that lead to other groups?

S: We know there's plenty of claims that sport and physical activity are really significant and there's a lot of grand claims made in that regard that we don't necessarily have a strong evidence base for. That makes coming to any form of evaluation quite problematic, complex and (I think) sometimes hard to manage. We do have to find an 'evidence base' but in some ways a 'healthist discourse' already significantly determines that – not surprisingly really in a public health context. What if we ask different questions? For instance, what happens to (accounting for) dance as an aesthetic practice where people like doing it because it is a fluid, embodied activity as opposed to activity that is codified and 'sportified' type of PA?

C: Yes, it is useful to try and pull that together and to look at what is the relationship? Currently physical activity thinking is dominated by two main areas – active travel, the walking and cycling thing, and sports – and public health is about as broad as you can get around physical activity. Another thing is something about the quality of dance that you (S) were just saying – that dance is very holistic, it's very social, it's very much got that fun, well-being, joy thing within it. And that's not to say that can't exist within sport, it does exist in sport but it is qualitatively different, the quality of the connection that people get through dancing together. (...) Yet we're so far away from that being a reality, thinking strategically and at government level they go 'oh gosh, I never thought about dance, that's a really good idea!' That's why it's important from a policy perspective. [...] I can give an analogy. In the current position it would be, if you flipped it, on every strategic board dealing with PA you would have lots of people representing different forms of dance and then you'd have one person there from, let's say tennis, meant to represent the whole of sport. That would be the equivalent of what it's like now for dance!

Dance, PA and PH

C: The way we frame PA agenda at the moment and this is pretty sort of uniform in the public health world is, we talk about active travel, so walking and cycling, active living, so like taking the stairs, then we talk about active recreation and then, sometimes we include sport in that and sometimes we have sport as a separate thing but generally active recreation is where I would see us talking about sports and dance and would make a lot of sense. (...) Public health is really about wider issues and how we think about them and priorities change. Like childhood obesity. Money went with childhood obesity and of course we didn't want to lose DAZL so it became an 'obesity reduction' programme. Now it's all about PA and health so it becomes 'ooh, it's a physical activity programme'.

G: Perhaps we need a reframing or shifting the discourse around health and PA? As you say C there appear to be two dominant discourses: the one about 'active travel and active living' and the other about 'sport' and, as we've been talking about, dance is not sport. So what if we challenge or reframe the discourse to ask: is dance active recreation? Or is it something more than that? Is it about getting people off the sofa and being active or is it about links into community; that is, is it about getting people out and meeting other people?

D: It is also about financial hardships and the fact a lot of our participants have to walk to DAZL sessions because they can't afford to get a bus and don't get lifts. [...] So it's about bringing it back into the context within which they live and their environment and not just about PA levels. And it's interesting because if you'd asked us about the programme even 5 years ago we would have said the social side is really important, like inclusion, but in a way we don't talk about that anymore. We talk about PA and we kind of dismiss that (social connection) side.

C: I think one of the biggest and powerful things DAZL does is to work with young people who often lack aspiration. And don't really have a great deal of drive to do anything. Or only in terms of passive consumption, whether that's consuming TV, consuming poor food, consuming benefits – I'm being very strong in presenting a dependency model there – but there is an element of that in the areas where DAZL works.

D: Yeah, you're not exaggerating. That would be probably about 80% of people in terms of where they are. That's why I keep saying it's about where people are at, understanding their needs and responding to their needs and that is the model.

Our conversation illustrates how the emphasis of programmes shifts in the context of changing priorities and wider policy discourses of health. It points to how the DAZL dance programme needs to be understood in relation to its 'life course' set within a shifting political landscape. Pawson (2003) states that 'good' evaluation is both retrospective and prospective and encourages programmes to generate dissent and new 'institutional memory' (2003, p. 487). He also states that evaluators cannot address everything and need to be comfortable and confident working from that position. It is where we would argue that academic research can help policy makers and practitioners, acting as what Fieldhouse *et al.* (2014) refer to as 'trusted friends'.

In a health context, some commentators have argued that a distinct 'health politics' (political science of health) is required to acknowledge power and the ideological context of resource allocation, including those within PH (Bambra *et al.* 2005). There is limited research and knowledge about dance, PA and PH and where some exists, conclusions are not always positive about the PA impacts of dance (Cain *et al.* 2015, Sebire *et al.* 2016). This research is also paradigmatically distinct from other studies focused on young people and dance, e.g. where potential social transformation (as opposed to increasing PA) is the goal (Gladstone-Barrett and Hunter 2015). Arguably, critical engagement with the political context of health and PH resources is lacking in much of the discourse in circulation. A focus on value for money with regards programmes and interventions can take precedence over tackling health inequalities and attempts to increase activity amongst young people (Arnold *et al.* 2016). This raises concerns for us regarding a neoliberal ideology in which health and wellbeing are increasingly individualised and regarded as a matter of personal responsibility (Bambra *et al.* 2005). Arts funding is also informed by this discourse; a shift evidenced in the language of present and forthcoming investment priorities (ACE 2018–22). Our conversations did not directly address power in decision-making but it is implicit when we look across a range of comments about shifting emphasis and emerging agendas.

C: Dance has a unique place in the PA framework. (...). If we look at horizon scanning at where public health policy is going there is some sign that we're going to be more interested in that much more holistic view. That social connectedness which I think you were also talking about because, well, we've spent a fortune on gym memberships (exercise prescriptions) where people have been dragged, de-motivated and overweight to go into a gym on their own, and they haven't been effective. A dance programme would be just so, so, much more potentially engaging, more enjoyable, less threatening, if it's done right. (...) Recently I presented at a dance and health event, focused on trying to bring the dance and health sector together and the Director of Public Health from that region was talking about the 5 ways to wellbeing, the New Economics Foundation model on wellbeing (NEF 2008) – and she said dance captures them all, holistically – so connecting with others, being active, keeping learning, taking notice (that sort of mindfulness approach, coming back to what you were saying about that embodied experience) and giving. (...) But the Chief Medical Officer did come out with questioning the evidence behind it but it's being used in the health world in making assessments and it's used in a social marketing campaign.

S: If we think about trends and developments in discourses around health, be they policy ones or academic then what you are saying is researchers need to think a bit more about that? And if we are suggesting that dance and PA have a meaningful connection it still needs some explaining – does it involve some risk taking then, to stake a case for dance?

C: It's a really good question. I think it's really hard to prove. If you take the DAZL model we've got kids pitching up and doing one or maybe two dance sessions a week as part of the whole picture of their lives. To try and simply pick that out and 'prove' that that is significantly impacting on their PA is really very hard to do because it's so multi-factorial.

G: I like the idea of turning the bag inside out, not just drawing from what's already inside it in terms of available discourses or ideas. We can say actually if we look at the relationship between PA and dance, or PA, sport and dance we can ask 'what does it point us towards?' Dance is an affective, emotional and embodied experience. It is social and cultural, it is about mental health and well-being. It is about the broader horizons and if we try to flip the discourse then it's not 'does dance and PA allow us to address this question of health', it allows to look at a whole lot more.

S: Yet we've still got to find a way to demonstrate effectiveness and it is a real challenge. There's something about models and frameworks isn't there and how we 'measure against' or 'measure up to' them.

Demonstrating that PA has positive impacts on social and emotional well-being is a difficult task (Lubans *et al.* 2012) and when what seems like promising conclusions are reached about potential impacts (in relation to youth and antisocial behaviour in this case), the actual type of activity is not always a significant factor (Morris *et al.* 2003).

C: D and I very much want to demonstrate that DAZL is effective so from a researcher's perspective that's always a bit of a tension because if I was in a more, purely academic place then I would be happy whatever the outcome. But if we then had to turn around and say we've invested x amount a year in running DAZL for 15 years and we can't prove anything, we can't prove what it does which I know, we know it does lots across all sorts of indicators it would be pretty devastating!

S: I think its immensely important to hear young peoples' views on the dance programme and we have lots of data covering things such as 'I like this space, this is a good space, I feel valued and I would come again and it is a place for people like me'. Alongside the participation rates and the sheer numbers of people who attend and the number of sessions that are provided and so on. So we seem to be in agreement about mixed methods having a place.

D: I think that's why we focus on the PA levels because of the sheer engagement level, so from a PH point of view you've got all those people moving. The numbers are important in showing evidence.

C: We know very concretely that currently Public Health England are producing promising practice guidelines of programmes that they're going to encourage commissioners around the country to commission on the basis of the Nesta level 3 and 4 data research design which is more or less controlled trials. So we have a very strong steer telling us that the only evidence they want to listen to is an RCT which is hugely powerful in sending a message that that's what we have to do. (...) It's quantifying PA absolutely and it's really focused and that's coming at you. You know they (Public Health England) are the leading, the major overarching organisation if you like that I as a commissioner work to and it's hard to ignore that. Their promising practice models that inform guidelines to increase PA are mostly sport and in relation to that discourse, particularly in relation to dance and sport, sport has worked really hard and have done a really good job at 'proving' that sport interventions can make people more physically active. If you look at the promising practice models that have come through they are mostly sport or gym based.

D: All sport, yeah.

C: There isn't a single dance one in there.

D: Nothing.

What this exchange highlights is how sport is seen to dominate, with dance seemingly excluded, despite the fact that the Public Health England 'Identifying what works for local physical inactivity interventions' (PHE 2014) incorporates sport and PA, where dance might well be occurring. Despite that, the perception at least is that dance is not recognised in its own right and is not easily 'measured' within or alongside the Nesta 'standards' of evidence (Puttick and Ludlow 2012). Meanwhile, the discursive context for gathering an evidence base on children and young people's activity levels remains one that is based upon medical models (Griffiths *et al.* 2013) that arguably further excludes dance. At the same time, what the PHE document and the Nesta hierarchy of measuring intervention and programme delivery demonstrate is an increased 'professionalisation' of evidence-based research.

S: But what if, as we're looking at it, dance doesn't readily fit a PA model?

C: But there's another hugely important reason to get together a case, one good strong controlled trial which 'proves' that dance can get people more active because otherwise we've got no case. And currently that's it. I mean I'm very frustrated by the fact that we've already proven a whole host of things about the health benefits of physical activity (...) As a PH commissioner I've very much gone down a sport science, physical activity route because for me I'm looking for an evidence base that will speak better to the health and well-being world and that seems to be the key area. However, horizon scanning and seeing the bigger picture and mental health and emotional well-being coming through it could be, indeed one of the things might be that we need a mixed methods, that we absolutely need to do both and we need to show we're getting inactive people active and we need to show the emotional stuff because that's where dance really has a USP (unique selling point). I'm not saying sport doesn't do that, in fact there's no doubt that it does so – team sport activity is hugely connecting, in many ways people connect very strongly. But it's a different kind of connection.

S: I think that's a useful tension or rather it's useful to expose that tension. I was thinking about the bag analogy

> G. If we were pulling out 'chips' to see what we've got then there's 'arts and health' and 'sports and health' and then 'dance'. What's wrong with what's in that bag at the moment is it's one or the other.

Stuckey and Nobel (2010) assert that how the arts improve 'health status' is not well understood. Their systematic review highlights how evaluation of arts programmes draws on predominantly psychological well-being and there is something of a push and pull for dance here in terms of it 'proving' itself. Is it 'best' in relation to PA and 'sports and health' in an embodied, literally physical context and/or a more mindful, emotional context? There is a danger of further dichotomising positions within health research, similar to concerns raised about a qualitative/quantitative split as opposed to working across divisions (Baum 1995, Allender *et al.* 2006) and there is a need to establish workable criteria that capture complexity and rigour (Rychetnik *et al.* 2002). There is limited work on specifically dance and PA and PH (Sebire *et al.* 2016) and attempts to review this as a body of evaluative research reflect the range of disciplines that might (or might not) be included in assessing what works and what counts (Burkhardt and Brennan 2012).

> S: For us as researchers, we need to look really carefully at what makes an evidence base. So it's not to dismiss RCTs but seeking to quantify something as complex as the DAZL model is limited. Equally you could say let's have a qualitative approach that's based on narrative and descriptive accounts and you could arguably see that funders are going to say that's not really enough evidence, it's not demonstrating that it's impactful. (…) And as C pointed out, people in sport are historically established in positions of (cultural and economic) power and therefore if they see there's money to be had well they will continue to draw that down.
> C: We're all rebranding, that's what's going on here yes. I mean I go into the dance sector and say you don't have to change what you're doing, do what you always do just rebrand yourselves, you're now about physical activity and well-being.
> D: They're just changing the language really.

Concluding possibilities: different dances

The purpose of this paper has been to explore critical conversations that shared the worldviews of the stakeholders and researchers involved in shared research, with an evaluative focus, on youth community dance programmes, in this instance DAZL. Through these conversations, we have asked how different worldviews of dance, sport, PA and health contour and constrain the kinds of knowledge that 'count' as evidence, and how such knowledge is produced, via research. In the tensions shared above, C is clearly straddling numerous borderlines between worlds – e.g. dance as community-orientated, locally specific practice and dance as a standardised national model for delivering PA and health. To this, C adds:

> C: But what we also do want to capture is creativeness and artistic element because we haven't mentioned that and it is another USP around dance, that creative, expressive form [...] if we only measure dance in terms of PA then we're in danger of missing another big area where, although obviously it isn't very big in terms of government policy and everybody knows, creativity is getting knocked on the head in schools and in terms of arts funding generally.

Evidently 'incommensurability', as our worldviews intone, seems to frustrate our attempts to locate dance as a meaningful sociocultural activity, *and* as sporting/physical pastime *and* as PH/well-being practice. We are, in equal turns, excited and exasperated by questions raised of how dance 'fits' with sport, PA and health. In terms of 'evidence' of dance's effectiveness, we are equally frustrated: for example, when arguing that dance is important as expressive embodied experience, its PA qualities risk being left out. Equally, when dance is reduced to primarily 'healthy' outcomes, its sociality and community context is downplayed. Additionally, the kinds of research that 'count' in measuring the effectiveness of dance keep us questioning our own 'footwork', and the conversation is riven between paradigmatic tensions over 'objective' measures (e.g. RCTs), and concerns not to lose sight of people (Baum 1995, Popay and Williams 1996). In sum, in attempting to locate dance, we have ourselves 'danced' in many ways, dazzled by the almost prismatic characteristics of dance as a kind of 'lens' through which sport, PA and health can be viewed. Thus, we express caution towards views that valorise dance as only a means to an end (e.g. dance will lead to health) rather than celebrate dance as an end in itself (i.e. 'leisure', see Arai and Pedlar 2003, Parr and Lashua 2004). Yet, we are aware that dance is also always 'more than' dance. That is, dance can lead to important 'benefits'; however, it is important that dance sits at the centre of such a configuration:

> G: The thing that strikes me as we've talked about worldviews and about PA, sport and PH, is that where we started out with 'well, what's a PH worldview and what is meant by PA?' and 'where do these things fit with dance?' is a kind of paradigmatic-worldview boundary. Maybe what we need to offer is that dance is a worldview in and of itself: what happens if dance is a worldview? Well, maybe it means that not only can we pay attention to health and PA but also we can pay attention to creativity and to connectedness and to communities and to emotional geographies, etc. You know, the range is big but it means that, it's starting from a position that isn't asking 'how does dance fit into these other things?' but 'how do those other things fit into dance?'

Our discussions suggest that dance needs to resist and to some extent retaliate against attempts to 'fit it into' dominant discourse premised upon quantifiable units of PA. Dance is somewhat unique in PH because of its multifaceted nature; it could and perhaps should aspire to 'dance to its own tune' a little more confidently. It is hard to 'plot' in policy terms currently and that requires further investigation. In relation to generating an evidence base that is taken seriously by policy makers, then it can effectively engage with multiple, interdisciplinary understandings or 'programme theories' and it may well be an exemplar for innovative and dare we say, impactful, mixed method-based research. Our critical conversations, shared openly in this present discussion, result in more questions than answers at this stage, not least because of paradigmatic differences across dance, PA, PH and sport. It is acceptable to us to 'generate dissent' (Pawson 2003) in engaging with questions of 'what works' in the context of evaluation-based research (Lub 2015) and not simply accept or conform to models of evaluation that operate within dominant discourse. We are confident that dance makes a difference, yet many questions about its 'impacts' and how to 'measure' these remain. One obvious way forward is to scrutinise the policy contexts, only sign-posted here, in relation to dominant discourse, powerful lobbying and decision-making processes and broader political/ideological 'circuits' that dance moves within. The interpretation of those policies will of course be greatly influenced by the disciplinary backgrounds, academically and practitioner speaking, of those undertaking such a project and that could be very different to the choreography of the conversations represented here.

Disclosure statement

No potential conflict of interest was reported by the authors.

References

Allender, S., Cowburn, G., and Foster, C., 2006. Understanding participation in sport and physical activity among children and adults: a review of qualitative studies. *Health education research: theory & practice*, 21 (6), 826–835. doi:10.1093/her/cyl063

Arai, S. and Pedlar, A., 2003. Moving beyond individualism in leisure theory: a critical analysis of concepts of community and social engagement. *Leisure studies*, 22 (3), 185–202. doi:10.1080/026143603200075489

Arnold, J., *et al.*, 2016. Mapping and evaluation of physical activity interventions for school-aged children. *Public health*, 136, 75–79. doi:10.1016/j.puhe.2016.02.025

Arts Council England Investment, 2018–22. Available from: http://www.artscouncil.org.uk/our-investment-plans-2018-22/report-and-our-response [Accessed July 2016].

Bambra, C., Fox, D., and Scott-Samuel, A., 2005. Towards a politics of health. *Health promotion international*, 20 (2), 187–193. doi:10.1093/heapro/dah608

Baum, F., 1995. Researching public health: behind the qualitative-quantitative methodological debate. *Social science & medicine*, 40 (4), 459–468. doi:10.1016/0277-9536(94)E0103-Y

Burkhardt, J. and Brennan, C., 2012. The effects of recreational dance interventions on the health and well-being of children and young people: a systematic review. *Arts & Health*, 4 (2), 148–161. doi:10.1080/17533015.2012.665810

Cain, K.L., *et al.*, 2015. Physical activity in youth dance classes. *Pediatrics*, 135 (6), 1066–1073. doi:10.1542/peds.2014-2415

Cake, S.A., *et al.*, 2015. Narrative as a tool for critical reflective practice in the creative industries. *Reflective practice*, 16 (4), 472–486. doi:10.1080/14623943.2015.1064384

Coalter, F., 2010. The politics of sport-for-development: limited focus programmes and broad gauge problems? *International review for the sociology of sport*, 45 (3), 295–314. doi:10.1177/1012690210366791

Dagenais, C., Laurendeau, M.-C., and Briand-Lamarche, M., 2015. Knowledge brokering in public health: a critical analysis of the results of a qualitative evaluation. *Evaluation and program planning*, 53 (2015), 10–17. doi:10.1016/j.evalprogplan.2015.07.003

Fieldhouse, E., Widdop, P., and Bunglawala, Z., 2014. *Knowledge exchange trials: pilot programme. Bridging the academic-policy divide*. Report prepared by Knowledge Exchange Group ESRC, knowledge.exchange@esrc.ac.uk

Freshwater, D., *et al.*, 2010. Qualitative research as evidence: criteria for rigour and relevance. *Journal of research in nursing*, 15 (6), 497–508. doi:10.1177/1744987110385278

Gildersleeve, R.E. and Kuntz, A.M., 2011. A dialogue on space and method in qualitative research on education. *Qualitative inquiry*, 17 (1), 15–22. doi:10.1177/1077800410389440

Gladstone-Barrett, P. and Hunter, V., 2015. The power of dance to transform the lives of disadvantaged youth. *In*: S. Clift and P.M. Carnic, eds. *Oxford textbook of creative arts, health, and wellbeing: international perspectives on practice, policy and research*. Oxford: Oxford University Press, 227–234.

Griffiths, L.J., *et al.*, 2013. How active are our children? Findings from the Millennium Cohort Study. *BMJ open*, 3 (8), 1–10. doi:10.1136/bmjopen-2013-002893

Guba, E.G., ed., 1990. *The paradigm dialog*. London: Sage Publications.

Harvey, A., 2016. Funding arts and culture in a time of austerity. New Local Government Network. Available from: http://www.artscouncil.org.uk/sites/default/files/download-file/Funding%20Arts%20and%20Culture%20in%20a%20time%20of%20Austerity%20(Adrian%20Harvey).pdf [Accessed July 2016].

HM Government, 2015. *Sporting future: a new strategy for an active nation*. London: Cabinet Office.

Kaur, M., 2016. Application of mixed method approach in public health research. *Indian journal of community medicine*, 41 (2), 93. doi:10.4103/0970-0218.173495

Kuhn, T.S., 1996. *The structure of scientific revolutions*. 3rd ed. Chicago: University of Chicago Press.

LeBesco, K., 2011. Neoliberalism, public health, and the moral perils of fatness. *Critical public health*, 21, 153–164. doi:10.1080/09581596.2010.529422

Local Government Association, 2016. Public health funding briefing note. Available from: http://www.local.gov.uk/documents/10180/11493/Briefing+-+Public+health+funding+in+2016-17+and+2017-18/981d88ec-b8d2-4461-99b8-a893494783cc [Accessed July 2016].

Lub, V., 2015. Validity in qualitative evaluation: linking purposes, paradigms, and perspectives. *International journal of qualitative methods*, 2015, 1–8.

Lubans, D.R., Plotnikoff, R.C., and Lubans, N.J., 2012. Review: a systematic review of the impact of physical activity programmes on social and emotional well-being in at-risk youth. *Child and adolescent mental health*, 17 (1), 2–13. doi:10.1111/camh.2011.17.issue-1

Milton, S., Petticrew, M., and Green, J., 2014. Why do local authorities undertake controlled evaluations of health impact? A qualitative case study of interventions in housing. *Public health*, 128, 1112–1117. doi:10.1016/j.puhe.2014.10.009

Morris, L., *et al.*, 2003. Sport, physical activity and antiscoial behaviour in youth. *Australian Institue of Criminology: trends and issues in crime and criminal justice*, 249. [online]. Available from http://www.aic.gov.au/media_library/publications/tandi_pdf/tandi249.pdf accessed July 2016).

NEF, 2008. *Five ways to wellbeing* [online]. Available from: http://www.neweconomics.org/publications/entry/five-ways-to-well-being-the-evidence [accessed July 2016].

Oliver, K., Aicken, C., and Arai, L., 2013. Making the most of obesity research: developing research and policy objectives through evidence triangulation. *Evidence & policy: a journal of research, debate and practice*, 9, 207–223. doi:10.1332/174426413X662617

Parr, M.G. and Lashua, B.D., 2004. What is leisure? The perceptions of recreation practitioners and others. *Leisure sciences*, 26 (1), 1–17. doi:10.1080/01490400490272512

Pawson, R. 2002. Evidence-based policy: In search of a method. *Evaluation*, 8 (2), 157–181.

Pawson, R., 2003. Nothing as practical as a good theory. *Evaluation*, 9 (4), 471–490. doi:10.1177/1356389003094007

PHE - Public Health England, 2014. Everybody active everyday: an evidence based approach to physical activity. Available from: https://www.gov.uk/government/uploads/system/uploads/attachment_data/file/353384/Everybody_Active__Every_Day_evidence_based_approach_CONSULTATION_VERSION.pdf [Accessed July 2016].

Popay, J. and Williams, G., 1996. Public health research and lay knowledge. *Social Science & Medicine*, 42 (5), 759–768. doi:10.1016/0277-9536(95)00341-X

Puttick, R. and Ludlow, J., 2012. *Standards of evidence for impact investing*. London: Nesta.

Roe, D. and Lysaker, P.H., 2012. Concerns and issues that have emerged with the evolution of evidenced-based practice. *Journal of mental health*, 21, 427–429.

Rossi, P.H., Lipsey, M.W., and Freeman, H.E., 2004. *Evaluation. A systematic approach*. 7th ed. Thousand Oaks, CA: Sage.
Rychetnik, L., *et al.*, 2002. Criteria for evaluating evidence on public health interventions. *Journal of epidemiology & community health*, 56, 119–127. doi:10.1136/jech.56.2.119
Sebire, S.J., *et al.*, 2016. Process evaluation of the Bristol girls dance project. *BMC public health*, 16, 349. doi:10.1186/s12889-016-3010-4
Sport England, 2016. *Towards an active nation* [online]. Available from: https://www.sportengland.org/media/10629/sport-england-towards-an-active-nation.pdf [Accessed September 2016]
Stuckey, H.L. and Nobel, J., 2010. The connection between art, healing, and public health: a review of current literature. *American journal of public health*, 100 (2), 254–263. doi:10.2105/AJPH.2008.156497
Watson, R., Tucker, L., and Drury, S., 2013. Can we make a difference? Examining the transformative potential of sport and active recreation. *Sport in society*, 16 (10), 1233–1247. doi:10.1080/17430437.2013.821258
Wight, C., 1996. Incommensurability and cross-paradigm communication in international relations theory: 'what's the frequency Kenneth?'. *Millennium-journal of international studies*, 25 (2), 291–319. doi:10.1177/03058298960250020401

Examining the integration of sport and health promotion: partnership or paradox?

Laura Misener and Katie E. Misener

ABSTRACT

Cross-sector partnerships between public health agencies and non-profit sport organisations may offer an effective approach to health promotion given their mutual interest in facilitating opportunities for individual and community well-being. The study draws on conceptual framing from the public non-profit partnership literature to understand the potential role of sport organisations in health promotion partnerships and the factors associated with engaging these cross-sector partners. The research involves a case study of a local, cross-sector partnership for health promotion aimed at increasing physical activity through strategic marketing campaigns. Data were gathered through semi-structured interviews with representatives from partner organisations in the sport sector and members of the partnership executive committee, as well as active-member participant observation. The results suggest that despite congruent organisational priorities and policy imperatives that link sport and health-based organisations, there was evidence of misalignment in the partners' capacity to collaborate. There was also notable incongruence in the discourses related to sport and health and the norms and values underpinning the partnership of public health and non-profit community sport. The implications of the research suggest that despite higher-order policy agendas emphasising partnerships as a means to advance health outcomes, there are significant constraints in local capacity for collaboration to meet these policy goals.

Introduction

> During this Year of Sport in Canada [2015] ... we are committed to providing opportunities for Canadians of all ages and all abilities to engage in sport and physical activity, because we know that embracing the power of sport leads to healthier, stronger communities.
>
> –The Honourable Bal Gosal, Former Canadian Minister of State (Sport)

Building towards 2015 as the 'Year of Sport' in Canada, there were many claims about the relationships between sport, physical activity, and public health. The 2010 Canadian Health Survey indicates that the majority of Canadian adults' waking hours are spent in sedentary activities, and those that are engaging in physical activity are doing so in inadequate proportion and intensity to gain health benefits (Statistics Canada 2010). Rising concerns about physical inactivity and related health problems have resulted in the development of new and innovative means of promoting healthy lifestyles (Canadian Fitness and Lifestyle Research Institute 2005, WHO 2010). Reducing the prevalence of population-wide physical inactivity is a priority of many public health services throughout the world (e.g. Sparling *et al.* 2000). Yet, there is a poor understanding of the determinants of physical inactivity and a lack of strategic interventions to address the concerns. In a similar vein, rates of participation in organised sport have been steadily declining for many years (Berger *et al.* 2008, Guèvremont *et al.* 2008) despite the increased attention agenda in global sport policies to the diverse outcomes of participation such as social capital, community development, and healthy lifestyles (e.g. Tremblay 2012, Aggestål and Fahlén 2015). Despite these political claims, there is a general lack of coordinated effort among public health agencies seeking to engage people in sustained physical activity, and sport-based organisations whose mandates also reflect their desire to provide participation opportunities (Donaldson and Finch 2012).

Sport and physical activity are purported be important instruments for marketing and promoting healthy lifestyles and tackling health concerns (Kelly *et al.* 2010). In addition to the central mandates of community sport and recreation organisations seeking to deliver recreation and competitive sport opportunities, they also provide an opportunity for physical activity, fitness, and individual well-being (Wankel 1994). As such, local sport and recreation organisations can play a key role in the development and coordination of physical activity strategies in health promotion.

While there is a clear philosophical alignment between sport and health organisations in terms of promoting health outcomes, little is known about the nature of these partnerships and how community sport organisations might be engaged alongside local health-based agencies to promote health outcomes. This is perhaps surprising given the policy mandates focusing on the need for organisations to work together to increase their profiles and reach new target audiences. A growing body of literature on partnerships for sport organisations is evidence of the need for connectivity and collective action of organisations for broader social outcomes (Casey *et al.* 2009a). However, the majority of the research related to partnerships in community sport has examined how partnerships impact specific sport organisations and their ability to provide sport services or build their own organisational capacity (e.g. Misener and Doherty 2012, 2013). There is little research that has examined the engagement of a wide range of sport and recreation organisations in partnerships that promote healthy and active lifestyles more broadly, without being limited to specific membership-based involvement (cf. Casey *et al.* 2009b).

Through a case study of a local, cross-sector partnership for health promotion aimed at increasing physical activity through strategic marketing campaigns, we sought to identify how sport organisations and public health providers are partnering around a specific policy agenda to deliver a meaningful and sustained contribution to health promotion. In doing so we provide an overview of policy alignment between sport and health, and discuss how the policy agenda is reflected in local implementation. We draw on the conceptual framings of public non-profit partnerships (e.g. Salamon 1987, Young 2000, Brinkerhoff 2002) to examine factors that might impact or constrain a cross-sector partnership in its pursuit of common policy objectives. As part of this process, we problematise the notion of 'partnering' through highlighting the discrepancy in the capacity and values underpinning collaboration in this context.

Partnerships in sport and health

Joint initiatives between educational, health, and social institutions using sport and leisure to address quality of life issues have emerged as important policy agendas (Frisby *et al.* 2004). Research by Thibault and colleagues showed that partnerships foster the development of a shared vision for sport and leisure services, enhance organisational effectiveness and efficiency, and reduce duplication of programmes (Thibault *et al.* 1999). Notably, working together, rather than in 'silos' is a central pillar of the Canadian Sport Policy (2012) where enhanced interaction is claimed to be critical for increasing sport participation, and ultimately achieving desired health outcomes. Best *et al.* (2003) have argued that narrowly targeted, less collaborative approaches to health promotion are not as effective in building capacity, rather comprehensive, participatory, and collaborative approaches are a more advantageous avenue. Despite these benefits, many challenges also persist as organisations attempt to work cooperatively, especially when partners represent various sectors (i.e. non-profit, for-profit, public).

For example, research on sport and recreation organisations and their various partners has demonstrated that unequal resources, power asymmetries, time demands, and competing agendas may compromise the potential outcomes of cross-sector partnerships (e.g. Alexander *et al.* 2003, Shaw and Allen 2006, Misener and Doherty 2012). With the proliferation of partnership arrangements for physical activity promotion, research is needed to understand the complexities and challenges of meeting the goals of partners from across the various sectors.

Health in sport policy – sport in health policy

From a policy perspective, health-related outcomes are entwined in both health and sport policy agendas. In 2003, the World Health Organisation issued a technical report entitled 'Health and Development through Physical Activity and Sport' (WHO 2003) emphasising the importance of regular physical activity, active play and sports to achieve positive health outcomes. The recognition of sport as an important contributor to positive health outcomes was an important step to moving towards a more integrated understanding of overall physical well-being.

Governments around the world have become increasingly invested in sport, recognising that sport is a powerful means of enhancing society's health and well-being. In Australia, the policy link between sport and health sectors has been institutionalised since the early 2000's. For example, Casey *et al.*'s work examining how VicHealth built partnerships and alliances with key bodies in the sport and recreation sector with the aim of improving health outcomes for Victorians is an example of the type of policy strategies being implemented (Casey *et al.* 2009a, 2009b). In the Canadian context, the agenda of partnerships to tackle complex issues has filtered down to a number of policy domains in the sport and health sectors. From the perspective of perceived sporting outcomes, the 2012 Canadian Sport Policy (CSP 2.0) emphasised a shift away from only focusing on high performance outcomes to a more holistic approach where sport should be contributing to individual health and well-being, and furthering socio-economic outcomes leading to overall well-being of communities. Further, the goals of CSP 2.0 articulate 'all Canadians have the opportunity to participate in structured and unstructured sport, for the purposes of fun, *health*, socializing and relaxation, delivered in a manner that maximizes community-building impacts' (p.1, emphasis added, Canadian Heritage 2012).

Given the rising concerns about physical inactivity and health-related co-morbidities, sport has been identified as a means to contribute to overall *population health*, community building, social development, nation building, and civic engagement (Canadian Heritage 2012). Sport's perceived ability to make a contribution to lifelong health and well-being through the provision quality programming across all contexts of participation has become a key policy driver. This vision advocates for sport as a driver of Canada's economic development and prosperity by *contributing to the health* and civic engagement of individuals in their communities. Thus, there is significant emphasis on the potential to leverage sport for broader societal goals of health and well-being.

Critical to the aims of policy perspectives at the provincial and National level, ensuring opportunities to participate in structured and unstructured sport, for the purposes of fun, *health*, socialising and relaxation, delivered in a manner that maximises community-building impacts has been at the core of the policy approaches. As a result, much emphasis has been placed on developing strong linkages and partnerships across sectors to facilitate barrier-free and relevant sport programming that can help to realise the intended outcomes of improved physical health, mental health, and psychological well-being. In fact, the first Canadian Sport Policy (2001) emphasised capacity and interaction as an approach to partnering, however in CSP 2.0 (2012), partnerships are more clearly articulated as a means of addressing the needs of the various sectors:

> The vision emphasizes a commitment to learning and implementing best practices in the pursuit of sport's objectives in an ever-changing environment. This includes building collaborative partnerships and linkages within the sport system as well as with other sectors such as education *and health*, with municipalities and community organizations, and with schools, recreation providers and the private sector. (Canadian Heritage 2012, p. 6)

Thus, an emphasis has been placed on sport providers seeking out partnerships with other sectors – 'most importantly with Education, Health, Recreation and Infrastructure' (Canadian Heritage 2012, p. 10, emphasis added). Despite the policy rhetoric for more collaborative approaches to public health, government initiatives with supporting capacity and resources have may not materialised in these sectors to support the policy claims. As a result, health agencies and public organisations have developed innovative partnership approaches to meet the broader health interests.

From the health sector, there has also been some recognition of the role that sport can play in influencing health outcomes. In 2005, the Public Health Agency of Canada developed the Pan-Canadian Healthy Living Strategy to support the fundamental importance of promoting healthy living behaviours through coordinated partnerships and sustained action focusing of healthy eating and active lifestyles. The aim of the policy was to increase the proportion of Canadians who are physically active, eat healthily, and are at healthy body weights by 20% by 2015. This target has clearly not been met and continues to be on the policy agenda. Many provinces in Canada have developed specific health policies to address the territorial health needs. In 2004, the Ontario Ministry of Health Promotion developed a policy strategy focusing on physical activity and sport for broader health-related outcomes. ACTIVE2010 (Ministry of Health and Long Term Care 2010) was aimed at creating a more cohesive relationship between the sport and physical activity sectors to improve the health and quality of life of all Ontarians. The approach was situated on the premise that no one sector can bring about significant change in Ontario alone, and thus in order to address the apparent physical inactivity and related health concerns, collective action of provincial organisations, stakeholder groups, and communities would be necessary.

Donaldson and Finch (2012) argued that sport is an ideal setting for promoting social good, particularly health, and for delivering health promotion messages. In order for this to occur in an effective way, partnerships between sport and health sectors are necessary. Wanner *et al.* (2011) described a successful nationwide programme in Switzerland to promote physical activity through sport involving a strong partnership from the health promotion sector and federal sports agencies. The emphasis on partnerships for promoting health outcomes has been underscored as a way to create the desired outcomes, but few have studied the mechanisms associated with these collaborations. The work of Casey and colleagues on the partnerships between the state department, VicHealth and sport clubs is an interesting example of the process of partnership formation and institutionalisation (Casey *et al.* 2009b). One of the aspects that Casey *et al.*'s work highlights is the need for further research to understand the capacity issues associated with these partnerships in order to effectively develop change strategies. Our study extends from this work to examine the potential role of sport organisations in health promotion partnerships, in order to better understand the factors associated with engaging sport partners in health promotion. Thus, we draw upon the public non-profit partnership literature to further inform our investigation.

Conceptual framing

Public non-profit partnerships are an important mechanism for mobilising resources beyond what may be available to one sector alone, and bringing together expertise and distinctive advantages to solve complex problems (Andrews and Entwistle 2010). Early theorisation of government non-profit partnerships evolved from the deficiencies of single-sector services where one sector must step in where another falls short (e.g. theory of government failure, voluntary failure theory, cf. Salamon 1987). This early work sets the foundation for understanding how one sector's weaknesses may align closely with another sector's strengths. For example, while government agencies may be in a stronger position to generate reliable resource streams and set priorities based on a democratic political process, voluntary organisations may be able to personalise the provision of services, and permit some degree of competition among service providers in order to adjust offerings to particular clients or groups. Collaboration between the two is therefore a 'theoretically sensible compromise' (Salamon 1987, p. 43).

Others have advocated that government non-profit sector relations must be understood as a multilayered phenomenon rather than one of solely substitution or compensation (Salamon 1995, Young 2000). Drawing on different strands of economic theory, Young (2000) offered that multiple views of non-profit organisations: '(a) operate independently as supplements to government, (b) work as complements to government in a partnership relationship, or (c) are engaged in an adversarial relationship of mutual accountability with government' (p. 149). Young (2000) posited that because of the complexity of roles and relationships of actors in each sector, partnerships might evolve and shift among these patterns.

Public non-profit partnerships have also been conceptualised within a broader framework of public–private partnerships, which are 'working arrangements based on a mutual commitment (over and above that implied in any contract) between a public sector organization with any other organization outside the public sector' (Bovaird 2004, p. 200). This framing highlights the centrality of a commitment to a shared goal or mutual dedication to achieve a joint outcome, as well as the additional, non-contractual value within the relationship (Brinkerhoff 2002, Gazley 2008). Further defining elements of a public–private partnership include mutuality (mutual dependence through joint commitment to the partnership's goals, equality in decision-making) and organisation identity (the distinctive competences brought by each partner and the organisation's ability to maintain commitment to its mission and core values, Brinkerhoff 2002). While these aspects may be seemingly incompatible, Birkenhoff and Birkenhoff (2011) noted that these two dimensions can be defined 'as a matter of degree' (p. 4), where the fullest expression of a partnership would involve both high organisation identity and high mutuality. In other words, an ideal partnership should strive for joint commitment to the partnership's goals and balance in decision-making, while remaining consistent and committed to each organisation's mission and core values.

Scholarly literature on partnerships involving sport organisations has been primarily conceptual in nature, advancing more fluid conceptual understanding of the factors impacting various stages of relationships rather than explicit theoretical categorisation between concepts. This conceptual approach has permitted multiple lenses from various authors in order to generate new understandings of a given phenomenon (cf. Skille 2015). The sport partnership literature has outlined some of the defining elements of cross-sector partnerships through their initiation/formation, process or partnership management, as well as desired and achieved outcomes (e.g. Frisby *et al.* 2004, Babiak and Thibault 2008, 2009, Casey *et al.* 2009b, Misener and Doherty 2012). At the heart of these stages are the ideology, values, and norms that inform all partnership interactions and influence motivations and behaviours. Within partnerships that cross-sector boundaries, values may clash resulting in differing expectations and priorities (Carroll and Steane 2000, Babiak and Thibault 2009). The alignment of values also tends to precede resource flow as it enhances the legitimacy of an organisation in the eyes of partners and other stakeholders, and as a result, values may influence the sustainability of the partnership. While values of each partner do not necessarily need to be completely mutual or shared, there must be at least a certain degree of complementarity and compatibility and a recognition of any diverse values (Frisby *et al.* 2004). Consistency, trust, balance, and engagement represent highly valued aspects of the relationship process that may be complementary among cross-sector agencies despite their service to diverse clientele (Misener and Doherty 2012). These elements are thus a normative expectation of partnerships in the community sport context, which can impact their own organisational capacity related to programme/service delivery, operations, and presence in their communities (Misener and Doherty 2012, 2013).

Sport organisations face considerable pressure to partner with other organisations, yet the research suggests that they may struggle to collaborate effectively given particular limitations related to partnership formation and management (Babiak and Thibault 2008, Casey *et al.* 2009b). Research shows that interorganisational relationships involve more than basic transactions and require diverse operational and relational competencies (Babiak and Thibault 2008, Misener and Doherty 2013). Within the community sport context, particular relationship management competencies have received greater attention for partnerships with commercial organisations (e.g. sponsors; Misener and Doherty 2013), yet the capacity of sport organisations to collaborate with public agencies has received less attention (cf. Frisby *et al.* 2004).

Research context

Given our interest in examining a specific case that could offer insights into how sport-health partnerships are functioning, we focused our work on a partnership for health promotion aimed at increasing physical activity through a strategic marketing campaign. We focused on this community-based partnership to promote healthy and active living in a midsized Canadian community of approximately 420,000 people, in order to further understand the nature of sport-health partnerships as they are becoming a focus within various policy arenas. *Active City* (pseudonym), is a partnership approach that focuses on a comprehensive, community-based health promotion strategy aiming to have all citizens make regular physical activity part of their daily lives. This community-based partnership was developed in 2008 as a way to ingrain understanding and health behaviour changes into the culture and fabric of the community. *Active City* is one of eight localised programmes that were all part of a national franchising strategy developed in response to decreased levels of physical activity in Canada, and a lack of federal messaging related to the importance of physical activity and nutrition to promote healthy lifestyles. While the various franchises adhere to the same mission and core activities, they operate independently within their individual community contexts and have little integration with one another. As such, the nature of the actual franchise 'partnership' was not a focus for the current study. Rather, each local unit has it's own Steering Committee and autonomy to customise their programming to suit local needs and interests. As a health promotion partnership, *Active City* has applied marketing and communication principles to influence target audiences to adopt regular physical activity in their daily lives for health benefits. *Active City* focuses on public awareness, education, and motivation strategies (e.g. Active City Challenge App) in combination with targeted audience strategies and constant evaluation to reach all corners of the community. The overarching goal of the strategy is to build Canada's most active community, doing so through partnerships in all sectors of the community. The central pillars of the strategy focus on physical activity and healthy eating in order to reduce the chances of preventative chronic diseases, achieve a healthy body weight, and reduce stress among the public at large. The strategy acts as a wide-spread messaging and educational campaign using partnerships in the community, targeted strategies, research and evaluation, and social media.

The public health unit within the local municipality in partnership with the local University purchased the rights to the initial franchising agreement and put together the initial framework for the strategy. As part of the package for the development of the strategy, a facilitator from the national office guided an initial partnership framework for a working relationship among community partners in a day-long capacity building workshop. From there, a steering committee was formed that meets on a monthly basis guiding the overall goals and promotional strategies. All participating organisations including public health representatives, university researchers, sport and recreation organisations, and other partners meet on a yearly basis at annual partnership forum. This range of non-profit and public sector partners have committed to the vision, mission, and operating principles/values of health promotion as either official supporters of the brand, or as partners in an official partnership agreement. Since the inception of the local partnership, there have been changes in the organisations involved in the partnership, but there has been a noticeable decrease in sport organisations involved in the partnership. At the initial strategy meetings, there were 12 sport/recreation organisations involved; as of October 2015, there are only three.

A centrepiece of the strategy has been the monthly challenge for community members to participate in 31 days of physical activity in the month of October. Through an in-depth examination of the various partnerships involved in the strategy, the case provides us with a context to understand the challenges and opportunities related to how sport organisations can partner with other community health partners to provide a meaningful and sustained contribution to health promotion.

Data collection

Given our primary interest in sport-health partnership, we employed an instrumental case study design (Stake 2003). This methodology encourages insight on an issue or is used to refine conceptual ideas through scrutinising a focal case, rather than because the case itself is of intrinsic interest (Stake 2003). While the theoretical underpinnings of case study research can vary widely, the current study is grounded in an interpretivist stance recognising the subjective nature of knowledge and the extensive interaction between the researchers and the case. The case study is developed through a relationship between the researcher and participants whereby the interest is not only the case itself but also the wider implications of the findings.

All data were collected over the course of a year of involvement by the lead author with the focal organisation. As per Yin (2014), we drew upon multiple sources of data for the case study. First, documents (n = 12; ~250 pages) were gathered from the Active City Steering Committee including meeting minutes, contracts, by-laws, government documents, etc. The purpose of the document analysis was to understand the community context, history of the partnership, and policy context in which it was developed. This informed the interview guide used for both health and sport partners and served as a foundation for discussion and reflexive practice among the researchers. Second, the lead researcher conducted observations at monthly steering committee meetings for 12 months as an active-member researcher (Adler and Adler 1987). At each meeting or event, the researcher took focused observation field notes, and reflected upon these notes post-meeting in relation to the interviews (~100 pages of handwritten notes). As per Brannick and Coghlan (2007), insider researchers can face issues of access, preconceptions of knowledge, role clarity, and organisational politics. In order to help mitigate any potential limitations, ongoing discussions with the second author and reflexivity were incorporated throughout the data collection. The observational data were also used to triangulate the document analysis and interview data. Lastly, semi-structured interviews with steering committee members and sport organisation partners (Club Presidents or representative). At the time of the study, there were 54 total community partners involved in the initiative, with eight being from the sport sector. Given that our focus was on the 'sport' partners (some now former partners), we invited a representative from each of the sport partner organisations to participate in an interview, and all accepted our invitation. Further, 10 semi-structured interviews were completed with members of the Steering Committee and sport partners (See Table 1 denoting sectors and role). The purpose of these interviews was to understand perceptions of the role of sport organisations in health promotion among non-sport partners. The same open-ended interview guide was used for both sport and health partners. We probed for perspectives related to organisational priorities, decision-making strategies, and involvement levels of sport partners within the coordinated planning process as well as perceived

Table 1. Interviewees identification.

Role and sector (SC denotes Steering Committee Member)	Pseudonym
City Sport and Recreation Director (SC)	SPORT Municipal
Health Care Professional (SC)	HEALTH Care
Manager Public Health (SC)	HEALTH Public1
Director Community Sport Club	SPORT Club1
President Community Sport and Recreation Organisation	SPORT Club 2
Community Health Promotion Officer (SC)	HEALTH Public2
President Multisport Organisation	SPORT Club3
Project Manager Health Promotion and City Sport Manager (SC)	HEALTH/SPORT Municipal
Community Health Education Partner (SC)	HEALTH Education
Project Manager Health Promotion (SC)	HEATLH Community

challenges and benefits of involvement in the initiative. Interviews lasted approximately 1 hour and were subsequently transcribed verbatim.

Data analysis

In order to analyse the data, we undertook an emergent coding process involving several stages. First, each researcher went through the textual data including interviews, documents, and observation notes independently for full iterative coding, and created independent coding schemes in relation to our research purpose. The researchers then came together and shared their codes, thought processes, and discussed the interpretations each presented. There was initial agreement on more than two-thirds of the codes. Following discussion, each researcher then undertook another round of independent coding with support of NVivo software to allow for greater levels of sharing the information and the development of coding schema. The researchers then came together again to discuss their coding schema and refine the structure. Changes were made accordingly to code titles and categories based on agreed definitions informed by the conceptual framework discussed previously, and identified new areas for exploration within the data (Krippendorff 2004). The researchers then worked together to refine the categories and themes relevant to the partnership literature and overall objective of the project. After refining of the codes based on our reflexive discussions, we reduced the agreed upon eleven codes to two themes to be discussed in this paper: Congruence and Capacity to Collaborate.

With any qualitative research, and particularly research involving active membership, it is important to recognise researcher positionality in order to promote reflexivity and recognise that the meaning-making process of data collection and analysis is interactive and embedded within social, cultural, and relational contexts. Both of the researchers share a passion for sport and physical activity both scholarly and personally and as such, engaging in reflexivity throughout the research process enabled us to examine and share our own assumptions and preconceptions with the other research participants in order to promote a more open interpretive process rather than attempting to distance ourselves from the data (Dupuis 1999).

(Mis)Alignment of sport and health partners

A central issue arising throughout the research process has been about alignment and whether organisations operating within different sector boundaries can share common language, understand one another's agenda, and work together towards a shared purpose within the partnership. Overall, this partnership demonstrates a clear power imbalance where the health sector partners have more control over the resources and mission of the group, and sport/recreation organisations have limited ownership and decision-making authority. Thus, two central themes related to potential alignment emerged throughout our analysis and provided insight into the role of sport organisations in health promotion partnerships. The first theme involved aspects of *partnership congruence* between the partners, which impacted their ability to work together towards the partnership's overall goal of increasing physical activity levels. Sub-themes include the varying discourses of sport and health as well as (mis)alignment of partnership values and norms. The second main theme emerging from the data involved the partners' *capacity to collaborate*. The related sub-themes invoke issues of capacity in regards to resource mobilisation and organisational readiness. These themes represent both constraints and opportunities for potential alignment between the organisational and the overarching policy objectives. The findings for each area of (mis)alignment will be presented below and integrated with discussion of the literature.

Partnership congruence

While the organisations involved in the partnership were seemingly interested in the supporting the overall goal of promoting health through physical activity, there were clearly issues of congruence or misalignment in discourse and values that were creating tensions in realising the objectives of this partnership. The findings also highlight a significant discrepancy in what Brinkerhoff and Brinkerhoff (2011) term the 'normative dimensions' of public–private partnerships. This includes the values, shared understandings, equity, and representativeness of each partner within the relationship. While the value congruence between sport and health might exist at an ideological level (e.g. Casey *et al.* 2009b), the findings of this case study highlight the incongruence of values and misaligned assumptions about what defined each others' sector. This was emphasised in the way that each sector discussed the other as a community partner for the health promotion.

Discourses of sport and health

A key issue that arose throughout the interviews, policy documents, and in observations of meetings was the discrepancy in language, and discourse related to 'sport' and 'health'. For sport organisations, the understanding of sport was comprehensive focusing on the spectrum of recreational, play-based participatory sport all the way up to elite-level competitive sport. As described by the Sport Manager of the City, 'Our definition of sport is very broad, its kind of building basic physical skills to allow people to evolve into different activities as they choose, all they way up to focused activities of sport, you know soccer, hockey, baseball ...'. In this sense, the sport organisations most engaged with this partnership saw sport as a broad context and one that could make people feel comfortable moving and confident to participate, 'a notion fundamental to health' (City Sport Manager). There was a clear belief from these organisations that participation in sport is about fostering a range of health outcomes through the involvement from social to physical well being. As one representative from a sport club noted, '... sure its about meeting and being with people, but we are also being proactive towards health outcomes' (Community Sport Club1). These organisations articulated a clear role for sport in fostering health outcomes, but often described a lack of knowledge in understanding whether they were actually able to make an impactful health difference.

Contrary to this inclusive definition of sport that would be beneficial for health outcomes, health sector representatives focused on a very narrow definition of sport with a tendency to emphasise the detrimental effects associated with involvement. As described by the Project Manager for City Health Promotion, 'sport is about philosophies of competition, sportsmanship, long-term athlete development, and of course health' (HEALTH Public2). Further to this, one Community Health Professional described the problems associated with over competitiveness of sport which foster negative health outcomes:

> The [Public] Health Unit really became involved in violence in sports, Violence in Hockey it was called. And there was a lot of tension, a lot of conflict with the sporting hockey community not recognizing it as violence and seeing it as part of the game. And the messaging that goes out there, I think it's a different messaging. And it really depends on ... I think that parents need to become more engaged in understanding that and knowing that, so when they're engaging their son and daughter that they recognize what's the ultimate goal? Is it just to play and have fun and do the activity and learn it or is it about winning at all costs. So I think there is a lot of tension because for us it's about health which isn't necessarily what sport is about – it's about individual success and the winning piece of things (HEALTH Public1).

There was also a significant disconnect in the language used to describe the role of physical activity for health versus sport for health. As described by a Community Health Promotion officer, 'I would see a distinction between physical activity as more broad overview of things with [health] outcomes, versus sport. Sport is something organised and classified' (HEALTH Community). This perspective was shared by other health partners who described a stronger link with health from prescriptive exercise or physical activity than from sport. Overall, this was consistent with health sector views that sport was more closely and narrowly aligned with competition and elitism, rather than mass participation, whereas sport sector partners used the language of sport from the spectrum of physical activity onwards as contributing to health outcomes. In essence, these health professionals are missing what Lawson (2005) calls the 'social work' of sport and exercise contributing to overall well-being and health-related outcomes.

Health organisations emphasised a competitive or high performance understanding of sport, focusing on the problematic health-related outcomes such as concussions, overtraining, and injuries. Yet, the sport organisations saw themselves as providers of a range of sport and physical activity opportunities leading to improved health outcomes. Rather than viewing their differences as a way to potentially complement or supplement their own expertise or shortcomings (cf. Young 2000), they were focused on how their differences could be potentially damaging to the overall success of the partnership. This misalignment in language is not only prevalent in cross-sector partnerships but also within partnerships between sport organisations at different levels (e.g. mass participation vs. high performance) where misalignment and asymmetrical power relations also exist (Grix and Phillpots 2011). Where health organisations are privately funded with substantial resources dictated by strict policy agendas, sport organisations tend to exist more in the non-profit sector relying on fluid resources and lacking stability, making them more reliant on the support of external partners. This was illustrated by a community sport partner who noted: 'We are working hand-to-mouth to get our stuff done, where they have loads of people and money to make it happen' (Community Sport Club 1).

(Mis)Alignment of partnership values and norms

Similar to the lack of congruency between the language used among partners, there was notable misalignment in the underlying values, or conceptions of what is important among sport and health sector organisations. Relatedly, the data also revealed that there was discrepancy in the social norms or expectations for behaviour between the sport and health partners. While values and norms are both social constructions that are intricately linked and often used interchangeably, it is important to distinguish between: (1) the central values each partner holds; (2) perceptions of the value of each partner's contribution to the partnership itself; and (3) the social norms or expectations of the partnership that result from these values.

One almost universally accepted value connected to physical activity policy is that sport and exercise are positively linked to health. This dominant ideal of 'healthy living' through active movement is reflected in the broader policy agenda of improving population-level physical activity in *Active City*. This shared belief in the positive impact of physical activity for health represented a foundational value of both sport and health partners and a key area of alignment. Further to this, partners also valued the idea of a partnership approach to address the physical activity messaging 'clutter' that was prominent in the sector with the proliferation of messaging about healthy lifestyles. This supports Mansfield *et al.* (2010) articulation that policy and strategy connected to physical activity (and sport) and health tends to share the values and assumptions reflective of a positive active lifestyle. Despite this synergy, there was a notable misalignment in perceptions of the value of each partner's contribution to the partnership itself.

Generally, there were some doubts about whether sport organisations can be effectively integrated into a programme such as Active City, despite the potential to act as an important site for achieving positive public health outcomes. For example, during Steering Committee meetings, sport was only referred to in terms of the high-level competitive aspects, with little reference to the participation level and related health outcomes. In fact, one member of the Steering Committee from the nursing sector commented during a discussion of potential new partners to bring on board, 'I don't know why sport organizations would want to be part of this initiative because it just doesn't fit with their competition agenda' (HEALTH Care). Despite policy agendas guiding the possibility of sport for broader health outcomes through mass participation (e.g. WHO 2003), representatives of non-sport organisations still viewed sport in an elite and potentially detrimental light. Health sector partners had difficulty articulating the potential health outcomes associated with sport involvement, suggesting the competitive values might actually be incongruent with the health promotion perspective and offered their perspective of what they should be doing. Most sport interviewees had a broader perspective on the role of their sector within the Active City, although they also recognised that sport organisations, even at the community level, often placed significant emphasis on high performance perspectives, which might compromise the value of their contribution to the partnership.

Some of the sport partners also viewed the competitive aspects of sport and the related assumptions regarding unhealthy behaviours to be problematic and detract from how they wanted to be perceived by others in the community. This challenge has been identified by others such as Murphy and Waddington (1998) who discussed the administrative complexity of managing sport and health policy for sustainable implementation strategies. Shaw and Allen (2006) have also noted how diverse values and perceptions of others may impact the functioning of a partnership, and this was evident in multiple ways within the current case. The (in)congruence in values within the partnership clearly impacted on their ability to fulfil their health promotion mandate. Our findings reflect that while setting an agenda through policy aims might be strategic, it does not necessarily translate into action (May *et al.* 2013). Further, disparity in values and the value of partnering itself may be more evident with partners rooted in different sectors given the inherent differences in motivation, structure, resources, and stakeholder demands (Gazley and Brudney 2007).

The (mis)alignment in values and understanding of one another's contribution also influenced the norms that were discussed in terms of expected activities or behaviours from each partner. Participants referred to several social norms that stem from the perceived value of each partner and could be viewed as instructional for how each partner should behave and contribute.

> I think they [sport] should have more of a role than they currently do in the promoting the health side of things. I think we get all hung up on the here and now and not the long term and I think health is much more of a long-term kind of outcome of sport and activity, but I know a lot of sport organizations focus on now. I'm winning games or getting participants now and not thinking about sustainability of that activity and that sport long term. (SPORT Club3)

Given that the values of the sport partners seem to align with high performance outcomes even at the community level, it often means that little attention is being paid to potential health outcomes. This certainly also links to capacity issues for these organisations where work is often done with small budgets and limited human resources. But others did see the opportunity to bring together the perceived values of sport as a way to clearly link the discourses of sport and health:

> I think that the Aussie Model really merges that sort of competitive aspect of sport with the social aspect of sport and strikes a much greater balance and therefore I think has a potentially greater role in health promotion than the competitive does. (SPORT Municipal)

Misalignment was also evident in the norms or expectations regarding the actual implementation of Active City and the contributions of each partner in the processes needed to deliver the campaign. The whole idea of *Active City* is about a social marketing campaign, and as articulated by the City Sport Manager, 'some partner organizations were used to programming kinds of things because that's what they are really good at, for example the sport sector, but what we [Active City] are about is social marketing which is very different' (SPORT Municipal). Further to this, a sport sector member who recently left the partnership commented, 'we spent all our time designing a pamphlet, there was no objectives or no direction in regards to doing recreation or in regards to doing sports' (SPORT Club1). This is clearly a disconnect in terms of the expected norms where health sector members understood the value of social marketing for social change, yet sport partners wanted more concrete programming. Thus, it was evident that there was incongruence in the narratives of each sector in terms of a common language and set of values and norms for which to continue this partnership. These findings also demonstrate the complexity in setting policy agenda that links sport and health without clear understanding of local implementation practices and the values that inform these practices (c.f. Mackintosh 2011). It is perhaps not surprising, though, that the salience of values and norms emerged as important themes within the partnership context as value congruence has been identified as central to sport organisation functioning and deep rooted norms and values are also critical in shaping the conditions under which we can expect convergence in sport policy (Houlihan 2012).

Together, the findings related to values and norms challenge the very notion of 'partnering' in this context. Given that the *Active City* partnership was initiated by the public sector, and that the resources to purchase the licensing agreement were provided exclusively from that agency, the ownership and investment in the partnership was inherently skewed, and thus lacked a central feature of public-private partnerships: mutuality (Brinkerhoff 2002). This was also demonstrated through the decrease in sport partners over the 'life' of the health promotion projects and the lack of engagement in leadership roles from sport organisation representatives. This imbalance may be expected given that the central purpose of the partnership (health promotion) is more closely aligned with the mission of the public health agency rather than the mandates of the various sport partners whose central purpose is to provide direct and accessible sport services in the community. Therefore, the discrepancy in bringing together partners with imbalanced resources and varying degrees of strategic interest may actually represent paradox rather than partnership (cf. Forsyth 2010).

Capacity to collaborate

Casey *et al.*'s (2012) research demonstrated that sport organisations with the financial and human resources to support change could implement health promotion programmes but that formalised and systematic efforts were needed to achieve significant changes in culture and systems. Essentially, both sport and non-sport organisations in the current case lacked a strategic focus in terms of how to integrate sport within the health promotion partnership and related social marketing tactics, thus relying on the partnership as a catalyst for alignment rather than relying on their own strategic planning and capacity to shape their strategic involvement. This led to a key issue that seems to arise in all discussions of partnership – capacity related to the formation and sustainability of partnerships. In this case, the capacity issues were perhaps exacerbated by the differences across sectors where the health-based organisations and policy structures were embedded in private (commercial) or government funded entities (Public Health, University, Private Health Sector) versus the sport partners which were primarily non-profit (Community Sport Organisations) or municipal (City Sport and Recreation). Two central issues emerged related to capacity to collaborate are: (1) resource mobilisation, and (2) organisational readiness.

Resource mobilisation

In a time of such fiscal austerity, all public sector organisations are faced with challenges of limited financial resources. While the lack of resources can certainly give rise to opportunities for partnering where sharing of resources is possible, it can also have the opposite effect where organisations become protective about what little resources that they do have, contributing to negative consequences among partners (Frisby *et al.* 2004). In this case, there are two critical aspects for discussion that emerge around the issue of financial resources. First, the sport sector perceives the health sector to be abundant in resources and seems to have an expectation of getting something more than a social service mandate out of the partnership. The health sector partners also recognised and noted this dominant perception among the sport partners. This directly relates to the misperceptions about what each sector is about in a social marketing partnership venture and has led to a tension between the two sectors where sport organisations are likely not going to be engaged in the partnership because of the resource constraints. 'We have access to people and we have access to money – those are two big things that sport organizations want' (HEALTH

Community). Among the health sector, there was also a perception that sport organisations want something tangible from this type of partnership, which is not necessarily what the relationship was intended to provide or represent. As described by the Manager of Public Health, 'they're [sport organizations] are looking for something more tangible – what else am I going to get? Am I going to get any balls? Money is the big thing and if we don't have it, they walk away' (HEALTH Public1). The perception was that these community sport organisations have an expectation of gaining resources through the partnership opportunity rather than seeing the broader picture of overall capacity building through these relationships. 'I guess they want sponsors, not partners' (HEALTH Community2).

The gap in perceptions of capacity between the sport and health partners highlights an important issue for cross-sector partnerships in terms of alignment and education related to resource availability. The research to date has revealed that community sport organisations reach out to cross-sector partners for multiple reasons and to mobilise both tangible and intangible resources including enhancing their programmes and services, improving operations, and building their community presence (Misener and Doherty 2012, 2013). However, these studies have not isolated outcomes from specific public sector partners where the stability of funding sources, and formalised decision-making processes may influence perceptions of resource mobilisation.

Another key area of resource capacity that became apparent in the discussions was human resources in that health sector personnel are paid staff, whereas typically sport organisations are run by volunteers. Herein the knowledge, time, and overall human capacity to sustain a partnership becomes even more difficult for sport organisations relying on volunteers. In relation to the idea of this being a social marketing campaign, the President of a Community Recreation and Sport Organisation described it best:

> I think at the most local level those sporting organizations, they're most worried about registration processes, getting kids on the right teams, finding volunteer coaches, securing facilities for the kids to play and participate at. And this is all largely done at a volunteer level. So who owns promotion and how do they really drive the behaviours that are going to be needed for it to be successful? (SPORT Club2)

There was also some tension between the sectors about the perspective of the paid staff with the knowledge and resources available to participate fully in the partnership. At one steering committee meeting, the Chair commented on the 'rolling cast of characters' coming to the meetings due to the volunteer turnover rate in many of the partner organisations. This was viewed as prohibitive in moving the Active City agenda forward. The expectation was that sport organisations needed stronger human capital and expertise to be more involved and fulfil their function as partners in the campaign: 'I think sport organizations should have someone who knows health promotion and can be involved in these aspects' (HEALTH Public2). As such, the volunteer-paid staff divide was a perceived constraint or under-mobilised resource.

The mobilisation of volunteers and participants was discussed as a strength and key resource for the Active City agenda. Particularly, sport organisations' access to a large network of volunteers was complemented by the health unit's access and reputation among a large population/participant base. Further, the availability and willingness of key local sport personalities has always been a resource for all promotion opportunities in the city and Active City was no exception.

> I can imagine that sport organizations would love our distribution network, and I know we would love theirs. They have people, they have what we often refer to as "cool role models", so they have connections to motivational levers which is key for the health sector. (HEALTH/SPORT Municipal)

Thus, the opportunity to use and build on the strengths of one another's existing networks created a new form of resource mobilisation among the partners. Further, the opportunity for cross-promotion was a key strength of the partnership and how it could be strengthened for both sectors' benefit. In fact, some saw the lack of resources as an opportunity to get creative about the way that health and sport are conceptualised. The City Sport Manager indicated that 'from the point of social capital as it were invested in organizations, the fact that people [in sport] are already linked, that they've got networks of people, I think that is a real resource'. While traditional resources of financial and human capital might not be in abundance, some saw the ongoing potential of the partnership more about the opportunity created from the linkages.

These findings support the notion of leveraging one another's assets or strengths to build further capacity and secure resources scarcest for the respective sector (Gazley and Brudney 2007). These actions demonstrate a willingness to work interdependently as both parties become more engaged in the initiative, and share resources in pursuit of mutual benefit. This exchange is central to the sustainability of a government non-profit partnership (Gazley and Brudney 2007).

Organisational readiness

Part of the constraints of the partnerships has been about whether the organisations were really ready to take on the task of working together to promote health in the broadest sense. In some respects, interviewees and members of the steering committee at the meetings expressed a concern about the fast tracking of initiatives that were not yet ready. At an early steering committee meeting, the Chair commented on how some of the principles that came from the national strategy seemed for the 'policy-folks' and not those actually working in health promotion and sport. This speaks to the organisational readiness of the partners to work together, and aligns with the literature suggesting that readiness is a key aspect of overall capacity building among sport and non-profit organisations (Casey *et al.* 2012). As indicated by a representative whose role in the city overlaps sport and health, 'Don't forget we're all social services folks, so we're warm and fuzzy, we like to dream big, and then we often run into resource and capacity issues, but it doesn't stop our enthusiasm and our motivation' (HEALTH/SPORT Municipal). So it would appear that while there may be good intentions behind working together on promoting health outcomes, numerous capacity constraints continue to hinder partner readiness to participate fully.

For many of the partners, the policy agenda of health promotion through physical activity and sport and vice versa is poorly understood if known at all. References to the sport policy agenda focused on issues related to high performance outcomes rather than the health outcomes that are apparent in the policy trajectory. In asking about the policy perspectives, only one partner from the municipality who had been a recreation specialist for many years could speak to the policy agenda in relation to the overarching agenda:

> I think the Canadian sport strategy and the coaching models and the various initiatives underway now really are helping change the fundamental understanding of how we should be approaching lifelong activity, and I think it's recognizing the social benefits of sport and all that stuff. So as a distribution point, as a way to get messages out to people, I think they could do a better job at just providing recreational activity versus competitive activity, and address the health outcomes desired. (SPORT Municipal)

Part of the potential lack of readiness from the partners could stem back to the initial formation of the group to lead the strategy. The public health unit and the local university partnered in bringing the franchise to the city. 'We were looking for something that would create an overarching brand' (HEALTH Municipal). Yet, it was unclear for many of the sport organisations as to why the idea of a brand was needed, suggesting that perhaps they do not see the same need to create these partnership opportunities. 'Given our already stretched resources, this was one more thing to think about, and we did not really know what it was all about, in fact, I'm still not sure I get it' (SPORT Club3). Given the lack of understanding, it is not surprising that sport organisations were not prepared to engage in an official partnership agreement, but rather remained partners through supporting the brand. Many of the organisations also talked about the high rates of turnover and not knowing who might be able to part of the health promotion agenda over the longer term. 'Someone needs to be the champion in the organization, and I'm not sure whom that would be if I left' (SPORT Club2). These findings offer further empirical evidence to Casey *et al.*'s (2012) prior research which demonstrated that organisational readiness, and particularly climate and capacity, is central for the success of programme implementation or capacity building initiatives. Indeed, Millar and Doherty's (2016) model of capacity building in community sport highlights the critical role of readiness as a component of successful organisational change and a way of explaining barriers to sustainability among sport-related organisations. In the current case, the different understandings and agendas of the sport and health partners also served as barriers to readiness in pursuit of a greater/joint objective.

In looking forward to the future agenda of the social marketing campaign, members felt optimistic about the opportunity to revitalise the partnership, 'I'm hoping that as our Active City challenge evolves, we have a sport champion or sport champions in the city that can say let's get sport organizations involved in thinking about how they can reach out and help embrace that whole public health kind of message' (Health/Sport Municipal). The Steering Committee discussed at many meetings, and used the opportunity of the Partner Forum, ways to attempt to reconnect with sport partners now that they might be a stage of readiness to be more involved, as the specific social marketing aspects were more established. In some respects, sport organisations might be 'more interested in being involved now that much of the early leg work is completed because they really weren't prepared to take that part on' (HEALTH Municipal). In effect, these findings demonstrate some misalignment in terms of multiple sectors contributing to a broad health promotion partnership, but also highlight the potential and opportunity to embrace a more collaborative policy-led perspective of health promotion (Casey *et al.* 2009b).

Conclusions and implications

This case demonstrates that while there may be a policy agenda driving the connection between the sport and health sectors, there are clearly numerous factors constraining the implementation of the partnership. For example, due to the limited capacity and scarce resources of community sport organisations, the basic question expressed by one participant, 'are we going to get any balls?', speaks to their primary concern for resource acquisition (i.e. sport equipment) through partnerships in order to improve the quality of their programme or their basic operations. These desired partnership outcomes are consistent with the findings of previous research in the community sport context (e.g. Casey *et al.* 2009a, Misener and Doherty 2012, 2013). The findings also provide new insight for the partnership literature in the community sport context that has previously focused on the qualities of the relationship process and dynamics between partners (e.g. trust, consistency, balance) amidst inter-organisational relationships that serve a utilitarian purpose for the sport organisation and a given partner (e.g. Misener and Doherty 2012, 2013). In those cases, the focal sport organisations sought out or were sought by specific partners that had a clear understanding of the sport organisation's mission and were able to align with and/or offer a particular desirable outcome. The findings of the current study draw attention to the importance of understanding a partner's values (cf. Shaw and Allen 2006), and how diverse values may impact the functioning of the partnership when in pursuit of a shared or common objective versus their respective or independent goals.

Our results further suggest that despite an overarching policy imperative from both the federal and provincial levels, the focus of policy rhetoric tends to be on outcomes with little groundwork done to ensure that either sport or health agencies at the local level are ready and able to collaborate on health promotion. While Young (2000) provides multiple views and degrees of interaction between non-profit and public organisations within a partnership, the current case does not reflect any of the supplementary, complementary, or adversarial models that Young (2000) outlines. Instead, the current case illustrates that public non-profit partnerships may also take the form of complaisant collaborations, where organisations continue to be involved because they see the value of being part of something that addresses an overall goal of interest to them, but lack the specific rationale, resources, or particular capacity elements that would enable them to collaborate more effectively.

Casey *et al.*'s (2009b) claim that for sport and recreation organisations participating in health interventions, 'pragmatic programmes that build on the core business of each participating organization, irrespective of whether they share a common mission, is important' (p. 129) is mirrored in our case. The findings provide insight for the local policy and practice communities who continually position partnerships as a panacea for involving cross-sector actors to address mutually concerning social issues (cf. Forsyth 2010). As Best *et al.* (2003) argued, closing the gap between health promotion research, policy, and practice involves comprehensive planning and sustained ongoing dialogue between partners in order to find common ground in an approach to community partnering.

The Public Health Agency of Canada recently had a call out for *Multisectoral Partnerships to Promote Health Living and Prevent Chronic Disease* (PHAC 2015), demonstrating the continued interest in developing partnerships to promote health outcomes. In the call for action, sport is specifically identified as an avenue for increasing health outcomes and demonstrating a continued policy commitment to the ideas of sport as a driver of health promotion. However, recognising that partnerships are complex and rapidly evolving and changing, the attributes identified here may change over time and create even further complexity in engaging partners for broader health outcomes. This exploratory work provides insight into an under-represented context of sport-based partnerships, which may contribute to public benefit. However, we also recognise that the notion of 'public benefit' is subjectively defined and highly political and therefore further research is needed to provide theoretical insights and policy alternatives that move beyond the rhetorical use of 'partnership', in order to advance a more nuanced understanding of local deliberation of sport and health. For example, participatory action research involving multiple stakeholders and researchers would provide new insight into building local adaptive capacity among the sport and health sectors. Other empirical examples that follow a partnership through from initiation to evaluation would help uncover specific tensions that occur during various phases or stages of working together. A multi-method examination of how sport and health are being integrated in policy and practice at all levels within the planned call from the Public Health Agency of Canada provides an opportunity for rethinking partnerships and providing actual evidence of the sport-health connection. If strides are to be made towards a more aligned approach to addressing health concerns where sport becomes an integral part of this agenda, then an integrated and coordinated approach will be needed.

Disclosure statement

No potential conflict of interest was reported by the authors.

References

Adler, P. and Adler, P., 1987. *Membership roles in field research*. Newbury Park, CA: Sage.

Aggestål, A. and Fahlén, J., 2015. Managing sport for public health: approaching contemporary problems with traditional solutions. *Social inclusion*, 3 (3), 108. doi:10.17645/si.v3i3.197

Alexander, J.A., *et al.*, 2003. Sustainability of collaborative capacity in community health partnerships. *Medical care research review*, 60 (4), 130S–160S. doi:10.1177/1077558703259069

Andrews, R. and Entwistle, T., 2010. Does cross-sectoral partnership deliver? An empirical exploration of public service effectiveness, efficiency, and equity. *Journal of public administration research and theory*, 20 (3), 679–701. doi:10.1093/jopart/mup045

Babiak, K. and Thibault, L., 2008. Managing inter-organisational relationships: the art of plate spinning. *International journal of sport management and marketing*, 3 (3), 281–302. doi:10.1504/IJSMM.2008.017193

Babiak, K. and Thibault, L., 2009. Challenges in multiple cross-sector partnerships. *Nonprofit and voluntary sector quarterly*, 38 (1), 117–143. doi:10.1177/0899764008316054

Berger, I.E., *et al.*, 2008. Determinants of sport participation among Canadian adolescents. *Sport management review*, 11, 277–307. doi:10.1016/S1441-3523(08)70113-X

Best, A., *et al.*, 2003. An integrative framework for community partnering to translate theory into effective health promotion strategy. *American journal of health promotion*, 18 (2), 168–176. doi:10.4278/0890-1171-18.2.168

Birkenhoff, D.W. and Birkenhoff, J.M., 2011. Public-private partnerships: perspectives on purposes, publicness, and good governance. *Public administration and development*, 31, 1–10.

Bovaird, T., 2004. Public-private partnerships: from contested concepts to prevalent practice. *International review of administrative sciences*, 70 (2), 199–215. doi:10.1177/0020852304044250

Brannick, T. and Coghlan, D., 2007. In defense of being "native": the case for insider academic research. *Organizational research methods*, 10 (1), 59–74. doi:10.1177/1094428106289253

Brinkerhoff, J.M., 2002. Government – nonprofit partnership: a defining framework. *Public administration and development*, 22, 19–30. doi:10.1002/(ISSN)1099-162X

Canadian Fitness and Lifestyle Research Institute, 2005. *Physical activity monitor*. Ottawa: CFLRI.

Canadian Heritage, 2012. *Canadian sport policy*. Ottawa, ON: Government of Canada.

Carroll, P. and Steane, P., 2000. Public-private partnerships: sectoral perspectives. In: S. P. Osborne, eds. *Public-private partnerships. Theory and practice in international perspective*. London: Routledge, 36–56.

Casey, M.M., Payne, W.R., and Eime, R.M., 2009a. Building the health promotion capacity of sport and recreation organisations: a case study of Regional Sports Assemblies. *Managing leisure*, 14 (2), 112–124. doi:10.1080/13606710902752588

Casey, M.M., Payne, W.R., and Eime, R.M., 2012. Organisational readiness and capacity building strategies of sporting organisations to promote health. *Sport management review*, 15 (1), 109–124.

Casey, M.M., *et al.*, 2009b. Engaging community sport and recreation organisations in population health interventions: factors affecting the formation, implementation, and institutionalisation of partnerships efforts. *Annals of leisure research*, 12 (2), 129–147. doi:10.1080/11745398.2009.9686815

Donaldson, A. and Finch, C.F., 2012. Sport as a setting for promoting health. *British journal of sports medicine*, 46 (1), 4–5. doi:10.1136/bjsports-2011-090743

Dupuis, S.L., 1999. Naked truths: towards a reflexive methodology in leisure research. *Leisure sciences*, 21 (1), 43–64. doi:10.1080/014904099273282

Forsyth, T., 2010. Panacea or paradox? Cross-sector partnerships, climate change, and development. *Wiley interdisciplinary reviews: climate change*, 1 (5), 683–696.

Frisby, W., Thibault, L., and Kikulis, L., 2004. The organizational dynamics of under-managed partnerships in leisure service departments. *Leisure studies*, 23 (2), 109–126. doi:10.1080/0261436042000224482

Gazley, B., 2008. Beyond the contract: The scope and nature of informal government–nonprofit partnerships. *Public administration review*, *68*(1), 141–154.

Gazley, B. and Brudney, J.L., 2007. The purpose (and perils) of government-nonprofit partnership. *Nonprofit and voluntary sector quarterly*, 36 (3), 389–415. doi:10.1177/0899764006295997

Grix, J. and Phillpots, L., 2011. Revisiting the 'governance narrative': 'asymmetrical network governance' and the deviant case of the sports policy sector. *Public policy and administration*, 26 (1), 3–19. doi:10.1177/0952076710365423

Guèvremont, A., Findlay, L., and Kohen, D., 2008. Organized extracurricular activities of Canadian children and youth. *Health reports /Statistics Canada, Canadian Centre for health information*, 19 (3), 65–69.

Houlihan, B., 2012. Sport policy convergence: a framework for analysis. *European sport management quarterly*, 12, 111–135. doi:10.1080/16184742.2012.669390

Kelly, B., *et al.*, 2010. Examining opportunities for promotion of healthy eating at children's sports clubs. *Australian & New Zealand journal of public health*, 34 (6), 583–588. doi:10.1111/azph.2010.34.issue-6

Krippendorff, K., 2004. Measuring the reliability of qualitative text analysis data. *Quality & quantity*, 38, 787–800. doi:10.1007/s11135-004-8107-7

Lawson, H.A., 2005. Empowering people, facilitating community development, and contributing to sustainable development: The social work of sport, exercise, and physical education programs. *Sport, education and society*, 10 (1), 135–160.

Mackintosh, C., 2011. An analysis of County Sports Partnerships in England: the fragility, challenges and complexity of partnership working in sports development. *International journal of sport policy and politics*, 3 (1), 45–64. doi:10.1080/19406940.2010.524809

Mansfield, L., Weed, M., and Dowse, S., 2010. Rethinking the role of values in Olympic/Paralympic legacy planning using the London 2012 games to get the nation moving. *In*: B. Barney, J. Fosyth, and M. Heine, eds. *ICOS symposium papers: rethinking matters olympic: investigations into the socio-cultural study of the modern Olympic movement*. London, ON: Western University, 412–426.

May, T., Harris, S., and Collins, M., 2013. Implementing community sport policy: understanding the variety of voluntary club types and their attitudes to policy. *International journal of sport policy and politics*, 5 (3), 397–419. doi:10.1080/19406940.2012.735688

Millar, P. and Doherty, A., 2016. Capacity building in nonprofit sport organizations: development of a process model. *Sport management review*. doi:10.1016/j.smr.2016.01.002

Ministry of Health and Long Term Care, 2010. *ACTIVE2010*. Toronto: Government of Ontario.
Misener, K. and Doherty, A., 2013. Understanding capacity through the processes and outcomes of interorganizational relationships in nonprofit community sport organizations. *Sport management review*, 16 (2), 135–147. doi:10.1016/j.smr.2012.07.003
Misener, K.E. and Doherty, A., 2012. Connecting the community through sport club partnerships. *International journal of sport policy and politics*, 4 (2), 243–255. doi:10.1080/19406940.2012.674962
Murphy, P. and Waddington, I., 1998. Sport for all: some public health policy issues and problems. *Critical public health*, 8 (3), 193–205. doi:10.1080/09581599808402907
Public Health Agency of Canada, 2015. *Multisectoral partnerships to promote health living and prevent chronic disease*. Government of Canada. Available from: http://www.phac-aspc.gc.ca/fo-fc/mspphl-pppmvs-eng.php
Salamon, L.M., 1987. Of market failure, voluntary failure, and third-party government: toward a theory of government-nonprofit relations in the modern welfare state. *Nonprofit and voluntary sector quarterly*, 16 (1–2), 29–49. doi:10.1177/089976408701600104
Salamon, L.M., 1995. *Partners in public service*. Baltimore, MD: Johns Hopkins University Press.
Shaw, S. and Allen, J.B., 2006. "It basically is a fairly loose arrangement … and that works out fine, really." Analysing the dynamics of an interorganisational partnership. *Sport management review*, 9, 203–228. doi:10.1016/S1441-3523(06)70026-2
Skille, E.Å., 2015. Community and sport in Norway: between state sport policy and local sport clubs. *International journal of sport policy and politics*, 7 (4), 505–518. doi:10.1080/19406940.2014.940998
Sparling, P.B., *et al.*, 2000. Promoting physical activity: the new imperative for public health. *Health education research*, 15 (3), 367–376. doi:10.1093/her/15.3.367
Stake, R.E., 2003. Case studies. In: N.K. Denzin and Y.S. Lincoln, eds. *Strategies of qualitative inquiry*. 2nd ed. Thousand Oaks, CA: Sage, 134–164.
Statistics Canada, 2010. *Canadian community health survey*. Ottawa, ON: Statistics Canada.
Thibault, L., Frisby, W., and Kikulis, L.M., 1999. Interorganizational linkages in the delivery of local leisure services in Canada: responding to economic, political and social pressures. *Managing leisure*, 4 (3), 125–141. doi:10.1080/136067199375805
Tremblay, M.S., 2012. Major initiatives related to childhood obesity and physical inactivity in Canada: the year in review. *Canadian journal of public health. Revue canadienne de sante publique*, 103, 164–169.
Wankel, L.M., 1994. Health and leisure: inextricably linked. *Journal of physical education, recreation & dance*, 65 (4), 28–31. doi:10.1080/07303084.1994.10606894
Wanner, M., *et al.*, 2011. Allez Hop, a nationwide programme for the promotion of physical activity in Switzerland: what is the evidence for a population impact after one decade of implementation? *British journal of sports medicine*, 45 (15), 1202–1207. doi:10.1136/bjsm.2009.070201
World Health Organization, 2003. *Health and development through physical activity and sport*. Geneva: WHO.
World Health Organization, 2010. *Global recommendations on physical activity for health*. Geneva: WHO. Available from: http://www.who.int/dietphysicalactivity/factsheet_recommendations/en
Yin, R.K., 2014. *Case study research: design and methods (5th ed.)*. 4th ed.. Thousand Oaks, CA: Sage Publications.
Young, D.R., 2000. Alternative models of government-nonprofit sector relations: theoretical and international perspectives. *Nonprofit and voluntary sector quarterly*, 29 (1), 149–172. doi:10.1177/0899764000291009

OPEN ACCESS

Resourcefulness, reciprocity and reflexivity: the three Rs of partnership in sport for public health research

Louise Mansfield

ABSTRACT

This paper explores the dynamics of research–policy–practice (RPP) partnerships in sport. Such partnerships, involving a diverse range of groups, have emerged as a response to: (1) a contemporary political prioritisation in the use of sport for health and wellbeing and (2) a parallel requirement for robust evidence of effectiveness and cost-effectiveness. A conceptual framework for understanding such RPP partnerships is proposed and discussed in relation to three overlapping characteristics; resourcefulness, reciprocity and reflexivity. The paper concludes that understanding these three Rs of RPP partnerships is a way to demythologise the role of sport in public health and present theoretically informed analyses about processes of knowledge production, dissemination and use. It is a conceptual framework which might also further an understanding of, and make public, issues concerning the legitimation of some forms of evidence over others, and potentially maximise the impact of the co-production of knowledge about sport for public health and wellbeing.

Introduction

In the wake of the London 2012 Olympic and Paralympic Games, the sport sector is currently a priority area for increasing population rates of physical activity for public health in the UK (Sport England 2012, DCMS 2015). Sport England, the Department of Health and Public Health England is represented on the Moving More, Living More cross government group which promotes the role that sport can play in helping people to become more active, more healthy and make a positive contribution to public health (Mansfield *et al.* 2015). This conspicuous articulation of sport for public health affixes sport to health as a contemporary UK welfare policy issue and legitimates sport as an antidote to the health problems of contemporary societies claimed to be associated with inactivity.

Public health refers to a range of approaches in research, policy and practice which aim to prevent disease, promote health and prolong life in a population as a whole (WHO, 2007). Public health is a dynamic sphere involving the surveillance of populations, evolving approaches to policymaking, policy implementation and policy enactment, and diversity of interventions and programming. Public health involves many different professionals delivering a multitude of initiatives in a wide range of settings, all of which are intended to contribute to the welfare of people (Douglas *et al.* 2007). Increasing levels of participation through sport is not a new public health or welfare policy issue. The historical development in the sport/health dynamic is well documented (Hargreaves 1986, 1994/2002, Waddington 2000). Participation in sport produces not just sporting abilities but, more broadly, an ability to care for and know one's own body in accordance with dominant ideals about health and hygiene. In other words, sport is part of a therapeutic technology of the body. Sport has always been a mechanism for the application of corporeal rules, practices and expectations typical of a given time and space. In sport and public health sectors, 'the notion of a direct, immutable and unproblematic link between sport and health' prevails (Mansfield and Malcolm 2014, p. 188). Sport can also be thought of as a relatively cheap and malleable policy tool which helps to explain its continued appeal as a simple solution to complex, deeper-seated social problems like health inequalities. Yet knowledge, understanding, experiences and beliefs about the relationship between sport and health improvement are complex and contested than is reflected in policy documents and Government promotional campaigns.

Little is known about the design, management and marketing of sport for the promotion of enhanced public health outcomes (Chalip 2006). Despite the well-established links between physical activity and health improvement (see Hillsdon *et al.* 2005), there is a cursory understanding about the precise mechanisms by which sport might contribute to improved public health. There are few studies evaluating the effects of interventions delivered though sporting organisations to increase participation for health outcomes (Priest *et al.* 2008). Cavill et al's. (2012) review of research and practice on improving health through participation in sport identifies that the evidence base for the contribution of sport to physical activity and health is underdeveloped and relatively weak. Despite a commitment to boost levels of physical activity to improve the general health of the UK population being a core aspect of the London 2012 Olympic and Paralympic legacy strategy, findings illustrate that there is no evidence base upon which to claim increased levels of participation from which positive health outcomes could be assumed (Weed *et al.* 2009, 2012). It appears that sports advocacy and political rhetoric are currently dominant forces in the legitimation of sport for health.

This political and academic backdrop raises questions about what counts as evidence in sport for health policy and practice; how evidence can and should be produced; the manner in which evidence is used and consumed; and the impact of the evidence–policy–practice agenda in the sport sector. Herein lies the broad purpose of this paper; to explore the relationship between evidence building, policymaking and delivery of community sport for health outcomes but with a particular focus on one increasingly prominent mechanism for developing and implementing effective research–policy–practice (RPP) strategies, that of partnerships. Rather than focusing on describing types of research partnerships, outlining their underpinning rationales and overviewing guidance on implementing partnerships, the discussion is written with a more nuanced framework of analysis in mind. It explores the complex processes and structures of RPP partnership working and considers competing and converging interests in the roles, responsibilities and values that shape them.

I begin with a brief overview of theoretical approaches to partnerships in public health and sport policy. The paper examines the relationship between partnership working and evidence building in the current sport for health policy agenda with a particular focus on the status and generation of knowledge. It explores the nature of partnership relations by articulating the processes of interdependence and power that characterise them. I then propose and discuss a conceptual approach to understanding the sociodynamics of partnerships which I identify as the three Rs of RPP partnerships; a potential way of examining the relationships between the everyday politics of partnership working and the broader socio-cultural structures of power that influence the partnership enterprise. This is a conceptual essay in which I draw on experiences of working on a range of RPP projects, and provide examples from a diversity of scholarly work related to partnership working in sport, policy and public health to illustrate my thinking. I invite other scholars to develop and improve the conceptual approach discussed.

What are partnerships?

Partnerships represent formal organisational arrangements whereby people are required to coordinate their activities towards a common goal. Yet conceptually partnerships remain quite a vague concept (Houlihan and Lindsey 2008). Partnerships appear to be a ubiquitous discourse in politics and social life, pervading government agendas, policy and practice in education, business, the environment, international development, transport, energy, defence, justice, public health and culture, media and sport. There is a long history of partnership working in local, national and global contexts. In the UK, partnership approaches have been in existence in various forms since before the advent of the welfare state. However, since the late twentieth century, partnership working has been underpinned by: a response to divided working practices between government, local authorities and service deliverers; the fragmentation of welfare services as a result of market forces; and an attempt to develop synergies that could lead to more effective, equitable and democratic decision-making, raise the quality of provision of a range of national and local services, and provide value for money in a public sector continually facing resource constraints (Balloch and Taylor 2001). It was under New Labour's modernising agenda that there was a renewed enthusiasm for the acclaimed virtues of partnerships which have become enshrined as a central operating system for effective service delivery of almost any kind (McDonald 2005). Partnerships are variously described as cross-sector organisations, inter-agency collaboration, joint initiatives, holistic services, coalitions and networks, and there is no one single partnership type. Partnerships reflect an array of organisational structures and working practices, are implemented for a diversity of reasons, and are marked by varying degrees of cooperation, coercion and coordination (Mackintosh 1992). Furthermore, partnership relationships are complex and dynamic with parties more usually than not finding themselves with intricate challenges to negotiate in the act of fostering agreements or finding common ground throughout the lifetime of the partnership (Lowndes and Skelcher 1998). Notwithstanding such diversity in partnership working, perhaps one common feature of partnerships is the logic of coordination; a strategic approach to co-governance which is rooted in the idea that a collaborative approach is a more effective, democratic and cost-effective alternative to traditional state-centric arrangements of government (Johnson and Osborne 2003). Yet such a wider perceptible 'culture of partnership' in the UK political, policy and practice spheres (Lewis 2005, p. 121) is paralleled by definable cultural characteristics of specific partnership arrangements. The precise nature of a partnership is driven by the dynamics of their unique relationships in which roles and responsibilities are carved out and where, as I noted earlier, there are fluctuations, tensions and convergences in the values by which different parties see themselves and articulate their objectives and purpose. A more detailed discussion of such complexities is the subject of the latter half of this paper. Here, it is worth explaining a little further some of the particularities of partnerships outlined above in the context of public health and sport policy.

Understanding partnerships in public health and sport policy

Arguably, one of the most significant policy areas in which partnerships have become advanced is in public health and particularly in health service provision. Balloch and Taylor (2001) provide a synopsis of the UK government white papers and strategy documents, published during the 1990s, which concisely illustrates a focus on developing integrated health care services through partnerships primarily focused on improving the quality of service delivery through pooled funding and performance management. More recently, *Healthy Lives; Healthy People* (Department of Health 2011, p. 31) set out a strategy for public health in England that reiterated partnership approaches for health improvement through the acclaimed Public Health Responsibility Deal; a strategy emphasising a 'partnership approach through life'. The emphasis was on a cross-government framework and local community engagement to improve health and reduce health inequalities. Specific reference was made to the promotion of sport for health through a number of government departments and initiatives including; the contribution of the Department for Education in ensuring access to high quality physical education in schools, the development of Change4Life sports clubs by the Department of Culture, Media and Sport, and the significance the Department of Transport's 'Bikeability' programme.

In the UK, the discourse of partnership working for public health outcomes through sport is recast most recently in the UK Department of Culture, Media and Sport (DCMS) publication *Sporting Future: A Strategy for an Active Nation (2015)*. Partnerships are defined by a universalising cross-government approach emphasising that government departments should engage in joined-up working towards shared public health and social value outcomes for sport. Collaborative arrangements have been emphasised in funding, delivery, and monitoring and evaluation. The realisation of multi-agency partnerships to achieve sport for health outcomes is linked to the devolution of public health from the UK National Health Service (NHS) in 2013, which broadly sought to locate public health where it could be most fully and effectively coordinated (Phillips and Green 2015). Health and wellbeing, including sport and physical activity, is now the responsibility of local authorities who have been directed to work with national bodies like Sport England and Public Health England and local organisations (e.g. community sport clubs, voluntary community agencies and clinical commissioning groups) in achieving health and wellbeing outcomes. Despite this increased responsibility, the parallel imposition of budgetary cuts has resulted in government extending its influence and regulation rather than reducing it. As in health, this appears to be fragmenting sport and physical activity provision locally. Still, DCMS (2015, p. 13) emphasises local responsibility and local delivery in collaborative arrangements where local councils are significant in 'bringing schools, voluntary sport clubs, National Governing Bodies of sport (NGBs), health and the private sector together to forge partnerships, unblock barriers to participation and improve the local sport delivery system'. Moreover, cultivating acclaimed 'natural synergies' (p. 14) between the sport sector and arts, heritage, housing and employment services is proposed as way of driving up physical activity unquestioningly associated with health benefit. There is an explicitly identified partnership role for communities and individuals in promoting and achieving health improvements through sport and physical activity thus shifting power and decision-making to local community contexts as a way to create a more democratic, equitable model of health provision. Involving communities and the people for whom health services are designed may have some potential for improving delivery and service evaluation by genuinely listening to and working with stakeholders (Popay *et al.* 1998, Barber *et al.* 2011). Yet, through both intended and unintended consequences, community collaborations can serve to protect the status quo and limit the role of diverse community-based leadership (Chavis 2001, Smith *et al.* 2008). Moreover, a pervasive discourse of healthism remains the dominant framework in public health policy that seeks to promote lifestyle change (including sport) as a means of improving the health of the nation (Crawford 1980; Lee and Macdonald 2010). In other words, the idea that health can be unproblematically achieved through individual and community effort, personal responsibility and self-discipline through sport or any other means is neither challenged nor erased in current strategies, including the promotion of partnership working for sport, health and wellbeing.

I do not intend to provide a detailed discussion of the history and development of partnerships in sport; others have done this in detail and to great effect (see for example, Houlihan and Lindsey 2008). However, it is worth noting that existing scholarship on sport partnerships has variously focused on managerial structures and processes and the organisational dynamics within a range of multi-agency contexts including: public sector sport and leisure services (Frisby *et al.* 2004, Thibault *et al.* 1999; Shaw and Allen 2006); elite sport development (Green and Oakley 2001); county sport partnerships (Mackintosh 2011); sport in international development (Lindsey and Banda 2011, Kay *et al.* 2015); school sport (Smith and Leech 2010, Flintoff *et al.* 2011) and community sport (Frisby and Millar 2002; Miesner and Doherty 2009, 2012). Alongside a focus on the more functional aspects of implementing and working in partnerships, further research has raised critical questions about the contested nature of partnership arrangements in sport in conceptual, applied and case study accounts of the policy context and politics of partnerships (see for example, Green and Houlihan 2004, McDonald 2005; Green 2007, Hayhurst and Frisby 2010, Mansfield and Killick 2012). Scholarly analyses of partnership theory and practice in policy work, including sport, has led to the articulation of partnership models identifying the organisational structures, roles and responsibilities of actors in particular inter-agency collaborations including: strategic and communicative models in county sport partnerships (McDonald 2005); advocacy coalition frameworks (ACF) in elite sport development contexts (Green and Houlihan 2004); and empowered franchising in the UK Netball Superleague (Mansfield and Killick 2012). There have also been critiques of the political rhetoric purporting that there is any inherent progressive capacity to partnerships. Such work has tended to highlight the paradox of partnership approaches challenging the acclaimed association between partnerships and inclusiveness, effectiveness and empowerment, and identifying the reality of partnerships as exclusive, ineffectual and ultimately autocratic (Grix and Phillpots 2010, Lindsey 2014). Yet partnership working rarely results in either positive relationships and outcomes or entirely negative ones. I agree with McDonald (2005) that partnerships are contextual, changeable and contradictory. In order to move beyond determining simply how to make partnerships work, we need an approach to exploring and understanding how they work, in what contexts and for whom. This is about examining the power relations that are inherent in the social interaction of actors in the partnership which serve to shape a complexity of negotiated relationships and lead to a range of expected and rather more unforeseen consequences; an issue I explore further on in the paper. Also important in the context of exploring RPP partnerships specifically is an understanding that the constitution of evidence, its use and impact is a contested terrain and one that is politically directed. The next section examines the contemporary quest for evidence in the sport-public health domain before turning to a discussion of the sociodynamics of RPP partnerships as one specific partnership approach to the acquisition, analysis and articulation of evidence on sport and public health.

Sport, public health and the quest for evidence

That sport is being extensively sanctioned for improved public health outcomes in the UK is coupled with an expansion and deepening of monitoring, assessment, measuring and an overarching research-based approach to the evaluation of the sport sector's capability to effectively deliver sport services to public health outcomes (Österlind 2016). An explicit concern for providing evidence of the effectiveness of sport in achieving health outcomes is part of an evidence-based approach to sport policy that has emerged during the latter half of the twentieth century alongside a wider focus on evidence-based policymaking in a number of sectors, including health, welfare and education (Coalter 2010). Such developments in accountability are characterised by a number of interlocking processes, including the growth of a well-informed public, an emphasis on productivity at local, national and international levels, the expansion and accessibility of data, and the development and rise of a professional research population (Davies *et al.* 2000; Thomas *et al.* 2010). In the UK, political motivations to fix policy and practice to rigorous, high quality evidence emphasise optimum delivery of policy goals through effective and efficient means (Coalter 2010).

RPP partnerships involving different academic, managerial, delivery and citizen organisations are a fundamental feature of public health where evidence-based policy and practice has become a universally accepted strategy for determining priorities, organisational structures, service delivery and surveillance mechanisms (Petticrew *et al.* 2004). Long-term processes have raised the status and employment of, and approaches to, evidenced-based policymaking. However, a contemporary take-off point in the discourse of evidence for decision-making emerged in the 1990s as a challenge from clinicians immersed in evidence-based medicine and signalled a directive for policymakers to ensure their work was founded on the findings of rigorous, high quality research (Black 2001). Evidence-based practice is directly drawn from evidence-based medicine which focuses on integrating clinical expertise with the best research evidence into decision-making about patient care (Sackett *et al.* 1996). The key principles of any evidence-based strategy are effectiveness; the achievement and measurement of stated outcomes, and efficiency; delivery with minimum resource wastage (Thomas *et al.* 2010). A focus on these tenets has led to the dominance of quantification of outcomes, an evaluation approach wedded to the management of cost such that evidence-based policy and practice has become the strategy for controlling health and health care costs. Successful interventions which are cost-effective are those deemed to be efficient (Thomas *et al.* 2010).

The authority of objective measurement of effectiveness and efficiency in public health has produced and reproduced a knowledge economy defined narrowly by the status and generation of predominantly quantitative data on which to base decisions about health. Debates abound regarding the proliferation of quantitative measures of effectiveness. Allied to such discussions is a critique of the applicability of an established hierarchy of evidence for assessing the relevance, significance, rigour and quality of evidence on which to make decisions about health; one which ranks a range of study designs in order of internal validity and thus credibility (Petticrew and Roberts 2003). Despite the trend towards evidence-based policy and practice, the enactment of it remains challenging as those charged with implementing it struggle to interpret and employ relevant methods with varying resource capacities. Several scholars examine and illustrate that the direct impact of research in policy–practice relations is somewhat lacking (Petticrew *et al.* 2004, Phillips and Green 2015). In discussing the reasons why research evidence has little impact on service, practice and governance policies in health, Black (2001) identifies three failings: (1) a failure of researchers to understand the environment of policymaking and the policymaking process; (2) a failure of funders to understand the complexities of research impact, especially in relation to the time it takes for impact to be realised, and the iterative nature of impact; and (3) the failure of policymakers to be more involved in the inception, design and delivery of research projects. There is a need to develop communities of researchers, policymakers, practitioners and participants in the production, mobilisation and translation of evidence; communities definable as RPP partnerships. In sport for health, such partnerships cannot be thought of as a simple extension of the practices of normative evidence-based medicine because this would reinforce the failings identified above. Furthermore, it would rely on a narrow conceptualisation of evidence connected to study design, excluding a full consideration of methodological aptness and additional evidence types that can be legitimate in making policy and practice decisions in public health (Rychetnik *et al.* 2002, Petticrew and Roberts 2003). Rather, an approach is needed that enables ongoing consideration of the values, goals, methods and objectives of all actors in the partnership as well as recognition of a range of sources of knowledge and types of evidence that can contribute to decision-making. Scrutiny of the processes by which evidence is produced and becomes legitimate is also needed. Such an approach may require levels of transparency not previously experienced in the sport sector. Furthermore, there may well be challenges in the extent to which sports organisations are able to be 'open' to methods which challenge their modes of delivery, find no evidence to support their work, or which are perceived by them to potentially have a detrimental effect on current delivery. However, given the identified weak evidence base for the contribution of sport to health and wellbeing, more rigorous evaluation is required. An analysis of the complexities of RPP partnerships is a fruitful starting point for developing RPP communities. Specifically, there is potential in considering the sociodynamics of research–policy–partnerships relations in terms of resourcefulness, reciprocity and reflexivity, issues which are discussed in the remainder of the paper.

Resourcefulness, reciprocity and reflexivity: the 3Rs of research–policy–practice partnerships in sport for public health

In the three Rs of RPP partnerships I am not outlining a typology, or proposing a model or best practice template or a set of guidelines for partnership implementation. Rather, I wish to articulate a conceptual framework for the analysis of RPP partnership working which identifies three key interrelated characteristics; resourcefulness, reciprocity and reflexivity. These characteristics are identifiable in the way RPP partnerships are conceived, implemented and developed and as they endure, mature, change, deteriorate and sometimes implode. These partnership dynamics are central to the organisation and structure within which RPP partnership working takes place and frame the processes by which such partnerships operate. Each characteristic has a strategic element to it, employed in various ways by partners as a means to achieving a goal, which may or may not be an agreed partnership goal. An understanding of the three Rs of RPP partnerships may advance knowledge about how and why RPP partnerships work, for whom and in what context and, indeed, why they do not work in the way that might be expected.

Resourcefulness

Resourcefulness in RPP partnerships refers to both the capacity and ability of partners to access and utilise the resources they require and will benefit from, and their predilection (intended or not) to withhold or block what other partners may require. Resourcefulness refers to the production and allocation of resources, processes of resource control and also to specifying the terms of ownership of resources. Resources vary and may relate to economic, sociocultural and/or political and ideological aspects of partnership work. Whatever the type of resources in question, resourcefulness can be understood in terms of the characteristic power dynamics of all partnership relationships. Several key sociological thinkers as well as those working specifically in the sociology of sport provide detailed discussions about the nature of power in human relations (Lukes, 1974, Elias 1978, Elias *et al.* 1998, Foucault 1980) and sport, leisure and lifestyle cultures (see, e.g. Elias and Dunning 1986, Hargreaves 1986, Tomlinson 1998, Howell and Ingham 2001, Sugden and Tomlinson 2002, Markula and Pringle 2006). For the purposes of understanding resourcefulness in RPP partnerships it is crucial to recognise 'that power is a relationship, a dynamic, and that the relationship involves human agents struggling over resources and outcomes' (Tomlinson 1998, p. 235). Whilst power relations operate within the domains of institutional structures, it is people that constitute those systems and who exercise power; a characteristic of all human relations (Elias 1978).

RPP partnerships represent interdependent, mutually orientated configurations of people whose social interaction is inextricably connected to the wider socio-economic and political environment in which RPP decisions and behaviours take place. As discussed earlier, the contemporary political endorsement of sport for public health improvement in the UK is paralleled by increasingly complex and expansive monitoring and evaluation requirements; the foundation upon which RPP partnerships emerge and develop. The requirement to work within more complex and extended RPP networks that involve a diverse range of groups reflects the history of organisational change in sports development more broadly (Bloyce *et al.* 2008). Relationships in RPP partnerships are never equal. The power dynamics of partnership relations mean that the benefits of partnership working are not received equally by partners. Thinking about the power relations that shape resourcefulness in RPP partnerships seems particularly pertinent in light of Newman *et al.* (2004) argument that the rhetoric of equality, communal values and collective trust in partnership discourse obscures constitutive differences of power and resources.

Some of the literature related to understanding resourcefulness or resource control has fruitfully drawn on the concept of the ACF in understanding the coordinated decision-making that takes place between people with different roles and responsibilities (Sabatier and Jenkins-Smith 1993). Green and Houlihan (2004) explore the role of the State in applying resource control to influence the context in which elite sport policy is made and remade. Examining the ways that established decision-making institutions in elite sport policy, through their funding arrangements, convey their own interests and combine and alter the preferences of other groups over time towards their own ends illustrates resource control of a financial kind at work. Over the period of a decade since the inception of the National Lottery in the UK in 1994, for example, there was evidence of a perceptible shift towards corporate and professional values and practices in elite sport through the allocation, control and management of funding a situation which continues to be reflected in UK elite sport policy. Green and Houlihan (2004, p. 393) explain that there are 'structural resource interdependencies' between policymaking and funding organisations and reconstituted national sports organisations as limited companies which exclusively focus on administering World Class Performance Lottery funds. Such structures and processes of resourcefulness serve to ensure that the organisational arrangements in elite sport policy compel actors to operate not only by the rules and regulations of the most powerful organisations in the network, but through their value systems which are increasingly focused on performance, professionalism and commercialisation. Financial resource interdependencies also operate between researchers and research funding agencies. As noted earlier the tendency towards the authority of objective assessment of effectiveness and efficiency in monitoring and evaluation of public health outcomes serves to reinforce the authority of quantitative data funded and produced by professional research organisations in both the public and commercial domain. Yet there have also been challenges to this linear hierarchical model of knowledge production and a shift, since the latter half of the 20th century, to the commissioning of more participatory approaches in understanding public health to evidence building and service delivery to include a wider range of stakeholders including users and practitioners to ensure that research findings are both useful and useable (Israel *et al.* 1998, Beresford 2002; Newman *et al.* 2004).

Resourcefulness is not only coupled with monetary control. In analysing community empowerment models in public health promotion and knowledge exchange, Labonte and Laverack (2001) identify the potential ability of communities to mobilise internal resources and to negotiate external resources as a central strand of partnership models. Resources in this context may be related to space, amenities, programmes and finances but might also be connected to information, knowledge and skills. Community-based resourcefulness in Labonte and Laverack's (2001) view can be thought of as a domain of capacity building in public health, something that is enabled and constrained by the dynamics of partnership relations between local communities, health promotion practitioners and the government and non-government organisations that shape policy values, provide funding and, thus influence the practices of particular programmes. Capacity building in RPP partnerships is a central tenet of Julier and Kimbell's (2015, p. 8) approach to maximising resourcefulness across academic, policy and practitioner networks for enabling 'research sprints'; agile, design oriented, cross-disciplinary and collaborative research for understanding social issues. There are economic, political and social resource opportunities and constraints that impact on the extent to which communities can participate in RPP partnerships and influence their outcomes. Community-based resource mobilisation is inextricably linked to the community capacity for participation, communication and critical reflection, leadership and programme design, development and management (Goodman *et al.* 1998). Furthermore, the flow of information, knowledge and material resources will be conditioned, constrained and facilitated by the nature of community alliances with local and wider agents (Labonte and Laverack 2001).

The idea of resourcefulness in RPP partnerships sheds light on a number of resource crises that occur in relation to differing motivations and values, outcomes and goals and methods of working that partners have. In partnerships where information building and exchange are central, resource crises also materialise in relation to time and timing. Temporal demands, expectations and indeed capacities differ amongst researchers, policymakers, practitioners and participants. Policymakers are often required to make decisions within short-time frames (days and weeks) without access to extensive research capacity. Practitioners and participants require information to inform programme design, delivery and participation within the duration of their projects (months) and do not have capacity for extensive information gathering. Researchers focused on methodological rigour and in-depth theoretical analysis most often work in the long term (years) and have working practices entirely devoted to knowledge production (Williams *et al.* 2005). Moreover, it has been argued that governments only use research at times when the findings match their assumptions and values (Weiss *et al.* 2008). Resourcefulness, then, is characterised by struggles over what is temporally, financially, sociologically, politically and ideologically feasible to different partners. The result of such struggles may be intended but could well be much more unplanned and concomitantly the consequences of resourcefulness may be conducive to the relative success of RPP partnership working and/or contribute to rather more ineffectual processes and results. Unintended consequences arise from the complex interweaving of intentional actions. Arguably the current focus, in the UK, on sport as a tool for non-sporting welfare outcomes, like public health, and the associated demands for monitoring and evaluating such outcomes, will unintentionally detract from increasing participation, the objective upon which non-sporting outcomes are predicated (Bloyce *et al.* 2008). It is also possibly that such demands might hinder provision of some community sport activities altogether. Linked to resourcefulness in RPP partnerships is reciprocity, an issue I turn to next.

Reciprocity

Reciprocity in RPP partnerships refers to the mutual exchange of information. This might be via a coordinated strategy on roles and responsibilities between researchers, policymakers, practitioners and participants or via more serendipitous and informal activities. Degrees and types of reciprocity occur in resource struggles of course but reciprocity extends to relationships that take shape in the production and consumption of knowledge in partnership working. Reciprocity is a concept that is grounded in philosophical discussions about the generation, status and ethics of knowledge production (Lincoln and Denzin 2000). Put simply, reciprocity is the give-and-take of partnership working but more particularly, reciprocity signifies the negotiation of meaning, power and identity in the partnership network. There are diverse theoretical perspectives concerning reciprocity and psychologists, economist, political scientists and sociologists have made contributions (Ostrom and Walker 2003). Lather (1986) argues that in research relations, reciprocity operates at two junctures; (1) the researcher and the researched and (2) theory and data. In RPP partnership terms the researched includes policymakers, practitioners and/or participants, and indeed the craft of research involves a two-way dialogue between theory and evidence in making sense of any topic under investigation (Maguire 1988). Reciprocal processes are evident in both theory-data relations and researcher-researched relations in RPP partnerships but more specifically and extensively they act in a wider range of decision-making situations in which mutuality shapes the nature and character of the processes and outcomes relating to: identifying and prioritising research agendas and topics; establishing project aims and outcomes; designing, promoting and delivering projects; agreeing research designs and managing data collection; analysing data; and reporting, translating and mobilising the findings. Reciprocity is also a central strand of the relationships that develop in the overall management of partnership projects which includes decisions and administrative requirements over funding and budgets, employment, intellectual property and other contractual arrangements. It should be emphasised that reciprocity is not isolated to any one of these aspects of partnership working rather a position or a 'stance of reciprocity' suffuses the partnership endeavour (Trainor and Bouchard 2013, p. 990). Several authors identify a link between reciprocity and trust (Harrison *et al.* 2001). Trust, at one level, involves an appropriate degree of respect and courteousness between those committed to work together on a project (Barber *et al.* 2011). Trust, cooperation and friendship, for example, are proposed as building blocks for collective action towards the promotion of a range of sport and non-sport-related outcomes in alliances between sport clubs and other community organisations (Misener and Doherty 2012)

Yet trust in RPP partnerships also operates at an ethical level in terms of confidentiality, consent and discretion. The relationship between reciprocity and trust then should be thought of as going beyond the boundaries of politeness and into the maelstrom of honesty and integrity which are framed by an open approach to partnership working; one which reflects a moral code of carefulness, exactitude and veracity no matter how difficult decisions might become. RPP partnerships are characteristically bureaucratic and it is often the case that different partners in the network have to adhere to their own complex governance processes which other partners may be unaware of (Johnson and Osborne 2003). Whilst working through the bureaucracy that comes with any RPP partnership is always challenging, a stance of reciprocity is likely to at least ameliorate any unduly obstructive approaches within the partnership and bring to bear more fruitful 'interpersonal relationships' which might realise the potential and address the problems inherent in an 'everyday politics' of partnerships, and help to develop a successfully coordinated collaboration based on honest negotiation (Phillips and Green 2015, p. 496). It might appear to some that by focusing on trust and honesty I am, myself, romanticising reciprocity. Some might argue that trust should be replaced with transparency and the principles of disclosure in decision-making so that all partners are held accountable for their decisions and actions. Indeed, accountability is an important feature of reciprocity. However, transparency can turn to political rhetoric and spawn a twinned characteristic; secrecy (Birchall 2011). Trust remains as important in RPP partnerships as openness and responsibility.

Mutuality is a matter of intent and extent (Lather 1986, Trainor and Bouchard 2013). There is a common intent in RPP partnerships in that all those involved wish to gather information on which to make decisions. However, the decisions being made and, thus, the specific information required as well as the requisite dissemination strategies differ amongst partners. Researchers tend to focus on data collection and analysis for academic publication, policymakers seek data that can inform guidance and procedural advice, practitioners need insights about best practice, and participants are interested in where and how they can access good quality, value-for-money services. Such diverse reasons for information gathering, alongside the complex negotiations of organisation and personal priorities, mean that degrees of reciprocity will vary according to the extent to which partners feel that the knowledge produced through the partnership is useful to them. RPP partnerships should go beyond the researcher habit of gathering more and better data; surpassing the collection and analysis of evidence solely as a means to efficient and effective service delivery outcomes (Labonte and Laverick 2001). RPP partnerships are well placed to embrace a concern with the production of information that can support a range of intentions in a partnership by maximising processes of reciprocity. Such an approach; one which has a research-praxis direction to it can potentially deliver more relevant information to a wider range of partners, augment the capacity of all those in the partnership to contribute, add value and benefit from the collaboration and perhaps have greater impact (Lather 1986, Gillies 1998, Labonte and Laverick 2001).

In the Health and Sport Engagement (HASE) project (Mansfield *et al.* 2015) a stance of reciprocity framed the involvement of researchers, policymakers (Sport England), sports coaches and public health professionals, and local people in the London Borough of Hounslow. Like Zigo's (2001) strategy for reciprocal research relations, the position of reciprocity in the HASE project was a cornerstone of the partnership from inception and design, to the development of methods and data collection, and data synthesis, analysis and dissemination. For example, 32 × 1 hour participatory focus groups were conducted in the planning phase of the project with identified inactive people for whom there were likely to be barriers to physical activity and who were interested in becoming more physically active through community sport. This method represented public or lay involvement in the project as a way of genuinely listening to those who wished to take part in community sport and gaining a deeper understanding of their views about inactivity, activity and local sport opportunities. The focus group findings were shared with sport coaches and public health practitioners and used by them to design community sport programmes tailored to the needs of previously inactive communities including considerations of types and intensity of sporting activity, scheduling of sessions, locations, venues, facilities and equipment, leadership and coaching and cost.

International alliances also have a place in the conceptualisation of RPP partnerships. For Kay *et al.* (2015) a long-term partnership strategy for developing local research capacity was underpinned by reciprocal learning in sport for development. Reciprocity in the collaborative research partnership between the commissioned researchers and Go Sisters girls' empowerment programme staff in Zambia enabled the evaluation to be framed by culturally relevant understandings, localised knowledge and the pursuit of decolonisation in research. For the researchers the reciprocal nature of the partnerships benefitted the quality and integrity of the evidence being produced and provided situations of co-learning about the local impacts of the programme particularly through verbal dialogues which were more detailed and insightful than anything written down. For the Go Sisters team, the reciprocal approach allowed them some flexibility in the research process and enabled them specifically to bring their expertise and voice to the development of research strategies and tools (Museke *et al.* 2015). This has supported the growth and development of their community sport projects but also aided their understanding of the successful and unsuccessful impacts of their projects.

While I have provided some rather affirmatory examples of reciprocity in RPP partnerships it should be emphasised that it is not an ingredient that leads to certain and automatic benefits for all communities. There is an inherent tension between the principle of reciprocity and the pursuit of interests particular to any organisation in a partnership (Beacom 2007). Power differentials that characterise RPP partnerships lead to the potential for research ends to dominate relationships. There is always a danger in lay involvement in research projects, for example, that research priorities become imposed and the social context of community is reified (Beresford 2002). Moreover, the demands of data collection cannot be underestimated for participants in community research projects (Carver 1997). Reciprocal relationships need to be negotiated and partners need to be respectful and flexible in understanding how relationships are working, in what contexts, and for whom so that meaning is negotiated and constructed with participants and not simply imposed upon them. This positions reciprocity as a guide to ethical practice in RPP partnerships (Maiter *et al.* 2008). I cannot claim to have achieved maximum reciprocity in any of the RPP partnerships I have worked within. However, what is important in RPP partnership is a conscious articulation of a position of reciprocity that creates a culture which can genuinely *value* the involvement of all actors in the production and validation of knowledge (evidence) in a respectful and ethical manner. Reciprocity occurs at many levels, is underpinned by various rationales and operates by degrees, and the particularities of taking a stance of reciprocity in any RPP partnership will shape the processes by which the collaboration operates and the outcomes are achieved. Taking a stance of reciprocity illustrates further the complex power dynamics that are central to the processes by which partnerships operate and which were also highlighted in the discussion of resourcefulness. There is a need to develop practices of reflexivity in RPP partnership working to explore the nature and mechanisms of both reciprocity and resourcefulness if research designs and evidence building is to go beyond tokenistic consultation and descriptive inquiry and employ partnership strategies that recognise and address the complexities of different objectives, values and practices. The final section of this paper examines the nature of reflexivity in RPP partnership working.

Reflexivity

Reflexivity in RPP partnerships refers to the systematic evaluation of the impact of oneself (the researcher) and the relationship dynamics of the partnership on the project. There are different versions and approaches to reflexivity and various outcomes. Reflexivity may be reinforcing and self-perpetuating, resistive and transformative, or incorporate processes of mediation and compromise. It is a well-established argument in the social sciences that contemporary social life is characterised by increasing forms of reflexive conduct (Adkins 2003) involving processes of hindsight and foresight about self-conscious as well as unconscious behaviours and habits (Elias 2000). In research terms reflexivity has its roots in qualitative traditions whereby researchers emphasise a need to assess their influence on the design, data collection, analysis and reporting aspects of projects. In this sense, it is commonly argued that reflexivity extends the act of simply thinking about something (reflection) to more critical self-awareness by the researcher (Finlay 2002a). Reflexivity in research, then, involves explicit, critical evaluation of the role of the researcher in knowledge production. Most often associated with qualitative research contexts reflexive acts are also married to assertions of integrity and trustworthiness in data collection, analysis and representation of findings. What is principally at issue here is the capacity and requirement in qualitative research to make appropriate and accurate claims to knowledge and to judge the adequacy of evidence being produced. This involves definitive strategies for exploring and managing the operation of power in the relationships between researchers and those who are researched (Alldred 1998).

The idea of reflexivity may well appear to be somewhat abstract, and indeed much of the literature is directed towards epistemological discussions of knowledge production and consumption. Theoretical foundations of reflexivity are important to understand but they are not divorced from the practice of reflexivity; from an application of reflexive analysis within the research process. Acts of reflexivity involving an examination of assumptions, behaviours, emotions and the impacts of actions are significant to understanding relationships in a range of contexts including research, management, professional and personal ones (Cunliffe 2004). The locus of reflexive analysis lies in striving for adequate balances of involvement-detachment at every level of RPP partnership work; from conception and design to delivery and evaluation (Mansfield 2007, 2008). The practicalities of reflexive practice are complex, ambiguous and often uncomfortable yet several authors in sport illustrate reflexive analysis as a detour to higher quality knowledge production and exchange. Brackenridge's (1999) analysis of managing her position as a white, middle-class lesbian researcher investigating sexual abuse in sport, illustrates the centrality of reflexivity in untangling the power dynamics of research relationships and the roles and impact of the researcher on the research. Sugden and Tomlinson's (1999, p. 386) strategies for accessing 'deep insider information' about sport, an approach to unpicking the complexities and contradictions of political relationships, emphasises the significance of being *in* the cultural scene of the research but simultaneously being semi-detached from the experience to employ an interpretive position in understanding the relationships between individual realties and the broader social and political milieu. Such research insights are significant in developing reflexivity in RPP partnerships.

In RPP partnerships there is no place for ceaseless immersion in the 'swamp of interminable self analysis and self disclosure'; the danger of reflexivity (Finlay 2002b, p. 212). Practices of reflexive analysis need only be exploited where there is a purpose for doing so within the RPP partnership. Where reflexivity is appropriate and required, Delamont (2005, p. 310) argues for it as a 'ruthless, relentless, continuous' process and an 'escape' from the problems of research via a positive 'attack' on those problems. There is merit in taking a structured approach to reflexivity (Barber *et al.* 2011). For Finlay (2002b) this involves processes of introspection, intersubjective reflection, mutual collaboration, social critique and discursive construction. In the context of RPP partnerships I work within and drawing on Grant's (2014) discussion, I contend that reflexive acts need to focus on four overlapping aspects of partnership working: (1) one's own personal and professional characteristics; (2) the status of people and relationships in a collaboration; (3) attending to expected and unexpected processes and outcomes in design, data collection, analysis, reporting and management aspects of RPP projects and (4) the various public and private impacts of partnership working.

Reflexivity in RPP partnerships is not the sole preserve of researchers. It can and should involve all actors in the partnership applying and articulating why and how they are involved in the RPP partnership and considering how their motivations, goals and methods impact on the work of others. In this sense there is a synergy between reflexivity and reciprocity. Indeed, Antonacopoulou (2006) surmises that reflexivity is a dynamic exchange between reflection and action which contributes to learning and adaptation. Mutual learning through reflexive and reciprocal exchange is perhaps a fundamental dynamic in RPP partnerships which seek to advance knowledge and build evidence for sport, public health and wellbeing. It is the central tenet of co-production. Co-production is most commonly associated with the delivery of public services in a democratic and reciprocal relationship between professionals and service users (Boyle and Harris 2009). However, it is an approach that applies to knowledge production and exchange partnerships and one which eschews hierarchical forms of knowledge production, seeks to go beyond a research focus on generating results for academic publication and embraces strategies for mutual engagement of a range of stakeholders in collaborative approaches to knowledge production, learning and dissemination.

Co-production, co-learning and co-researching are central tenets of the collaborative development work in the culture, sport and wellbeing project; a RPP partnership within the UK What Works Wellbeing Centre (whatworkswellbeing.org). In this project around 55 partner organisations from policy, commissioning and managing, service delivery, academic and public/citizen sectors have come together through face-to-face workshops, telephone conversations, email exchanges, seminar discussions and participatory activities. This has opened up opportunities for reflexive dialogue to develop knowledge about conceptualising and measuring wellbeing in culture and sport, and to express a consensus about focused topics and methods for identifying, assessing, synthesising, translating and mobilising evidence on the relationships between wellbeing and taking part in cultural and sport activities. Embracing a reflexive perspective and concomitantly taking a stance of reciprocity in this particular RPP partnership is not without its challenges. It requires ongoing, elaborate and extended negotiations about both personal and project politics (Grant 2014). Yet, there is some potential through a critical reflexive perspective to construct and reconstruct alternative possibilities for research and learning, decision-making and service delivery via an undoing of taken-for-granted, established rules and norms of knowledge production and partnership working. Alongside a stance of reciprocity that frames co-production, reflexivity can help confront a prevailing positivist hegemony in knowledge production and exchange and challenge traditional hierarchies of governance in research, policy and practice networks. The contemporary emphasis of partnership working already discussed in this paper and particularly the development of 'deliberative forums' seeking to engage the public in policy and decision-making, and I would add knowledge production and exchange, is a case in point (Newman *et al.* 2004, p. 205). In RPP partnerships I would argue that reflexivity presents the possibility of a more 'responsible politics' (Bourdieu and Wacquant 1992, p. 194). Critical reflexivity, then, enables a re-thinking of established, normative methods of working; advancing knowledge production, exchange, translation and mobilisation in innovative and possibly more impactful ways.

Conclusion

In the first editorial of the *International Journal of Sport Policy and Politics*, Houlihan, Bloyce and Smith (2009, p. 5) identified theoretically informed analysis of the 'evidential turn' in policymaking and the insistence on monitoring and evaluation as a central theme in developing the research agenda in sport policy. There appears to be a window of opportunity in the current policy focus in the UK on sport for health where the values of research, policy and practice are coinciding around evidence building. Partnership working and its alleged benefits are well established in public health and now sport appears to be a policy sector which is being shaped along similar lines. This poses opportunities and challenges of course. Thinking optimistically, there may be opportunities for knowledge exchange about RPP working between public health professionals and those in sport. Equally, sport scholars and professionals from a range of disciplines in the social and political sciences are well placed, and expertly trained to understand, develop, lead and work within complex, collaborative RPP partnerships that are emerging in the sport for health agenda particularly where the focus is on understanding sport and public health inequalities. They are also theoretically able to critically examine the politics of the RPP partnerships in which they might be involved.

One conclusion to the question about how collaborative partnership working in RPP networks can be successful is based on practical requirements such as an identified need to agree goals, methods of working and objectives and strategies for monitoring and evaluation before the implementation of partnership projects. The intention of such practical arrangements is to protect programme fidelity and increase the potential for service delivery effectiveness. Yet, such a view misses out an analysis of the complex sociodynamics that characterise partnership working and that are central to understanding how such partnerships work, for whom and in what contexts. An overlapping nexus of social interactions with actors engaging in varying degrees of resourcefulness, reciprocity and reflexivity marks out partner motivations and methods of working, shapes the processes by which partnership working takes place, and influences knowledge production and exchange. Understanding the dynamics of the three Rs in RPP partnerships has the potential to demythologise the role of sport in public health through an analysis of the way resources are allocated, used and owned, and by consideration and articulation of the relationship dynamics of partnership working. Such critical examination can further an understanding of, and make public, issues concerning; knowledge production, dissemination and use; the legitimation of some forms of evidence over others; and it can potentially maximise the impact of the co-production of knowledge.

Disclosure statement

No potential conflict of interest was reported by the author.

References

Adkins, L., 2003. Reflexivity freedom or habit of gender? *Theory, culture & society*, 20 (6), 21–42.

Alldred, P., 1998. Ethnography and discourse analysis: dilemmas in representing the voices of children. *In*: J. Ribbens and R. Edwards, eds. *Feminist dilemmas in qualitative research: public knowledge and private lives*. London: Sage.

Antonacopoulou, E., 2006. *The dynamics of reflexive practice: the relationship between learning and changing* (Unpublished Doctoral dissertation). University of Liverpool.

Balloch, S. and Taylor, M., 2001. *Partnership working: policy and practice*. Bristol: Policy Press.

Barber, R., *et al.*, 2011. Evaluating the impact of service user involvement on research: a prospective case study. *International journal of consumer studies*, 35 (6), 609–615. doi:10.1111/ijcs.2011.35.issue-6

Beacom, A., 2007. A question of motives: reciprocity, sport and development assistance. *European sport management quarterly*, 7 (1), 81–107. doi:10.1080/16184740701270386

Beresford, P., 2002. User involvement in research and evaluation: liberation or regulation? *Social policy and society*, 1 (02), 95–105. doi:10.1017/S1474746402000222

Birchall, C., 2011. Transparency, interrupted: secrets of the left. *Theory, culture & society*, 28 (7–8), 60–84. doi:10.1177/0263276411423040

Black, N., 2001. Evidence based policy: proceed with care. *British medical journal*, 323 (7307), 275. doi:10.1136/bmj.323.7307.275

Bloyce, D., *et al.*, 2008. Playing the game (plan): a figurational analysis of organizational change in sports development in England. *European sport management quarterly*, 8 (4), 359–378. doi:10.1080/16184740802461637

Bourdieu, P. and Wacquant, L., 1992. *An invitation to reflexive sociology*. Chicago, IL: University of Chicago press.

Boyle, D. and Harris, M., 2009. *The challenge of co-production*. London: New Economics Foundation.

Brackenridge, C., 1999. Managing myself: investigator survival in sensitive research. *International review for the sociology of sport*, 34 (4), 115–130.

Carver, C., 1997. You want to measure coping but your protocol' too long: consider the brief cope. *International journal of behavioral medicine*, 4 (1), 92–100. doi:10.1207/s15327558ijbm0401_6

Cavill, N., Richardson, D., and Foster, C., 2012. *Improving health through participation in sport: a review of research and practice*. Oxford: BHF Health Promotion Research Group.

Chalip, L., 2006. Toward a distinctive sport management discipline. *Journal of sport management*, 20 (1), 1–21.

Chavis, D., 2001. The paradoxes and promise of community coalitions. *American journal of community psychology*, 29 (2), 309–320. doi:10.1023/A:1010343100379

Coalter, F., 2010. The politics of sport-for-development: limited focus programmes and broad gauge problems? *International review for the sociology of sport*, 45 (3), 295–314.

Crawford, R., 1980. Healthism and the medicalization of everyday life. *International journal of health services*, 10 (3), 365–388.

Cunliffe, A., 2004. On becoming a critically reflexive practitioner. *Journal of management education*, 28 (4), 407–426. doi:10.1177/1052562904264440

Davies, H., Nutley, S.M., and Smith, P.C., 2000. *What works: evidence-based policy and practice in the social services*. Bristol: Policy Press.

DCMS, 2015. *Sporting future: a new strategy for an active nation*. London: Crown Copyright.

Delamont, S., 2005. No place for women among them? Reflections on the axe of fieldwork. *Sport, education and society*, 10 (3), 305–320.

Department of Health, 2011. *Healthy lives healthy people: a call to action on obesity in England*. London: The Stationary Office, Crown Copyright.

Douglas, J., *et al*., 2007. *A reader in promoting public health*. London: Sage.

Elias, N., 1978. *What is sociology? Translated by* Stephen Mennell and Grace Morrissey. London: Hutchinson, 5.

Elias, N. and Dunning, E., 1986. *Quest for excitement: sport and leisure in the civilizing process*, Vol. 288. Oxford: Blackwell.

Elias, N., Mennell, S., and Goudsblom, J., 1998. *On civilization, power, and knowledge: selected writings*, Vol. 1. University of Chicago Press.

Elias, N., 2000. *The civilising process: sociogenetic and psychogenetic investigations*. London: WileyBlackwell.

Finlay, L., 2002a. "Outing" the researcher: the provenance, process, and practice of reflexivity. *Qualitative health research*, 12 (4), 531–545. doi:10.1177/104973202129120052

Finlay, L., 2002b. Negotiating the swamp: the opportunity and challenge of reflexivity in research practice. *Qualitative research*, 2 (2), 209–230. doi:10.1177/146879410200200205

Flintoff, A., Foster, R., and Wystawnoha, S., 2011. Promoting and sustaining high quality physical education and school sport through school sport partnerships. *European physical education review*, 17 (3), 341–351. doi:10.1177/1356336X11416731

Foucault, M., 1980. *Power/knowledge: selected interviews and other writings, 1972-1977*. London: Pantheon.

Frisby, W. and Millar, S., 2002. The actualities of doing community development to promote the inclusion of low income populations in local sport and recreation. *European sport management quarterly*, 2 (3), 209–233. doi:10.1080/16184740208721923

Frisby, W., Thibault, L., and Kikulis, L., 2004. The organizational dynamics of under-managed partnerships in leisure service departments. *Leisure studies*, 23 (2), 109–126. doi:10.1080/0261436042000224482

Gillies, P., 1998. Effectiveness of alliances and partnerships for health promotion. *Health promotion international*, 13 (2), 99–120. doi:10.1093/heapro/13.2.99

Goodman, R.M., *et al*., 1998. Identifying and defining the dimensions of community capacity to provide a basis for measurement. *Health education & behavior*, 25 (3), 258–278.

Grant, J., 2014. Reflexivity: interviewing women and men formerly addicted to drugs and/or alcohol. *The qualitative report*, 19 (38), 1. Available from: http://nsuworks.nova.edu/tqr/vol19/iss38/2 [Accessed 14 June 2015].

Green, M., 2007. Governing under advanced liberalism: sport policy and the social investment state. *Policy sciences*, 40 (1), 55–71. doi:10.1007/s11077-007-9034-y

Green, M. and Houlihan, B., 2004. Advocacy coalitions and elite sport policy change in Canada and the United Kingdom. *International review for the sociology of sport*, 39 (4), 387–403. doi:10.1177/1012690204049066

Green, M. and Oakley, B., 2001. Elite sport development systems and playing to win: uniformity and diversity in international approaches. *Leisure studies*, 20 (4), 247–267. doi:10.1080/02614360110103598

Grix, J. and Phillpots, L., 2010. Revisiting the 'governance narrative': 'asymmetrical network governance'and the deviant case of the sports policy sector. *Public policy and administration*, 26 (1), 3–19.

Hargreaves, J., 1986. *Sport, power and culture. A social and historical analysis of popular sports in Britain*. Cambridge: Polity Press.

Hargreaves, J., 1994/2002. *Sporting females: critical issues in the history and sociology of women's sport*. London: Routledge.

Harrison, J., MacGibbon, L., and Morton, M., 2001. Regimes of trustworthiness in qualitative research: the rigors of reciprocity. *Qualitative inquiry*, 7 (3), 323–345. doi:10.1177/107780040100700305

Hayhurst, L.M. and Frisby, W., 2010. Inevitable tensions: Swiss and Canadian sport for development NGO perspectives on partnerships with high performance sport. *European sport management quarterly*, 10 (1), 75–96. doi:10.1080/16184740903554140

Hillsdon, M., *et al*., 2005. *The effectiveness of public health interventions for increasing physical activity among adults: a review of reviews*. London: Health Development Agency, 1–40.

Houlihan, B., Bloyce, D., and Smith, A., 2009. Developing the research agenda in sport policy. *International journal of sport policy and politics*, 1 (1), 1–12. doi:10.1080/19406940802681186

Houlihan, B. and Lindsey, I., 2008. Networks and partnerships in sports development. *In*: V. Girginov, ed. *The management of sports development*. Oxford: Butterworth-Heinemann, 225–242.

Howell, J. and Ingham, A., 2001. From social problem to personal issue: the language of lifestyle. *Cultural studies*, 15 (2), 326–351.

Israel, B., *et al*., 1998. Review of community-based research: assessing partnership approaches to improve public health. *Annual review of public health*, 19 (1), 173–202. doi:10.1146/annurev.publhealth.19.1.173

Johnson, C. and Osborne, S., 2003. Local strategic partnerships, neighbourhood renewal, and the limits to co-governance. *Public money and management*, 23 (3), 147–154. doi:10.1111/1467-9302.00362

Julier, G. and Kimbell, L., 2015. *Research sprints: doing agile, design-oriented, cross disciplinary research in relation to societal issues*. Final report for the developing participation in social design: prototyping projects, programmes and policies: AHRC, UAL, University of Brighton and the Victoria and Albert Museum.

Kay, T., Mansfield, L., and Jeanes, R., 2015. Researching with GoSisters Zambia: reciprocal learning in sport for development. *In*: L. Hayhurst, T. Kay, and M. Chawansky, eds. *Beyond sport for development and peace - transnational perspectives on theory, policy and practice*. London: Routledge, 214–230.

Labonte, R. and Laverack, G., 2001. Capacity building in health promotion, part 1: for whom? And for what purpose? *Critical public health*, 11 (2), 111–127. doi:10.1080/09581590110039838

Lather, P., 1986. Research as praxis. *Harvard educational review*, 56 (3), 257–278. doi:10.17763/haer.56.3.bj2h231877069482

Lee, J. and Macdonald, D., 2010. 'Are they just checking our obesity or what?' The healthism discourse and rural young women. *Sport, education and society*, 15 (2), 203–219. doi:10.1080/13573321003683851

Lewis, J., 2005. New labour's approach to the voluntary sector: independence and the meaning of partnership. *Social policy and society*, 4 (2), 121–131. doi:10.1017/S147474640400226X

Lincoln, Y.S. and Denzin, N.K., 2000. The seventh moment: out of the past. *In*: N.K. Denzin and Y.S. Lincoln, eds. *Handbook of qualitative research*. 2nd ed. Thousand Oaks, CA: Sage, 1047–1065.

Lindsey, I., 2014. Prospects for local collaboration into an uncertain future: learning from practice within labour's partnership paradigm. *Local government studies*, 40 (2), 312–330. doi:10.1080/03003930.2013.805690

Lindsey, I. and Banda, D., 2011. Sport and the fight against HIV/AIDS in Zambia: a 'partnership approach'? *International review for the sociology of sport*, 46 (1), 90–107. doi:10.1177/1012690210376020

Lowndes, V. and Skelcher, C., 1998. The dynamics of multi-organizational partnerships: an analysis of changing modes of governance. *Public administration*, 76 (2), 313–333. doi:10.1111/padm.1998.76.issue-2

Lukes, S., 1974. *Power: a radical view*, vol. 1. London: Macmillan.

Mackintosh, M., 1992. Partnership: issues of policy and negotiation. *Local economy*, 7 (3), 210–224.

Mackintosh, C., 2011. An analysis of county sports partnerships in England: the fragility, challenges and complexity of partnership working in sports development. *International journal of sport policy and politics*, 3 (1), 45–64. doi:10.1080/19406940.2010.524809

Maguire, J., 1988. Doing figurational sociology: some preliminary observations on methodological issues and sensitizing concepts. *Leisure studies*, 7 (2), 187–193. doi:10.1080/02614368800390161

Maiter, S., *et al.*, 2008. Reciprocity: an ethic for community-based participatory action research. *Action research*, 6 (3), 305–325. doi:10.1177/1476750307083720

Mansfield, L., 2007. Involved-detachment: a balance of passion and reason in feminisms and gender-related research in sport, tourism and sports tourism. *Journal of sport & tourism*, 12 (2), 115–141.

Mansfield, L., 2008. Reconsidering feminisms and the work of Norbert Elias for understanding gender, sport and sport-related activities. *European physical education review*, 14 (1), 93–121.

Mansfield, L., *et al.*, 2015. The Health and Sport Engagement (HASE) intervention and evaluation project: protocol for the design, outcome, process and economic evaluation of a complex community sport intervention to increase levels of physical activity. *BMJ open*, 5 (10), e009276. doi:10.1136/bmjopen-2015-009276

Mansfield, L. and Killick, L., 2012. The UK netball superleague: a case study of franchising in elite women's sport organisations. *European sport management quarterly*, 12 (5), 545–567. doi:10.1080/16184742.2012.734525

Mansfield, L. and Malcolm, D., 2014. 13 The Olympic movement, sport and health. *Health and Elite sport: is high performance sport a healthy pursuit?* 38, 187–204.

Markula, P. and Pringle, R., 2006. *Foucault, sport and exercise: power, knowledge and transforming the self*. New York: Routledge.

McDonald, I., 2005. Theorising partnerships: governance, communicative action and sport policy. *Journal of social policy*, 34 (4), 579. doi:10.1017/S0047279405009165

Misener, K. and Doherty, A., 2009. A case study of organizational capacity in nonprofit community sport. *Journal of sport management*, 23 (4), 457–482.

Misener, K.E. and Doherty, A., 2012. Connecting the community through sport club partnerships. *International journal of sport policy and politics*, 4 (2), 243–255. doi:10.1080/19406940.2012.674962

Museke, S., Namukanga, A., and Palmer-Felgate, S., 2015. Reflection on researching with GoSisters Zambia: reciprocal learning in sport for development. *In*: L. Hayhurst, T. Kay, and M. Chawansky, eds. *Beyond sport for development and peace - transnational perspectives on theory, policy and practice*. London: Routledge, 230–237.

Newman, J., *et al.*, 2004. Public participation and collaborative governance. *Journal of social policy*, 33 (02), 203–223. doi:10.1017/S0047279403007499

Österlind, M., 2016. Sport policy evaluation and governing participation in sport: governmental problematics of democracy and health. *International journal of sport policy and politics*. doi:10.1080/19406940.2015.1123755

Ostrom, E. and Walker, J., eds., 2003. *Trust and reciprocity: interdisciplinary lessons for experimental research: interdisciplinary lessons for experimental research*. New York: Russell Sage Foundation.

Petticrew, M. and Roberts, H., 2003. Evidence, hierarchies, and typologies: horses for courses. *Journal of epidemiology and community health*, 57 (7), 527–529. doi:10.1136/jech.57.7.527

Petticrew, M., *et al.*, 2004. Evidence for public health policy on inequalities: 1: the reality according to policymakers. *Journal of epidemiology and community health*, 58 (10), 811–816. doi:10.1136/jech.2003.015289

Phillips, G. and Green, J., 2015. Working for the public health: politics, localism and epistemologies of practice. *Sociology of health & illness*, 37 (4), 491–505. doi:10.1111/1467-9566.12214

Popay, J., *et al.*, 1998. Theorising inequalities in health: the place of lay knowledge. *Sociology of health & illness*, 20 (5), 619–644. doi:10.1111/1467-9566.00122

Priest, N., *et al.*, 2008. Policy interventions implemented through sporting organisations for promoting healthy behaviour change. *Cochrane database of systematic reviews* [Online], 3. Available from: http://www.cochranelibrary.com/ [Accessed 1 June 2013].

Rychetnik, L., *et al.*, 2002. Criteria for evaluating evidence on public health interventions. *Journal of epidemiology and community health*, 56 (2), 119–127. doi:10.1136/jech.56.2.119

Sabatier, P. and Jenkins-Smith, H., 1993. *Policy change and learning: an advocacy coalition approach*. Boulder, CO: Westview Press.

Sackett, D., *et al.*, 1996. Evidence based medicine: what it is and what it isn't. *British medical journal*, 312 (7023), 71–72. doi:10.1136/bmj.312.7023.71

Shaw, S. and Allen, J., 2006. "It basically is a fairly loose arrangement… and that works out fine, really." Analysing the dynamics of an interorganisationalPartnership. *Sport management review*, 9 (3), 203–228. doi:10.1016/S1441-3523(06)70026-2

Smith, A. and Leech, R., 2010. 'Evidence. What evidence?': evidence-based policy making and School Sport Partnerships in North West England. *International journal of sport policy*, 2 (3), 327–345.

Smith, E., *et al.*, 2008. Service user involvement in nursing, midwifery and health visiting research: a review of evidence and practice. *International journal of nursing studies*, 45 (2), 298–315. doi:10.1016/j.ijnurstu.2006.09.010

Sport England, 2012. *Creating a sporting habit for life: a new youth sport strategy*. London: DCMS.

Sugden, J. and Tomlinson, A., 1999. Digging the dirt and staying clean: retrieving the investigative tradition for a critical sociology of sport. *International review for the sociology of sport*, 34 (4), 385–397.

Sugden, J.P. and Tomlinson, A., 2002. *Power games: a critical sociology of sport*. London: Routledge.

Thibault, L., Frisby, W., and Kikulis, L.M., 1999. Interorganizational linkages in the delivery of local leisure services in Canada: responding to economic, political and social pressures. *Managing leisure*, 4 (3), 125–141.

Thomas, M., Burth, M., and Parkes, J., 2010. The emergence of evidence-based practice. *In*: J. McCarthy and P. Rose, eds. *Values-based health and social care: beyond evidence-based practice*. London: Sage, 3–25.

Tomlinson, A., 1998. POWER: domination, negotiation, and resistance in sports cultures. *Journal of sport & social issues*, 22 (3), 235–240. doi:10.1177/019372398022003001

Trainor, A. and Bouchard, K., 2013. Exploring and developing reciprocity in research design. *International journal of qualitative studies in education*, 26 (8), 986–1003. doi:10.1080/09518398.2012.724467

Waddington, I., 2000. *Sport, health and drugs: a critical sociological perspective*. London: Taylor & Francis.

Weed, M., *et al.*, 2009. *A systematic review of the evidence base for developing a physical activity and health legacy from the London 2012 Olympic and paralympic games*. Department of health. London: Crown Copyright.

Weed, M., *et al.*, 2012. Developing a physical activity legacy from the London 2012 Olympic and paralympic games: a policy-led systematic review. *Perspectives in public health*, 132 (2), 75–80. doi:10.1177/1757913911435758

Weiss, C.H., *et al.*, 2008. The fairy godmother—and her warts making the dream of evidence-based policy come true. *American journal of evaluation*, 29 (1), 29–47.

Williams, A., *et al.*, 2005. Establishing and sustaining community–university partnerships: a case study of quality of life research. *Critical public health*, 15 (3), 291–302. doi:10.1080/09581590500372451

World Health Organisation (WHO), 2007. *Working for health: an introduction to the World Health Organization*. Geneva: WHO.

Zigo, D., 2001. Rethinking reciprocity: collaboration in labor as a path toward equalizing power in classroom research. *International journal of qualitative studies in education*, 14 (3), 351–365. doi:10.1080/09518390110029094

Exercise on referral: evidence and complexity at the nexus of public health and sport policy

E. J. Oliver, C. L. Hanson, I. A. Lindsey and C. J. Dodd-Reynolds

ABSTRACT

Exercise on referral schemes (ERS) are recommended by the National Institute of Clinical Excellence for increasing physical activity in inactive patients with long-term health conditions. The current paper critiques a recent extension to ERS provision, specifically, schemes using sport as the primary delivery mechanism (sport-based ERS). We suggest attention should be given to how such schemes that operate across sport and public health sectors may have mismatched approaches to evidence and policy implementation.

Specifically, we highlight two current issues concerning ERS and consider the addition of sport-based schemes in respect to these. First, we argue that ERS-related public health policy and guidance is drawn from a limited evidence base, and is consequently vague. While this leads to opportunities for local innovation, the subsequent design, implementation and evaluation of ERS is diverse. 'Scaling-up' of effective interventions, desired by Public Health England, is therefore problematic, and likely to be further exacerbated by introducing sport-based ERS. Second, we contend that sport-based schemes are unlikely to overcome existing challenges concerning untargeted provision of ERS, and that funding would be better directed towards services for those who have complex barriers to successful engagement.

Introduction: the emergence of sport-based ERS

Exercise on referral schemes (ERS) are one of the most widespread physical activity interventions in the United Kingdom, with a sustained rise in number initiated since the early 1990s (Pavey *et al.* 2011). Usually commissioned via public health, they involve referral of patients with long-term conditions from primary care to a third party (typically a leisure provider), where a programme is provided that aims to encourage participants to increase their physical activity levels. There is, however, a lack of clear evidence about ERS' effectiveness in terms of changing physical activity behaviour and for whom different types of scheme are most effective (National Institute for Health and Care Excellence (NICE) 2014). Accordingly, NICE guidance (2014) proposes broad restrictions on ERS funding and use, recommending that referral is not appropriate where individuals are inactive or sedentary but are otherwise healthy. Furthermore, when schemes are commissioned, NICE recommends performance data be collected and made available to allow for assessment of effectiveness within population subgroups.

Despite the cautious approach recommended for public health commissioning of ERS, new schemes have recently been implemented with support from Sport England's 'Get Healthy, Get

Active' fund (Sport England 2014). One development of particular note has been the commissioning of ERS that use sport (as opposed to traditional gym or class-based activities) as the primary delivery mechanism, here called sport-based ERS. Funding sport pathways within established public health provision is a clear attempt to enact the recommendations of Cavill, Richardson and Foster's (2012) review, funded by Sport England, for sport to be fully integrated in service offers for health.

Targeting public health objectives through sport is not novel in itself. From the 1960s, sport has repeatedly responded to political impetus to contribute to various social policy objectives (Houlihan and White 2002). Policy documents from the turn of the century through to the most recent government strategy for sport have repeatedly advocated and sought to evidence the health benefits of sport as a form of physical activity (e.g. DCMS /Strategy Unit 2002, Carter 2005, DCMS 2010, HM Government 2015). However, the extent to which the implementers of sport programmes are themselves deeply committed to, and capable of, delivering on health agendas has previously been questioned (Bloyce *et al.* 2008). Nevertheless, current policies for sport (HM Government 2015) and public health (Public Health England 2014a) are aligned in identifying a need for cross-sectoral approaches to address physical inactivity. 'Everybody Active Every Day' (Public Health England 2014a) acknowledges existing networks between stakeholders from sport, leisure, social care and health, for example, and highlights an opportunity for sport and fitness professionals to deliver targeted health-based programmes for those with complex health issues. Such policies provide a clear steer for Sport England's funding for new programmes using sport to improve health.

Given this increasingly prominent overlap and coworking, exploring the potential for complementarity or conflict between sport and public health policy is both pertinent and topical. Here, we focus on the emerging use of sport-based ERS to highlight some of the difficulties in seeking a greater role for sport within public health. We briefly summarise existing problems with ERS policy, in terms of interpretation, delivery and evaluation, and consider implications for both sport and public health policy makers. First, we discuss how problems in evaluating ERS' effectiveness have previously limited the scaling-up of good practice in order to inform policy, and argue this also applies to sport-based ERS. Second, we consider whether current policy is appropriate in advocating a relatively untargeted approach to the prescription of ERS, and whether sport-based ERS will serve those neglected by or unable to access current schemes. We conclude by suggesting that these concerns represent a significant challenge for any continuing impetus towards sport-based ERS.

The problematic relationship between ERS evidence and policy

Rigorous systematic reviews encompassing extensive literature are required to inform NICE guidelines, including those applicable to ERS. For physical activity-based interventions sensitive to complex individual behavioural and social influences, this approach may limit broader understanding of what works, for whom and in what circumstances (Pawson *et al.* 2005). This is further exacerbated as PHE's (2014b) application of rigorous quantitative Nesta standards has resulted in criticisms of the ERS evidence-base in terms of sparse use of randomised control trials (RCTs), failure to establish causality (e.g. PHE 2014c) and considerable variation in data collection, analysis and reporting quality between schemes. Responding to these criticisms is a challenge for those involved in the delivery of ERS given the pragmatic nature of the schemes and service expectations of referrers. Similar constraints commonly apply to community-based physical activity interventions more broadly, and indeed also to sport-based interventions. Although some reviews attempt to adopt a balanced and inclusive approach to interpreting the diverse evidence-base for sport-based interventions (e.g. Taylor *et al.* 2015), determining the effectiveness of sport-based ERS may be problematic when examples and expertise of methodologies, such as RCTs, prioritised by public health policy makers are found even more rarely within the sport sector (Cavill *et al.* 2012).

With trial-based evidence taken to be the gold standard, assessments have indicated that the evidence for public health-based physical activity schemes is weak. This is reflected in Public Health England (2014b) findings that from 952 programmes, only 34 were sufficiently rigorous to be classified according to Nesta standards of evidence. No ERS interventions met standards for 'proven practice', or 'promising practice'; only 6 of the 28 programmes classed as 'emerging practice' were ERS-based. Since ERS are generally tailored to the requirements of the community in which they are based, scalability is a problem (PHE 2014b).

Given this, it is perhaps unsurprising that national policy and best practice guidelines that attempt to draw from the evidence-base are somewhat vague; for example, NICE (2014) are unable to define discrete subpopulations for whom an ERS pathway may be more effective, nor provide a single 'gold standard' in terms of programme structure. Such ambiguous policy, or guidance that lacks specificity, enables a myriad of interpretations in practice (Matland 1995). In the case of ERS, we suggest that one consequence has been continued diversity in terms of scheme delivery and evaluation quality (PHE, 2014b). While this might well be construed as positive in terms of allowing for local innovations in service provision, perhaps including the development of sport-based ERS, it does little to resolve uncertainties concerning the relative effectiveness of schemes or their components. In turn, this has impeded progress in terms of identifying, communicating and achieving the desired scaling-up (Public Health England 2014b) of best practice models for ERS. Recognition that there is insufficient understanding as to how national policies may effectively contribute to improving sport participation (Nicholson *et al.* 2011) suggests that the addition of sport-based ERS will exacerbate rather than clarify these problems. As such, while there is strong political impetus for linking sport and ERS, diversifying ERS delivery in this way may raise additional problems when seeking to summarise the evidence.

Broad or narrow: should policy advocate the more targeted delivery of ERS?

At present, NICE (2014) offer only a broad recommendation for ERS' eligibility criteria, namely individuals who are inactive or sedentary and have existing medical conditions. This approach fails to acknowledge emerging evidence suggesting schemes may be more, or only, effective or engaging for particular groups. While this does not yet reach a consensus (Campbell *et al.* 2015), extending the range of evidence considered by public health reviews may offer guidance for more targeted policy. For example, some ERS have been identified as more successful at engaging older individuals (Isaacs *et al.* 2007, Hanson *et al.* 2013), those living in a less deprived area (Gidlow *et al.* 2007) or those referred from specific disease pathways (Dugdill *et al.* 2005; Sowden *et al.* 2008; Hanson *et al.* 2013). At the least, guidelines should encourage attention to subgroup effects in both evaluations and by evidence users.

Exploring *why* subgroups do not initially engage with, or continue to attend, ERS will have value for informing more effective practice as well as future policy through enhancing understanding of the complex sociodemographic, environmental, economic and cultural barriers that may inhibit behaviour change. For example, previous work has linked factors, such as age, employment status, family type, household income and habitual location to physical activity (e.g. Bergman *et al.* 2008; Pan *et al.* 2009, Borodulin *et al.* 2016). Mixed methods approaches can highlight not only groups who may be poorly served by interventions, but also provide detail on how these barriers and interventions are experienced from the perspective of the individual. For example, qualitative data (Hanson 2015) identifies serious psychological barriers (e.g. low self-esteem, fear of change and body image disorders), impaired social circumstances (ranging from a lack of active peer role models to codependent or restrictive interpersonal relationships) or chronic negative experiences of exercise, often commencing in childhood, as factors influencing participants' ERS experiences.

For individuals who are affected by severe or multiple barriers, we argue that it is unrealistic to expect ERS to result in sustained change of habitual behaviours. Such participants may require a different or more intensive approach before change at the individual level can occur (e.g.

therapeutic approaches, support from multiple agencies or broader system change). These arguments, focusing on how individuals can be empowered for change, have begun to inform community sport interventions (e.g. Mansfield *et al.* 2015); they are also clearly relevant to the delivery of ERS. Although considering scheme inclusion and exclusion criteria at the point of referral would enable more effective provision, targeted towards individuals likely to benefit, we must be mindful that this approach would require alternative intervention pathways for those unlikely to engage with and adhere to current ERS provision. Of key relevance here, we must ask whether sport-based ERS are likely to present an attractive alternative for those who do not currently engage with or benefit from schemes, and if not, whether they are really an appropriate way of extending ERS provision.

In this last regard, there has been long-standing recognition (e.g. Collins and Kay 2003) that identified groups who are more likely (e.g. older adults, women) or less likely to engage (e.g. individuals from deprived backgrounds) in ERS are all amongst those less likely to engage with sport. More recent data from Sport England's (n.d.) Active People Survey reinforce the continuation and currency of these trends. It can be argued that the former groups are unlikely to be further engaged by the option of sport-based ERS and there can be little expectation of success for the latter when significant, if somewhat inconsistent, policy impetus and sport-based interventions have previously failed to significantly increase participation amongst those living in deprivation (Bloyce and Smith 2009). Further, sport-based schemes that *have* shown greater promise in engaging individuals from deprived backgrounds have tended to be those that adopt locally driven, bottom-up approaches to implementation (e.g. Walpole and Collins 2010), a direct conflict with the centralised guidance-driven approach favoured in public health guidelines.

Conclusions

We have argued that (i) enhanced quality and consideration of a broader range of evidence concerning ERS' effectiveness is needed before we can establish how they can best be delivered and developed, and (ii) provision for those who are not able to benefit from existing schemes is necessary. On the one hand, the limitations of evidence on public health ERS and the associated ambiguity in policy could be viewed as an opening for adding sport-based ERS to the diversity of current practices. On the other hand, and moving beyond such policy opportunism, there are a number of reasons for concern as to the long-term appropriateness of promoting sport-based ERS as interventions at the nexus of sport and public health policy.

Critically, allocating funding to sport-based ERS is unlikely to address either of the problems identified in this paper. First, the type of evidence desired in the public health sector to scale up interventions is not and has not been widely collected for sport-based interventions. Perceived weaknesses in the evidence-base for ERS are likely to also apply to sport-based ERS trials, resulting in continued ambiguity in national policy guidance. Second, there is little to suggest that sport-based ERS would offer an alternative well-suited to engaging those underserved by current schemes.

More generally, the complexity of issues that can be identified at the nexus of sport and public health requires greater recognition and more nuanced approaches on behalf of policy makers. Some groups, which ERS do not currently engage (e.g. younger adults) *are* more likely to participate in sport (Sport England, n.d.), and offering sport-based ERS may have a role to play in attracting and retaining such individuals. Critically, however, we propose that the more pressing issue is to identify and develop schemes that will work for those who are most in need and least likely to benefit from traditional ERS, that is, those with poor health and complex barriers to engagement.

Disclosure statement

No potential conflict of interest was reported by the authors.

References

Bergman, P., *et al.*, 2008. Adherence to physical activity recommendations and the influence of socio-demographic correlates – a population-based cross-sectional study. *BMC public health*, 22 (8), 367. doi:10.1186/1471-2458-8-367.
Bloyce, D. and Smith, A., 2009. *Sport policy and development: an introduction*. London: Routledge.
Bloyce, D., *et al.*, 2008. 'Playing the game (Plan)': a figurational analysis of organizational change in sports development in England. *European sport management quarterly*, 8 (4), 359–378. doi:10.1080/16184740802461637.
Borodulin, K., *et al.*, 2016. Socio-demographic and behavioral variation in barriers to leisure-time physical activity. *Scandinavian journal of public health*, 44 (1), 62–69. doi:10.1177/1403494815604080.
Campbell, F., *et al.*, 2015. A systematic review and economic evaluation of exercise referral schemes in primary care: a short report. *Health technology assessment* [online], 19 (60), 1–110. Available from: http://www.journalslibrary.nihr.ac.uk/hta/volume-19/issue-60#abstract [Accessed 30 October 2015].
Carter, P., 2005. *Review of national sport effort and resources*. London: DCMS.
Cavill, N., Richardson, D., and Foster, C., 2012. *Improving health through participation in sport: a review of research and practice*. Oxford: BHF Health Promotion Research Group.
Collins, M. and Kay, T., 2003. *Sport and social exclusion*. London: Routledge.
Department for Culture, Media and Sport (DCMS). 2010. *Plans for the legacy from the 2012 Olympic and Paralympic games*. London: DCMS.
Department for Culture, Media and Sport (DCMS) /Strategy Unit. 2002. *Game plan: a strategy for delivering government's sport and physical activity objectives*. London: DCMS/SU.
Dugdill, L., Graham, R., and McNair, F., 2005. Exercise referral: the public health panacea for physical activity promotion? A critical perspective of exercise referral schemes; their development and evaluation. *Ergonomics*, 48, 1390–1410. doi:10.1080/00140130500101544.
Gidlow, C., *et al.*, 2007. Socio-demographic patterning of referral, uptake and attendance in physical activity referral schemes. *Journal of public health*, 9, 7–13.
Hanson, C.L., 2015. *The Northumberland exercise on referral scheme; what works, for whom and in what circumstances?* Unpublished thesis. Durham University.
Hanson, C.L., *et al.*, 2013. An evaluation of the efficacy of the exercise on referral scheme in Northumberland, UK: association with physical activity and predictors of engagement. A naturalistic observation study. *BMJ open* [online], 3 (8), e002849. Available from: http://bmjopen.bmj.com/content/3/8/e002849.long [Accessed 30 October 2013].
HM Government. 2015. *Sporting future: a new strategy for an active nation*. London: Cabinet Office.
Houlihan, B. and White, A., 2002. *The politics of sports development*. Oxon: Routledge.
Isaacs, A., *et al.*, 2007. Exercise evaluation randomised trial (EXERT): a randomised trial comparing GP referral for leisure centre-based exercise, community-based walking and advice only. *Health technology assessment* [online], 11 (10), doi:10.3310/hta11100 [Accessed 30 October 2007].
Mansfield, L., *et al.*, 2015. The Health and Sport Engagement (HASE) Intervention and evaluation project: protocol for the design, outcome, process and economic evaluation of a complex community sport intervention to increase levels of physical activity. *British medical journal open*, 5 (10), e009276.
Matland, R.E., 1995. Synthesizing the implementation literature: the ambiguity conflict model of policy implementation. *Journal of public administration research and theory*, 5, 145–174.
National Institute for Health and Care Excellence (NICE). 2014. *Physical activity: exercise referral schemes (PH54)* [online]. Available from: http://www.nice.org.uk/guidance/ph54/resources/physical-activity-exercise-referral-schemes-1996418406085 [Accessed 7 February 2016].
Nicholson, M., Hoye, R., and Houlihan, B., 2011. Conclusion. In: M. Nicholson, R. Hoye, and B. Houlihan, eds. *Participation in sport: international policy perspectives*. Abingdon: Routledge.
Pan, S.Y., *et al.*, 2009. Individual, social, environmental, and physical environmental correlates with physical activity among Canadians: a cross-sectional study. *BMC public health*, 9 (1), 21. doi:10.1186/1471-2458-9-21.
Pavey, T.G., *et al.*, 2011. The clinical effectiveness and cost-effectiveness of exercise referral schemes: a systematic review and economic evaluation. *Health technology assessment* [online], 15. Available from: http://www.journalslibrary.nihr.ac.uk/hta/volume-15/issue-44 [Accessed 30 October 2015].
Pawson, R., *et al.*, 2005. Realist review - a new method of systematic review designed for complex policy interventions. *Journal of health services research & policy*, 10 (1), 21–34. doi:10.1258/1355819054308530.
Public Health England. 2014a. *Everybody active, every day: an evidence-based approach to physical activity* [online]. PHE publications gateway number: 2014432. Available from: https://www.gov.uk/government/publications/everybody-active-every-day-a-framework-to-embed-physical-activity-into-daily-life [Accessed 7 February 2016].
Public Health England. 2014b. *Identifying what works for local physical inactivity interventions* [online]. PHE publications gateway number: 2014432. Available from: https://www.gov.uk/government/uploads/system/uploads/attachment_data/file/374560/Whatworksv1_2.pdf [Accessed 7 February 2016].
Public Health England. 2014c. *Identifying 'what works' for local physical inactivity interventions. Tailored feedback for the Northumberland Exercise on Referral Scheme*. London: ukactive Research Institute.

Sowden, S.L., *et al.*, 2008. Do general practices provide equitable access to physical activity interventions? *British journal general practical* [online], 58, 1–8. Available from: http://bjgp.org/content/58/555/e1.long [Accessed 30 October 2008].

Sport England. 2014. *Get healthy get active: what we've learnt so far.* Available from: http://www.sportengland.org/media/397773/FINAL-Get-Healthy-Get-Active-what-we-ve-learnt.pdf [Accessed 14 October 2015].

Sport England. n.d. *Active people Interactive.* Available from: http://activepeople.sportengland.org/ [Accessed 7 February 2016].

Taylor, P., *et al.*, 2015. *A review of the social impacts of culture and sport.* London: Department for Culture, Media and Sport (DCMS).

Walpole, C. and Collins, M., 2010. Sports development in microcosm: braunston sport action zone. In: M. Collins, ed. *Examining sports development.* Abingdon: Routledge.

The world turned upside down: sport, policy and ageing

Michael Gard and Rylee A. Dionigi

ABSTRACT
Sport as social policy has reached a peculiar and somewhat paradoxical crossroads. Historically, sport has generally been seen as healthy for young people but ill-advised for older people. However, in the context of the twenty-first century's 'obesity epidemic', the rising 'risk' of lifestyle diseases and ageing populations, some scholars suggest that competitive and vigorous sports may not be the right kind of physical activity for young people because, they argue, it is not something they will be able to keep doing in later life. As a result, they argue that young people should be introduced to moderate intensity 'lifestyle' activities like walking and going to the gym which will hopefully improve their health and protect them from weight gain and ill-health as they age. At the same time, enthusiasm for sport participation as a policy setting to help older people maintain their independence and improve their general quality of life is growing. Sport participation also appears to be on the rise among older people and, as our research suggests, is becoming understood as a more 'normal' part of the ageing process in Western countries. In this article, we offer examples of these rhetorical shifts and argue that, as ever, sport emerges as an endlessly flexible discursive policy resource.

Putting to one side their medical significance, public health crises offer rich terrain for social scientists. For one thing, they invariably become the pretext for commentators to push their pre-existing agendas, hobbyhorses, biases and prejudices, regardless of how tangential they might seem to the problem at hand. For example, one public health crisis among many is the emergence of the 'obesity epidemic' from about the beginning of the twenty-first century onwards, which was seized upon by ideologues, academics and moral crusaders alike. Two broad camps centring on the obesity crisis are 'alarmists' who characterise it as a looming global health catastrophe and 'sceptics' who argue that the consequences of rising obesity levels have either been greatly exaggerated or are unclear (see Gard 2011a for a more complex account of the different groups that make up both sides of this debate). As a result, a rainbow of social phenomena – including but by no means limited to gay marriage, feminism, technology, poverty, affluence, urbanisation, fast food, rampant individualism, capitalism and socialism – have all been blamed for rising bodyweights (see Gard 2011b for an extended discussion of these different explanations). Other related public health risks are the social and economic 'burden' of the world's ageing population (Pike 2011) and the rise in so-called 'lifestyle diseases', such as diabetes and cardiovascular disease, of which inactivity has been labelled as a major contributing factor (see Confederation of Australian Sport 2014; Australian Sports Commission 2015).

A second but related dimension of public health crises is their tendency to generate a flurry of ameliorative responses, many of which enjoy little or no empirical foundation or track record of success. Three responses we will focus on are the *de-emphasis* on sport for young people, the increase in public money promoting sport in schools and the growing emphasis on sport for older people. Before discussing the relationship between sport policy and public health, however, we share examples of responses to the obesity epidemic more broadly to demonstrate that, above all, public crises tempt people to call for measures that might, were it not for the prevailing crisis rhetoric, seem unwise, heavy-handed or reactionary.

In the case of obesity, the construction of rising body weights as a public health emergency has licensed a strangely cavalier approach to public health policy and intervention. This is sometimes phrased as the need to act on the 'best available evidence' rather than waiting for the 'best possible evidence' (see Heart and Stoke Foundation of Canada 2005; see also Institute of Medicine 2013). In a striking recent example, Hodge *et al.* (2014) argued for a complete ban on American young people being sold or possessing sweetened beverages in public. Sweetened beverages, they claimed, should only be consumed by young people in their own home under the supervision of adults where nobody else can see them. In other words, when a matter of public health interest morphs into a 'crisis' in the way that childhood obesity has, extreme measures begin to look less extreme, at least in the eyes of some.

An apparently less extreme but more widespread line of thinking has emerged concerning the role of sport in the lives of young people. In this formulation, those involved in the promotion of physical activity among young people, such as physical educators and other active living or health promotion stakeholders, are being encouraged to *de-emphasise* sport (and focus on regular moderate to vigorous physical activity) in order to reduce population weight and obesity (Trost 2006, Harrington and Fullagar 2013). The reasoning here rests on a number of alleged shortcomings of sport. In particular, it is held that participation in school sport does not equate to 'adequate' physical activity levels among youth (see Hastie and Trost 2002), organised sport is not universally liked by young people, especially those who are more interested in less structured, non-mainstream lifestyle pursuits such as skateboarding, surfing and bicycle motocross or BMX (Kellett and Russell 2009, Breivik 2010, Wheaton 2010) and, most important of all, sport cannot be considered a 'lifetime' activity (Trost 2006). Instead, public health researchers, physical activity recommendations and government reports alike claim that young people need to be introduced to lifelong activities such as walking, jogging and going to the gym (see Department of Health and Human Services 2008, Hajkowicz *et al.* 2013, Department of Health 2014). As much as anything else, this seems an oddly dispiriting vision in which young people are instructed to prioritise the same forms of activity at age 15 as they might do when they are 70; a life sentence of moderate intensity, calorie-burning physical activity devoid of the emotional highs and lows of competition or physical risk that sport implies.

This trend is interesting for a number of reasons. First and most obvious, these claims are being made at exactly the same time as sports participation is being promoted and publically funded as an anti-childhood obesity policy and/or part of a preventative health strategy more broadly by governments in countries such as Australia, New Zealand and the United Kingdom. For example, Australia saw growth in the *Active After-School Communities* (AASC) programme from 21 schools participating in 2004 to 3270 schools and childcare centres by 2010 (Australian Sports Commission 2010). A total of $A262.7 million of the 2010–2011 Australian federal budget was committed to increasing sports participation (Department of Health and Ageing 2010). In 2011, a *National Sport and Active Recreation Policy Framework* was agreed upon by all Australian and State governments, which called for the 'systematic adoption of sport within all Australian schools' on the basis that it 'is central to achieving better education and health outcomes for Australian youth' (Australian Government 2011, p. 19), including the reduction of obesity levels. For instance, by 2015, the AASC had evolved into the *Sporting Schools* programme which 'is part of the Federal Government's commitment to tackle increasing levels of obesity, particularly among children' (see www.sporting

schools.gov.au/news/Playing-the-Game). This programme saw the Australian Government commit 100 million dollars 'to help schools to increase children's participation in sport, and to connect children with community sport' by primary/elementary schools partnering with endorsed National Sporting Organisations (see www.sportingschools.gov.au/).

It is also worth remembering that sport's critics are not limited to the epidemiologically or public health minded. It has also drawn criticism from feminist scholars who emphasise its oppressively sexist and overtly competitive dimensions (Wright 1995, 1999, 2001, Rich 2004, Enright and O'Sullivan 2010), physical educators who have long doubted its educational value (e.g., Tinning 1995), as well as scholars of youth culture who suggest sport may be an increasingly anachronistic imposition on young people who are moving towards more informal, cooperative and digitally mediated forms of recreation (Wright and Macdonald 2010, Gilchrist and Wheaton 2013). In sum, there is no shortage of researchers and commentators who doubt sport's appropriateness as the basis for a lifetime of meaningful and health-enhancing physical activity.

The divergence of opinion here could not be more stark; on the one hand, a significant amount of public money is being staked on sport's utility in controlling human body weight and managing chronic conditions, while it is being implicated as a serious obstacle on the other hand. This conclusion sits uncomfortably alongside what appears to be a shift away from obesity rhetoric towards an equally overbearing healthy and active ageing agenda and the growing popularity of competitive sports among older people in many parts of the world (Dionigi 2008, Weir *et al.* 2010, Dionigi *et al.* 2011). For example, approximately 30,000 people participated in the 2009 Sydney World Masters Games (WMG; a multisport and entertainment event with most athletes aged in their 40s, 50s and 60s, and a few aged over 100 years). In terms of participant numbers, the Sydney WMG was almost three times larger than the Beijing Olympics (Shephard 2010). Not only are the numbers of senior or 'masters' athletes growing, but sporting organisations, exercise scientists and government agencies now advocate for sport to promote 'healthy lifestyles' and 'active ageing' (see www.imga.ch/; van Uffelen *et al.* 2015) without clearly defining terms or presenting opposing viewpoints. For example, in the 2015 Victoria University report for the Australian Sports Commission, called *Active and Healthy Ageing through Sport* (van Uffelen *et al.* 2015), the authors did not offer a definition of 'active and healthy ageing' nor cite any of the sociological literature that has problematised the participation of sport for older people over the past 10 years (see Dionigi 2016 for a review of such literature).

By 'active ageing', we mean the dominant discourse in policy, the media and health promotion messages, and language used in gerontological and sport science literatures which generally encourages people to remain physically, socially and mentally active as they age. With respect to older people, the World Health Organization (WHO) focuses heavily on physical activity, while the European Union (EU) focuses on productivity and work-like activities (World Health Organization 2002, 2015, Pike 2011, Moulaert and Biggs 2013, Lassen and Moreira 2014). Other similar phrases include healthy ageing, productive ageing, positive ageing and successful ageing all of which have become particularly evident in health-related policy and practice since the 1990s (Dillaway and Byrnes 2009, Biggs 2014a, 2014b, 2014c, World Health Organization 2015). In this climate, sport and physical activity are positioned as crucial, not only in delaying age-related decline and reducing the risk of many chronic conditions (Tulle 2008), but also in keeping older people productive (Biggs 2014b, 2014c) and consuming (Gilleard and Higgs 2007). At the same time, older people who cannot or do not want to participate in sport or physical activity are stigmatised, victimised, medicalised and/or forgotten in health policy and practice (Dionigi and Horton 2012, Dionigi forthcoming).

Charting a way through these divergent ideas about sport's public health utility is difficult enough at the level of conceptual plausibility. However, the task becomes even more complicated when we factor in some empirical and contextual specifics. For example, conclusive evidence that sports participation causes, rather than is simply associated with, good health or 'normal' body weight in the short or long term is scarce. In fact, it is extremely difficult to mount a strong empirical case that sports participation in and of itself leads necessarily to measurable, durable and generalisable social, mental or biomedical outcomes (see Bailey *et al.* 2009, Green 2014, for extended discussions of this empirical challenge).

Another layer of complexity comes into focus when one considers that sport is not simply a form of physical activity but also an industry. Across the Western world, sporting organisations are looking for ways to maintain market share in the face of proliferating entertainment and recreational choice. Notably, in 2013, the Australian Sports Commission teamed up with market analysts, GfK Blue Moon, to conduct the *Market Segmentation Study* on sports participation trends among the Australian adult population (aged 14–65 years). In recognition that sporting club membership has stagnated across Australia, this study identified 10 consumer segments and resulted in recommendations about the types of products, messages and tone necessary to appeal to each segment, with an end goal of attracting and retaining increased club sport memberships (Australian Sports Commission 2013).

This trend is why many sporting organisations devote so much energy to establishing a presence in schools. For instance, the *Sporting Schools* programme in Australia supports *Nestlè* Athletics Australia, *Woolworths* AFL, *MILO* cricket programmes and many other corporate-sponsored sports organisations to deliver before, during and after school programmes to students (www.sportingschools.gov.au). This activity is routinely justified with platitudes and dubious claims about the obesity-busting and intelligence-boosting power of organised sport. This school-offensive currently being waged around the world is also being funded by sport's commercial sponsors who see sport as an efficient and convenient way of lifting awareness and goodwill towards their brand among young people (see Powell 2014 for more examples of school-based corporate 'solutions' to childhood obesity). The deeper truth, however, is that sporting organisations understand that grassroots participation is either withering in some contexts or must at least be nurtured and defended.

In the context of masters sport, international and national Masters Games events, like the WMG, have become a place where the market can use the 'sport for all' and 'active and healthy ageing' dogma to exploit and regulate financially comfortable middle-aged and older adults who have a desire for sport performance, travel, consumption and socialising (Dionigi and Litchfield forthcoming). Governments, too, increasingly see the sports industry as a driver of economic growth and a source of foreign investment and export income, a point which necessitates the development of new sports-related policies (for a discussion of the economic dimensions of government sports policies in Australia, see Hajkowicz *et al.* 2013).

Last, sport is both an ideology and a form of culture. That is, there are many who simply believe in their hearts, without the need for evidence, in sport's inherent moral and social goodness. For example, the latest document to increase sports participation from the Australian Government agency, the Australian Sports Commission (2015, p. 3), unequivocally claims that, 'Australians love sport.... And sport is good for Australians'. Coakley (2015) calls this the Great Sport Myth (GSM). For believers of the GSM, advocating for sport, whether for the young or the old, is a matter of straightforward common sense, a situation that makes it difficult for them to engage with, let alone understand, objections to their point of view.

These observations do not, we think, lead to an obvious end point. Rather, what we are inviting readers to consider is the convergence of social, cultural, economic, political and ideological forces that shape the way people think about the *usefulness* of sport. To emphasise our central argument, no clear-cut empirically supported reason for playing sport exists and interested parties can only, at best, engage in Foucauldian 'truth games' (see Foucault 1988) as they pick and choose the ideas and knowledge claims that best match their pre-existing motivations. In the case of older people, our research suggests that masters sport is both a burgeoning area of middle class consumption as well as a social context in which new understandings of the ageing process are being creatively stitched together out of familiar discursive odds and ends (Dionigi *et al.* 2014). Both old and new ideas about the unsuitability of competitive sport for older people are being turned upside down.

Sport for older people will neither reduce the pressure on national medical systems nor make ageing populations an easier social policy challenge for governments to deal with, but the idea that it might is spreading.

Organised codified sport and the idea that it could be put to premeditated social policy ends were born at a particular point in Western history. Presumably, they both will die somewhere in our future. In the meantime, the life of the idea of sport as a policy instrument reminds us that sport is an endlessly flexible discursive resource capable of meaning almost anything to anyone. Above all, what we have tried to suggest briefly here is that it is important to look beyond familiar or 'common sense' claims about the need for or the effectiveness of sport to solve problems. This is particularly true amidst 'crises' talk of an 'obesity epidemic', 'ageing populations' and rising 'lifestyle diseases' because, as we argued at the beginning of this article, these are fertile discursive conditions for exaggeration, hyperbole and self-interested reasoning.

Disclosure statement

No potential conflict of interest was reported by the authors.

Funding

This work was supported by the Social Sciences and Humanities Research Council of Canada [grant number 435-2013-0647].

References

Australian Government, 2011. *National sport and active recreation policy framework*. Canberra: Commonwealth of Australia.

Australian Sports Commission, 2010. *Active after-school communities program review*. Canberra: Australian Sports Commission.

Australian Sports Commission, 2013. *Market segmentation for sport participation – adults*. Canberra: Australian Sports Commission.

Australian Sports Commission, 2015. *Play.Sport.Australia: Australian Sports Commission's participation game plan*. Canberra: Australian Sports Commission.

Bailey, R., *et al.*, 2009. The educational benefits claimed for physical education and school sport: an academic review. *Research Papers in Education*, 24 (1), 1–27. doi:10.1080/02671520701809817

Biggs, S., 2014a. Adapting to an ageing society: the need for cultural change. *Policy Quarterly*, 10 (3), 12–16.

Biggs, S., 2014b. Precarious ageing versus the policy of indifference: international trends and the G20. *Australasian Journal on Ageing*, 33 (4), 226–228. doi:10.1111/ajag.2014.33.issue-4

Biggs, S., 2014c. The promise of a long life? Cultural adaptation to productive aging, spiritual empathy, and a sustainable future. *Journal of Religion, Spirituality & Aging*, 26 (2–3), 96–108. doi:10.1080/15528030.2013.855964

Breivik, G., 2010. Trends in adventure sports in a post-modern society. *Sport in Society*, 13 (2), 260–273. doi:10.1080/17430430903522970

Coakley, J.J., 2015. Assessing the sociology of sport: on cultural sensibilities and the great sport myth. *International Review for the Sociology of Sport*, 50 (4–5), 402–406. doi:10.1177/1012690214538864

Confederation of Australian Sport, 2014. *Maximising the potential of Australian Sport*. Canberra: Confederation of Australian Sport.

Department of Health, 2014. *Physical activity and sedentary behaviour guidelines for young people (13–17 years)*. Canberra: Australian Government.

Department of Health and Ageing. 2010. World first action on preventative health. *Media Release*, 11 May. Canberra: Australian Government.

Department of Health and Human Services, 2008. *Physical activity guidelines for Americans*. Washington, DC: Department of Health and Human Services. http://www.health.gov/PAGuidelines/pdf/paguide.pdf

Dillaway, H.E. and Byrnes, M., 2009. Reconsidering successful aging: a call for renewed and expanded academic critiques and conceptualizations. *Journal of Applied Gerontology*, 28 (6), 702–722. doi:10.1177/0733464809333882

Dionigi, R.A., 2008. *Competing for life: older people, sport and ageing*. Saarbrüecken: Verlag Dr. Müller.

Dionigi, R.A., 2016. The competitive older athlete: a review of psychosocial and sociological issues. *Topics in Geriatric Rehabilitation*, 32 (1), 55–62. doi:10.1097/TGR.0000000000000091

Dionigi, R.A. and Litchfield, forthcoming. The mid-life 'market' and the creation of sporting sub-cultures. *In*: R.A. Dionigi and M. Gard, eds. *Sport and physical activity across the lifespan: critical perspectives*. Basingstoke: Palgrave Macmillan.

Dionigi, R.A., forthcoming. Leisure and recreation in the lives of older people. *In*: M. Bernoth and D. Winkler, eds. *Healthy ageing and aged care in Australian communities*. Sydney: Oxford University Press.

Dionigi, R.A., Baker, J., and Horton, S., 2011. Older athletes' perceived benefits of competition. *The International Journal of Sport and Society*, 2 (2), 17–28.

Dionigi, R.A., *et al*. 2014. Sport as leisure for older adults: critical reflections and recommendations. *Paper presented at the 14th Canadian Congress on Leisure Research: our new leisure society*, 21–23 May, Halifax, NS.

Dionigi, R.A. and Horton, S., 2012. The influence of leisure on discourses of aging. *In*: H.J. Gibson and J.F. Singleton, eds. *Leisure and aging: theory and practice*. Champaign, IL: Human Kinetics, 27–39.

Enright, E. and O'Sullivan, M., 2010. "Can I do it in my pyjamas?" Negotiating a physical education curriculum with teenage girls. *European Physical Education Review*, 16 (3), 203–222. doi:10.1177/1356336X10382967

Foucault, M., 1988. Technologies of the self. *In*: L.H. Martin, H. Gutman, and P.H. Hutton, eds. *Technologies of the self*. Amherst: University of Massachusetts Press, 16–49.

Gard, M., 2011a. Truth, belief and the cultural politics of obesity scholarship and public health policy. *Critical Public Health*, 21 (1), 37–48. doi:10.1080/09581596.2010.529421

Gard, M., 2011b. *The end of the obesity epidemic*. London: Routledge.

Gilchrist, P. and Wheaton, B., 2013. New media technologies in lifestyle sport. *In*: B. Hutchins and D. Rowe, eds. *Digital media sport: technology, power and culture in the network society*. Abingdon: Routledge, 169–185.

Gilleard, C. and Higgs, P., 2007. The third age and the baby boomers: two approaches to the social structuring of later life. *International Journal of Ageing and Later Life*, 2 (2), 13–30. doi:10.3384/ijal.1652-8670.072213

Green, K., 2014. Mission impossible? Reflecting upon the relationship between physical education, youth sport and lifelong participation. *Sport, Education and Society*, 19 (4), 357–375. doi:10.1080/13573322.2012.683781

Hajkowicz, S.A., *et al*., 2013. *The future of Australian sport: megatrends shaping the sports sector over coming decades. A consultancy report for the Australian Sports Commission*. Canberra: CSIRO, Australia.

Harrington, M. and Fullagar, S., 2013. Challenges for active living provision in an era of healthism. *Journal of Policy Research in Tourism, Leisure and Events*, 5 (2), 139–157. doi:10.1080/19407963.2013.793519

Hastie, P.A. and Trost, S.G., 2002. Student physical activity levels during a season of sport education. *Paediatric Exercise Science*, 14, 64–14.

Heart and Stroke Foundation of Canada, 2005. *Interventions related to obesity: a state of the evidence review*. Ottawa, ON: Heart and Stroke Foundation of Canada.

Hodge, J.G., *et al*., 2014. A proposed ban on the sale to and possession of caloric sweetened beverages by minors in public. *The Journal of Law, Medicine & Ethics*, 42 (1), 110–114. doi:10.1111/jlme.12124

Institute of Medicine, 2013. Educating the student body: taking physical activity and physical education to school. *Recommendations*, May, 1–4. Available from: http://www.nationalacademies.org/hmd/~/media/Files/Report%20Files/2013/Educating-the-Student-Body/EducatingTheStudentBody_Insert.pdf [Accessed 15 January 2016].

Kellett, P. and Russell, R., 2009. A comparison between mainstream and action sport industries in Australia: a case study of the skateboarding cluster. *Sport Management Review*, 12, 66–78. doi:10.1016/j.smr.2008.12.003.

Lassen, A.J. and Moreira, T., 2014. Unmaking old age: political and cognitive formats of active ageing. *Journal of Aging Studies*, 30, 33–46. doi:10.1016/j.jaging.2014.03.004.

Moulaert, T. and Biggs, S., 2013. International and European policy on work and retirement: reinventing critical perspectives on active ageing and mature subjectivity. *Human Relations*, 66 (1), 23–43. doi:10.1177/0018726711435180

Pike, E.C.J., 2011. The active aging agenda, old folk devils and a new moral panic. *Sociology of Sport Journal*, 28 (2), 209–225.

Powell, D., 2014. Childhood obesity, corporate philanthropy and the creeping privatisation of health education. *Critical Public Health*, 24 (2), 226–238. doi:10.1080/09581596.2013.846465

Rich, E., 2004. Exploring teachers' biographies and perceptions of girls' participation in physical education. *European Physical Education Review*, 10 (2), 215–240. doi:10.1177/1356336X04044073

Shephard, R.J., 2010. The future of masters games: implications for policy and research. *In*: J. Baker, S. Horton, and P. Weir, eds. *The masters athlete: understanding the role of sport and exercise in optimizing aging*. London: Routledge, 186–193.

Tinning, R., 1995. The sport education movement: a phoenix, bandwagon or hearse for physical education? *ACHPER Healthy Lifestyles Journal*, 42 (4), 19–21.

Trost, S., 2006. Public health and physical education. *In*: D. Kirk, D. Macdonald, and M. O'Sullivan, eds. *Handbook of physical education*. London: Sage, 163–187.

Tulle, E., 2008. Acting your age? Sports science and the ageing body. *Journal of Aging Studies*, 22 (4), 340–347. doi:10.1016/j.jaging.2008.05.005

van Uffelen, J.G.Z., *et al.* 2015. *Active and healthy ageing through sport*. Report prepared for the Australian Sports Commission. Melbourne: Victoria University, Institute of Sport, Exercise and Active Living (ISEAL).

Weir, P., Baker, J., and Horton, S., 2010. The emergence of masters sport: participatory trends and historical developments. *In*: J. Baker, S. Horton, and P.L. Weir, eds. *The masters athlete: understanding the role of sport and exercise in optimizing aging*. London: Routledge, 7–14.

Wheaton, B., 2010. Introducing the consumption and representation of lifestyle sports. The representation and consumption of lifestyle sports. *Special Issue of Sport in Society*, 13 (7/8), 1057–1081.

World Health Organization, 2002. *Active ageing: a policy framework*. Available from: http://www.who.int/ageing/publications/active_ageing/en/ [Accessed 15 January 2016].

World Health Organization, 2015. *World report on ageing and health*. Available from: http://www.who.int/ageing/events/world-report-2015-launch/en/ [Accessed 15 January 2016].

Wright, J., 1995. A feminist post-structural methodology for the study of gender construction in physical education: description of a study. *Journal of Teaching in Physical Education*, 15 (1), 1–24.

Wright, J., 1999. Changing gendered practices in physical education: working with teachers. *European Physical Education Review*, 5 (3), 181–197. doi:10.1177/1356336X990053002

Wright, J., 2001. Gender reform in physical education: a poststructuralist perspective. *Journal of Physical Education New Zealand*, 34 (1), 15–25.

Wright, J. and Macdonald, D., eds., 2010. *Young people, physical activity and the everyday*. London: Routledge.

The sociopolitics of sport, physical education, and school health in the United States

James D. Ressler, K. Andrew R. Richards and Paul M. Wright

ABSTRACT

Evidence from global sources indicate that physical education (PE) has an integral role to play in the development of behaviours supporting lifetime physical activity. However, PE programmes in many countries fall short of accomplishing this charge. The marginality of PE in comparison to school-based athletic programmes, and inter-role conflict arising from concurrent performance of teaching and coaching roles contribute to this phenomenon. Grounded in role socialisation theory and drawing primarily from the United States context, we explore the social construction of PE teaching and athletic coaching roles in school environments. Different priorities and time demands can lead to conflict, and teachers/coaches often prioritise the role for which they are rewarded and held most accountable. These reward and accountability structures favour coaching in many schools, leading teachers/coaches to focus on coaching to the detriment of their teaching performance. Formal accountability and reward structures are reinforced by administrators, colleagues, children and community members who praise coaching prowess, but fail to acknowledge successes in teaching environments. Since only a small percentage of school children engage in interscholastic athletics, the complex relationship between teaching and coaching can inhibit physical activity and public health agendas that seek to enhance children's health through school-based programming. The content of PE at the secondary level, which replicates team sport environments and reinforces athletic achievement, also marginalises children who are not interested in traditional forms of sport. It is against this backdrop that we discuss opportunities and challenges for the future of PE as a public health intervention.

Introduction

Internationally, there is an increasing focus on the role physical activity plays in promoting public health. The World Health Organization (WHO 2012) identifies physical inactivity as the fourth leading risk factor for global mortality and endorses a population-based approach to preventing childhood obesity through systematic policies and interventions. The United Nations Educational, Scientific and Cultural Organization (UNESCO 2015) emphasises the critical role of school-based physical education (PE) in supporting a well-rounded education, the healthy development of individuals and serving public health aims related to disease prevention. As one example, due to increases in childhood obesity in recent decades a great deal of research and policy activity in the United States (US) has focused on the role of PE in childhood obesity prevention (Boehmer *et al.* 2008, Frieden *et al.* 2010).

Despite calls for policy intervention, research has revealed that legislative action intended to support PE is often ineffective. A recent study of PE policy changes at the high school level (Grades

9–12) in secondary education in the US identified several barriers to effective policy implementation (Amis *et al.* 2012). These barriers included the prioritisation of standardised testing, resource constraints, the marginalisation of PE, as well as the competing interests between PE and interscholastic sport. Unlike many countries that emphasise community-based 'club' sports for children and adolescents, in the US, interscholastic sport at the secondary level is extremely competitive. The perceived pathway to elite/professional levels begins with exceling at the high school level and then university. Given the popularity and intense pressure surrounding high school athletics in the US, its relationship to PE merits further exploration (Amis *et al.* 2012).

In this paper, we consider ways the interscholastic sport model in US schools may unintentionally, but systematically, interfere with the implementation of quality PE policy and the preventative school health initiatives (e.g. nutrition, chronic illnesses, obesity prevention, physical activity). At the heart of the precarious relationship between PE and interscholastic sport in the US is the PE teacher and/or coach, their role in the school and their place in the curriculum. Using role socialisation theory (RST; Richards 2015) as a guiding framework, we interrogate the assumption of a symbiotic relationship between PE and school sport. We argue that role conflict arising from skewed reward and accountability structures can work against a public health agenda by leading dual role teachers/coaches (T/Cs) to prioritise coaching over teaching roles (Richards and Templin 2012). We conclude with recommendations for appropriate practices in PE that supports the development of behaviours leading to a lifetime of physical activity.

RST and teacher/coach role conflict

RST (Richards 2015) blends elements of occupational socialisation theory and role theory to provide a theoretical framework for understanding the recruitment, training and ongoing socialisation of PE teachers within the occupational milieu of schools. The perspective adopts a dialectic approach to socialisation by acknowledging that individuals play an active role in negotiating with key stakeholders in their work and do not passively adopt the beliefs and attitudes held by others (Schempp and Graber 1992). The role of the PE teacher is socially constructed and bound to a particular school setting (Richards 2015), which explains why some contexts value the subject and others marginalise it (Lux and McCullick 2011).

Within a given school setting, the PE teacher negotiates expectations for performance with salient members of the school community, including other teachers, administrators, children and parents (Richards *et al.* 2013). When there is relative agreement on the way in which the PE teacher role should manifest across stakeholder groups, it can be performed without social barrier. In this situation, everyone is striving for and expecting the same role performance (Turner 2001). However, consensus is rare and individuals within the same school often hold differing expectations for performance, which can lead to role stress (Hindin 2007). In the US and other countries around the world, it is common for teachers to also coach extracurricular sports. In these contexts, one form of role stress that holds relevance to the work of physical educators is role conflict, which relates to tension that arises when performing the roles of PE teacher and coach concurrently (Richards and Templin 2012).

Related to recruitment into the field of PE, childhood experiences in sport and PE programmes predispose individuals to adopt orientations lying on a spectrum that ranges from teaching oriented to coaching oriented (Richards 2015). Those who adopt teaching orientations are more likely to view teaching as their primary motivation a career in the PE profession, whereas coaching-oriented recruits favour coaching school sports (Curtner-Smith 2001). When working in school settings, the construction of coaching 'as an expected extracurricular professional commitment for PE teachers' can perpetuate the preference for coaching held by coaching-oriented recruits, while challenging and frustrating those who favour teaching (Konukman *et al.* 2010: 19). In many settings, the roles of PE teacher and athletic coach are nearly synonymous with members of the school community holding the expectation that all PE teachers will also coach sports, even if they are not interested in doing so (Richards and Templin 2012). This relationship has evolved from the historical connection between PE and athletics, with the resulting assumption that all PE teachers should also coach (Figone 1994).

Reward and accountability structures related to teaching and coaching can further the pressures related to coaching (Konukman *et al.* 2010). Dual role T/Cs are often praised for their coaching prowess, and their jobs may depend on developing a culture of success. Rewards allocated for being a good PE teacher are by comparison somewhat minimal, and T/Cs are often not held accountable for teaching excellence (Richards and Templin 2012). This facilitates teaching mediocrity, which aligns with the expectations of coaching-oriented recruits. As a result, the social construction of the T/C role encourages time to be spent developing athletic success while enabling a structure in which the teaching role can be deprioritised without consequence. In some settings, expectations actually construct social barriers to developing quality PE programmes because prioritising the teacher role runs counter to the expectations of school stakeholders (Amis *et al.* 2012, Richards 2015).

A key outcome of the social pressure to prioritise coaching is that performance in the teacher role suffers (Konukman *et al.* 2010). Further, while some teaching-oriented recruits are able to persist in these environments, many are either forced out of the profession because of unsupportive school cultures, or encouraged to adapt their beliefs and practices to be more in line with the prevailing norms (Richards 2015). Given the preferences and perspectives of coaching-oriented T/Cs, the PE curriculum also tends to overemphasise team sports, which disadvantages children who are not interested in or skilled in these activities (Amis *et al.* 2012). Negative experiences in PE may even discourage participation in lifetime physical activities during and after graduation from school. Since only a small percentage of high school children engage in interscholastic athletics, the complex relationship between teaching and coaching can inhibit physical activity and public health agendas that seek to enhance children's health through school-based programming (Amis *et al.* 2012).

Supporting best practices in school-based PE in the US

In order to make more of a difference in the physical activity and promoting healthy schools in the US, the Society of Health and Physical Educators America (SHAPE America 2014) adopted new content standards for students in Grades K-12 (i.e. ages 5–18) that define what a student should know and be able to do. Each SHAPE America standard begins with the phrase, 'the physically literate individual' to emphasise an effort to prioritise teaching and learning across school contexts in K-12 schools in addition to balancing multiple domains of learning on display in a PE learning environment (e.g. psychomotor, cognitive, affective). The future of PE aspires to pursue themes central to the concept of physical literacy (Whitehead 2010), such as supporting student identities, valuing regular physical activity for all in school PE settings and advocating for physical activity as a regular and consistent function of one's lifestyle.

Physical educators are expected to document the achievement of their students using a range of informal and formal assessments to enhance learning. Regular (i.e. formative) monitoring and final evaluative measures (i.e. summative) approaches are expected in each domain with the intent to maintain a strong balance among the three listed above. Despite these suggestions, differences in instructional opportunities, communities and their priorities limit the execution of state- and national-level recommendations for effective PE programming. PE varies by region and can be very much driven by local and state policy. In local contexts, PE could be guided mostly by the norms of the school and the expectations established directly by the teacher.

State governments in the US exercise direct oversight of education at all levels while both national and state standards in the US guide PE professionals towards acceptable PE programming. The local, socially constructed norm of the PE teacher role should align with the effective teaching standards from national and state government. Unfortunately, the current set up perpetuates the considerable variance of programmes and their offerings (Kirk 2010). As a result, fewer examples of clearly aligned programmes exist – dodged because of inconsistent understandings of what is being taught and learned in schools – regardless of demographics and resources.

Organising a quality PE programme can greatly influence more broad school and public health agendas, but suggesting it to be the sole entity is insufficient. Attention towards school and non-school PE, physical activity and deliberate education on nutrition, family fitness and healthy practices for families are necessary considerations. Related specifically to PE, however, we recommend more purposeful and organised evaluation of PE teachers and PE programmes. This includes holding higher expectations of physical educators in relation to effective teaching standards and halting local, ineffective practices. Local administrators would shoulder the extra effort to assess effectiveness. Expectations for PE teachers should be consistent with those for other professional educators withstanding any coaching duties. Such expectations could be met in part through better acknowledgement of expected teacher behaviours and performances. Other recommendations include more specific expectations in PE settings for developing innovative cultures focused on the enactment of research-based practices and student learning. Lastly, in order to promote a stronger sense of T/C role balance, local administrators should develop protocols that support and hold PE T/Cs accountable for performance in teacher and coach roles.

Disclosure statement

No potential conflict of interest was reported by the authors.

References

Amis, J., *et al.*, 2012. Implementing childhood obesity policy in a new educational environment: the cases of Mississippi and Tennessee. *American journal of public health*, 102, 1406–1413. doi:10.2105/AJPH.2011.300414

Boehmer, T.K., *et al.*, 2008. Preventing childhood obesity through state policy. *American journal of preventive medicine*, 34, 333–340. doi:10.1016/j.amepre.2008.01.003

Curtner-Smith, M., 2001. The occupational socialization of a first-year physical education teacher with a teaching orientation. *Sport, education and society*, 6, 81–105. doi:10.1080/713696040

Figone, A.J., 1994. Origins of the teacher-coach role: idealism, convenience, and unworkability. *Physical educator*, 51 (3), 148–156.

Frieden, T.R., Dietz, W., and Collins, J., 2010. Reducing childhood obesity through policy change: acting now to prevent obesity. *Health affairs*, 29, 357–363. doi:10.1377/hlthaff.2010.0039

Hindin, M.J., 2007. Role theory. *In*: G. Ritzer, ed. *Blackwell encyclopedia of sociology*. Hoboken, NJ: Blackwell Publishing. Blackwell Reference Online.

Kirk, D., 2010. *Physical education futures*. London: Routledge.

Konukman, F., *et al.*, 2010. Teacher-coach role conflict in school-based physical education in USA: a literature review and suggestions for the future. *Biomedical human kinetics*, 2, 19–24. doi:10.2478/v10101-010-0005-y

Lux, K. and McCullick, B.A., 2011. How one exceptional teacher navigated her working environment as the teacher of a marginal subject. *Journal of teaching in physical education*, 30, 358–374.

Richards, K.A.R., 2015. Role socialization theory: the sociopolitical realities of teaching physical education. *European physical education review*, 21, 379–393. doi:10.1177/1356336X15574367

Richards, K.A.R. and Templin, T.J., 2012. Toward a multidimensional perspective on teacher-coach role conflict. *Quest*, 64, 164–176. doi:10.1080/00336297.2012.693751

Richards, K.A.R., Templin, T.J., and Gaudreault, K.L., 2013. Understanding the realities of school life: recommendations for the preparation of physical education teachers. *Quest*, 65, 442–457. doi:10.1080/00336297.2013.804850

Schempp, P.G. and Graber, K., 1992. Teacher socialization from a dialectical perspective: pretraining through induction. *Journal of teaching in physical education*, 11, 329–348.

Society of Health and Physical Educators, 2014. *National standards & grade-level outcomes for k-12 physical education*. Reston: Author.

Turner, R.H., 2001. Role theory. *In*: J.H. Turner, ed. *Handbook of sociological theory*. New York: Kluwer Academic/Plenum Publishers, 233–254.

United Nations Educational, Scientific, and Cultural Organization, 2015. *Quality physical education: guidelines for policy makers*. Paris: Author.

Whitehead, M., 2010. *Physical literacy: Throughout the lifecourse*. London: Routledge.

World Health Organization, 2012. *Population-based approaches to childhood obesity prevention*. Geneva: Author.

Index

Note: Page numbers in **bold** type refer to tables
Page number in *italic* type refer to figures
Page numbers followed by 'n' refer to notes

academic community 21
acceptance 107
access 47, 138, 143, 174
accountability 185, 216; structures 215
action 94, 106
active ageing 207
active lifestyles 10, 166
active living 96
active nation 40
Active People Survey (UK) 34, 35–36
activity: choices 28; lifetime 206; moderate intensity 68; physical 84; sedentary 163
actors, cross-sector 178
adaptation 192
administrative structures 53
adults 12, 68
adverse circumstances 20
aesthetics 97–98, 105–108
age-appropriate guidance 10–13
ageing 14
agency 18, 97
agenda 170
agenda-setting 173
alarmists 205
alignment 170
alliances, international 190
ambitions 84, 88, 152
anxiety 66
appearance 122
assessments 215
assets 176
assumptions 39, 102
At Least Five a Week: Evidence on the Impact of Physical Activity and its Relationship to Health (2004) 67
attitudes 29
attractiveness 121
austerity 174
Australia 131–145, 205–211
Australian Sports Commission (ASC) 132
autonomisation 81
awareness 31

Be Active, Be Healthy (England, 2009) 68
beauty 97, 122
behaviour: change 13–17, 96, 150; philosophy of 86; shaping 81
behavioural change model 102
beliefs 118, 172
benefits 85, 159
biocultural discourse 109
bioeconomic discourse 109
biological facts 108
biomedicalization 109
Bodet, G., Bretherton, P. and Piggin, J. 3, 77–92
body 46–47; beautiful 109, 110; docile 118; of exercise 103; ideal 98, 106–108, 122; looks of 97–98; management 117; projects 125
body image 106
body image distortion (BID) 107
bodywork 109
brand 168, 176
Bretherton, P., Piggin, J. and Bodet, G. 3, 77–92
bureaucracy 189

campaign 168
Canada 4, 93–111, 163–178
Canadian Active Living Guidelines (CALG) 93, 94, 102
Canadian Sport Policy: (2001) 165; (2012) 164
capacity, building 142, 188
care 143; ethic 125
case study 169
causality 200
causation, reciprocal 13
causes of causes 10
challenge 168
change, theory of 29, 33, 38, 40
Chief Medical Officer 67
Chikinda, J., and Markula, P. 3, 93–114
children and young people 11, 45, 62, 66, 78, 138, 142, 206
choice 72, 84, 102, 107, 108, 115, 117
civic pride 86
class structure 103

cleaners 115–127
Closing the Gap: Priorities for Change in Mental Health (2014) 64
co-learning 191, 193
co-researching 193
coaches 86
coaching 214
coding 135, 170
cognitivism 13, 14
collaboration 52, 183; capacity for 170, 174–177; community 184
collaborative working 4
collective action 56, 164
collectives 53
commercialisation 188
commitment 53, 54
common sense 209
communication 117; chain of 11
community: academic 21; well-being 165
community development model 150
community health approaches 16
community sport 133
community-building 165
competition 71, 173
competitive sport 68, 207, 208
competitiveness 138
complexity 154
conceptual framing 166
confessional 107
confidentiality 189
conflation 70
connection 157
connectivity 164
consent 189
constraints 123
content analysis 135
context 11, 29–34, 50, 71
control 55, 94
controlled designs 32
conversation 120, 151
convert 107
cooperation 80, 189
coordination 52, 53–56
cosmetics industries 107
creativeness 158
crisis, public health 205
critical conversation 151
critical thinking 98
cross-sector actors 178
cross-sectoral approaches 200
cultural geography 153
cultural sensitivity 117, 127
culture 118, 208, 215

Dance Action Zone Leeds (DAZL) 149, 152
dance projects 4
dancing 122
data 189; collection 190; quantitative 186; social statistical 19
debate 5
decision-makers 21
decision-making 156, 167, 184, 187
decolonisation 190
deep insider information 192
deliberative forums 193
demand 31, 37; latent 38
dementia 68
demonstration effect 80
Denmark 4, 115–127
dependency model 155
depression 62, 65–66, 68
deprivation 202
developed countries 131
Dionigi, R.A., and Gard, M. 3, 205–211
disability adjusted life years (DALYs) 62
disadvantage 19, 118
disadvantaged people 47
disciplinary base 21
disciplinary power 118
disciplinary techniques 96
discourses 95; biocultural 109; bioeconomic 109; discrepancy in 171; dominant 155; health 95; reward 85; risk 81, 84
discretion 189
discursive construction 78
disease: burden 9, 61; lifestyle-related 116
disinterest 54
dissent 159
diversity 108, 136, 139
doctors 123
documentary content 82
Dodd-Reynolds, C.J., *et al.* 2, 199–204
Duffell, T., *et al.* 3, 61–75

early years 11
eating 107, 166
eating disorders 107, 108, 111n2
economic instability 87
education 100
effectiveness 72, 185
efficiency 185
Eime, R.M., *et al.* 4, 131–148
elite sport 79, 132, 138, 143; policy 187
emergency, public health 206
emotion 157
empirical foundations 206
empowerment 23, 46, 202; community 188
energy 121, 125
engagement *140*, 152, 157, 202
England 61–73, **67**
enjoyment 123, 127
enthusiasm 152, 176
environment 104
environmental factors 87, 89
epidemic 106
ethical practice 191
ethnic identity 122, 124
evaluation 78, 182, 191; good 156; teacher 216
Everybody Active Every Day (England, 2014) 68, 200
evidence 30, 33, 40, 70, 72, 111, 154; best available 206; best possible 206; and policy 200–201; standards 38, 157, 200, 201; trial-based 200–201

evidence base 19, 154, 155; weaknesses in 200–202
evidence-building 4
evidence–policy–practice agenda 182
excuses 124
exercise: behaviour 96; healthy 95–97; leadership 102; prescription 95, 104, 110; on referral 2
exercise class: design 103–105; group 96
Exercise Theory manual (Fitness Leadership Certification Association) 95, 98
exhaustion 124, 125, 127
expectations 137, 140, 143
experiences 20; negative 201, 215
experts 21, 39, 42, 117, 123, 200

facilities, sport 37, 137, 138
family 122, 125, 136; situations 12
fan base 137, 139
fatigue 124, 125
female clients 106
feminine aesthetics 97–98, 106–108, 110
feminism 107, 207
festival atmosphere 86
financial crisis 87, 88
financial hardship 155
financial stability 13
fitness: instructors 3; levels 33
Fitness Leadership Certification Association (FLCA) 95, 99, 111; *Exercise Theory* manual 95, 98
Fitness Unit (Canada) 99
FITT formula 95
foresight 191
Foucault, M. 80, 117
fragmentation 51, 183
framing 166
France 2, 45–56; Departmental Directorates for Social Cohesion 48; Ministry of Health 50; Ministry of Sport 50; National Centre for the Development of Sport 51; Regional Directorates for Young People, Sport and Social Cohesion 46, 53; Regional Health Agencies 46, 53
freedom 119; to act 94
friends 156
friendship 189
fun 121, 123, 165
functionality 104
funding sources 175
Future in Mind: Promoting, Protecting and Improving Our Children and Young People's Mental Health and Wellbeing (England, 2015) 65

Game Plan: A Strategy for Delivering Government's Sport and Physical Activity Objectives (England, 2002) 69
Gard, M., and Dionigi, R.A. 3, 205–211
gaze 118
gender 3–4, 9, 14
Get Healthy Get Active 78
goals 72, 123, 159; shared 167, 177
government 80; agencies 166; intervention 2, 49; purpose of 94
governmentality 117
gratification, delayed 125
Great Sport Myth (GSM) 208
guaranteeing health 81
guilt 107

Hanson, C.L., *et al.* 2, 199–204
harm 40, 42
health: capital 47; movements 16; outcomes 171; politics 156; problems 163; risk 46; services 183
Health and Sport Engagement (HASE) project 190
Health Survey for England 34, 35–36
healthism 184
healthist discourse 155
healthy ageing 107
heroes 136
hindsight 191
homogeneity 105
Honta, M. 2, 45–59
Hospital–Patients–Health–Territories law (France, 2009) 48
Houghton, L., *et al.* 3, 61–75
human capital resource 142

identity 124; ageing 144; ethical 122, 124; national 143; negotiating 189; organisational 167; professional 55; social 144
ideology 67, 208
ill people 105
illness prevention 103, 105, 110
impact 157; evaluation 191
implementation 177; strategies 173
inactive people 2, 39, 42
inactivity 46, 47, 150, 163, 199, 213
incentives 123
inclusion 202
incommensurability 158
inconsistency 51
individual agency 18
individual behaviour, change 13–17
individualisation 104
individuals 72, 102; choice of 102; normative view of 16; responsible 46
indulgence 107
industry 208
influence, multiple levels of 13
informal conversations 120
information: deep-insider 191; exchange 189; policing 99
injury 71
inspecting gaze 98
inspection 55
inspiration 80, 85
institutional memory 156
instruction 103
integration 50
integrity 191
intentions 123, 176
interest 31, 38; overlapping 51–53
intergenerational opportunities 136
intermediary determinants 18
interscholastic sport 214

intervention: measuring 157; pathways 202
interviews **49**, 100, 119–120, 133, 169; guide 120
introspection 192
Investing in Mental Health: Evidence for Action (WHO, 2013) 63
investment 38–39, 126
involvement 152
involvement–detachment 192
irresponsibility 88

Jenkin, C.R., *et al.* 4, 131–148
Jones, J., *et al.* 3, 61–75
judgement 109

Kay, T. 2, 7–25
key performance indicators (KPIs) 150
knowledge 99, 121; alternative 110; community 21–22; dissemination 190; forms of 89; lack of 115; production 4, 188, 191; scientific 105; sharing 52; western-centric 118
knowledges 95

language 171
Lashua, B., Watson, B. and Trevorrow, P. 4, 149–161
latent coding 135
lay knowledge 22
laziness 124
leadership 102; community-based 184
learning 192; curve 51, 56
least active 28, 38, 42, 45
least healthy groups 10
legacy 3; agenda 20; effects 3; measurement 87; strategy 182
legitimacy 54, 72
Lenneis, V., and Pfister, G. 3, 115–130
less active 28, 38, 42
life: balance 102; expectancy 9, 63–64; quality of 104
life course approach 63
lifestyle: active 10, 166; collective 124, 126; correct 117; diseases 205; healthy 46; sedentary 47, 102, 116
lifestyle model 102
lifetime activity 206
Lindsey, I.A., *et al.* 2, 199–204
listening in 151
lived realities 127
local authorities 184
logic models 29
London Olympics and Paralympics (2012) 3, 77, 181
looking body 108
looks 97–98
low- and middle-income countries (LMICs) 9

magazines 107
magical properties 86
management 55, 107
Mansfield, L. 4, 181–197
marginalisation 120
marginality 72
market share 208
marketing 138, 143
Markula, P., and Chikinda, J. 3, 93–114
Marmot, Sir M. 8
meaning 152, 189; negotiating 191
meaningful research 151
measurement 42, 72, 78, 87, 89, 154, 157; objective 186
medical conditions 104, 105
medical expenditures 116
medicine 185
member diversity 136
men 9
mental health 3, 61–73, 110, 165
Mental Health Action Plan 2013–2020 (2013) 63
Mental Health Taskforce 65
mental, neurological and substance (MNS) disorders 61, 73n1
mental well-being 69
mentoring 136
messaging clutter 172
methodologies 200
migrant cleaners 4
minority ethnic groups 4
Misener, L., and Misener, K.E. 4, 163–180
missions 54–55
mixed methods approaches 201
mobilisations 53
modifications 104
monetary control 188
monitoring 107
moral obligation 118
moral technology 84
mortality risk reduction *30, 31*
motivational experts 96
motivations 38, 70, 192
muscles 108
Muslim women 118–119
mutuality 167, 174

National Lottery (UK) 187
national programming 2
National Sport and Active Recreation Policy Framework (Australia, 2011) 206
need 202; special 47
neo-liberal economics 109
neo-liberalism 72, 81, 94, 97
networks 52, 200
New Public Management 48
NHS Five Year Forward View (England, 2014) 65
No Health Without Mental Health: A Cross-Government Mental Health Outcomes Strategy for People of All Ages (England, 2011) 64
non-communicable diseases (NCDs) 9, 10, 61
non-participants 40
normalisation 105
norms: misaligned 172–174; oppressive 107
nudging 81
nutrition 49–50

obese bodies 97
obesity 84, 155; childhood 213; discourses 106

observation 169
older people 4, 12, 68
Oliver, E.J., *et al.* 2, 199–204
Olympic bidding 83
Olympic Charter 79
Olympism 86
opinions 121
opportunities 12, 85, 116, 126, 136, 138, 143; intergenerational 142
organic control 103
organisational capacity 142
organisational readiness 176–177
Organising Committee of the Olympic Games (OCOG) 78
othering 120

Pan-American Healthy Living Strategy 95
Panopticon 109
paradigms 153
parenthood, lone 12
participant observation 120
participation 35, 71; benefits of *140*; legacy 3, 20, 31, 79–80; mass 87; reasons for 123–124; shifts *37*; shifts in 36; targets 27–28, 82, 87–89; youth 78
participation barriers 31, 117, 124; psychological 40, 201; severe 201; structural 37
partnership 4, 49–51
path dependence 54
perceptions 28–29, 137, 140, 143
performance 188, 215
personal trainers 111n1
personalities, sports 175
Pfister, G., and Lenneis, V. 3, 115–130
physical activity, defining 84
physical education (PE), programmes 3
physical literacy 215
physiology 103
Piggin, J., Bretherton, P. and Bodet, G. 3, 77–92
player representation 138
playing: facilities 143; opportunities 138, 140, 143
policy: barriers 138–139; documents 82–83, **85**; problem 62–64; tools 182
policymaking process 186
political context 17
population: control 94; groups 9; management 81
positive ageing 207
Post-Traumatic Stress Disorder (PTSD) 66
poverty 11, 47
power 80, 86, 118, 156; differentials 191; disciplinary 118; dynamics 191; local 185; negotiating 189; relations 94, 185, 187
practice models 157
practitioners 39
pressure 106
prevention 65
principles, applied 104
priorities 137, 143
privilege 120
productive ageing 207
professionalisation 157
professionalism 188
programme theory 29
promotion opportunities 175
proportionate universalism 18, 63
provider acceptance 29, 38
public benefit 178
public health, objectives 200
Public Health England 7, 181
Public Health Responsibility Deal 183
public health unit 168
public services delivery 72

qualitative methodology 20
qualitative research 20, 21, 150
quality assurance 99
quantification 185
quantitative data 186

randomised control trials (RCTs) 157–158, 200
readiness 177
realist approach 135
realist view 152
reciprocity 189–191
recognition, mutual 49–53
recreational sport 68
recruitment 139
reference points 52
reflexivity 191–193
regeneration 79
regions 46, 50
relationships 136; interpersonal 190
relaxation 125, 165
religion 118, 124
representing health 10
repression 110
research: agenda 1; dissemination 190; impact 186; population 185; projects 186; qualitative 20, 21, 150; rigorous 32–33; sprints 188; use 22
researcher 189, 191
research–policy–practice (RPP) partnerships 4, 182, 185–193
resourcefulness 187–189
resources 50, 54–55, 126, 174; acquisition 177; allocation 154; control 187; crises 188; mobilisation 174; ownership 187; scarce 177
respect 189
responsibilisation 81, 84
responsibility 46, 82, 184; personal 94, 110, 117, 150; working 143
responsible politics 193
Ressler, J.D., Richards, K.A.R. and Wright, P.M. 3, 213–215
results 48
return on investment 150
revenue streams 137
reward: discourse 85; structures 215
rhetoric 88, 166, 177, 182
rhetorical strategies 89
Richards, K.A.R., Wright, P.M. and Ressler, J.D. 3, 213–215
risk: discourses 81, 84; management 138
role models 86, 97, 108, 136, 139

role socialisation theory (RST) 214–215
role stress 214

safe environment 98
salvation 107
sampling, purposeful 100
sceptics 205
schizophrenia 66
schools 206, 208, 215
scientists 8
screening 65
scrutiny 109
second shift 125, 126
secrecy 190
sedentary activity 163
sedentary lifestyles 47, 102, 116
self, healthy 97
self-acceptance 108
self-analysis 192
self-confidence 106
self-discipline 124
self-disclosure 192
self-esteem 68, 110
self-governance 84
self-regulation 117, 124
self-surveillance 96, 98, 121, 122
self-work 96
semantic coding 135
settings 70
silence 110
situatedness 120
sleep 68
slimness 121
Smith, A., *et al.* 3, 61–75
social actors 13
social capital 176
social change 79
social circumstances 201
social constructions 85
social critique 192
social determinants 63
social disadvantage 19
social ecological models (SEMs) 11, 13, 14, **15**, 19
social factors 14
social gerontology 144
social inequalities 61
social interaction 185, 187
social justice 47
social marketing campaign 173
social position 18
social pressure 215
social processes 72
social relationships 71
social responsibilities 79, 85
social sciences perspective 2
social structural factors 14
social work 172
socialising 165
societal expectations 137
Society of Health and Physical Educators America 215
socio-economic context 17
special groups 104
special needs 47
spending 39; cuts 87, 184
sponsors 208
sport, defining 84, 171
Sport England 7, 42, 69, 78, 150, 181, 200
sport equipment 177
Sport, Health and Well-being programme (France) 45–56
Sport Mega Events (SMEs) 77
Sporting Future: A New Strategy for a Sporting Nation (England, 2015) 69
Sporting Future: A Strategy for an Active Nation (England, 2015) 184
Sporting Mega Events (SMEs) 80, 89
sporting nation 77
sporting outcomes 165
Sporting Schools programme (Australia) 208
sports advocacy 182
Sports Council (UK) 36, 42n9
sports movement 27
sports organisations, capacity-building 133
staff: cutbacks 53, 56n3; paid 175
stakeholders, sport 39
standards, evidence 38, 157, 200, 201
Start Active, Stay Active: Report on Physical Activity in the UK (2011) 8, 10–13, 68
status 186; anxiety 72; special 85
steering committee 168
stepped care 66
stigma 118
strategies 34
stress relief 12
stressors 20
structural determinants 17
structural disadvantage 118
structural factors 14
struggles 188
subgroup effects 201
success: culture of 215; indicators 28; measuring 154
successful ageing 207
suicide 62
surveys 34, 35–36
Sustainable Development Goals (SDGs) 64
sweetened beverages 206
synergies 183; natural 184

tactics 81, 88, 89
Taking Part survey (UK) 34, 35–36
talent pool 79
target audience 52; young people 138, 142
target groups 40
teacher 214; evaluation 216
teams 140
tension 153–154
territorial delegation 48
textbooks 99
thematic analysis 83, 135
theory 189; of change 29, 33, 38, 40

This Girl Can campaign 31
thought, styles of 89, 94
time 124
time-series analysis 34
tone 108–109
Towards an Active Nation (England, 2016) 70
training 22
transferability 154
transparency 186, 190
treatment 65
Trevorrow, P., Watson, B. and Lashua, B. 4, 149–161
trickle down effect 80
trust 189
trusted friends 156
trustworthiness 191
truth 96, 107, 122; games 208
turnover rate 175

Uffelen, J.G.Z. van, *et al.* 4, 131–148
uncertainty 56
understanding 176, 177
uniqueness 85–87
United Kingdom (UK) 10, 28, 199–202; Department of Health 181; National Institute for Health and Care Excellence (NICE) 7, 68, 199; Office for National Statistics (UK) 19, *see also* England
United Nations (UN), Sustainable Development Goals (SDGs) 64
United States of America (USA) 3, 214
university 168, 176
urgency 117, 124

value 173; for money 150, 156
values 86, 118, 177; corporate 187; misaligned 172–174; professional 187
violence 71
virtuous cycle 79
vision 164
voluntary organisations 166
volunteer capacity 138
volunteering 136, 142
volunteers 140, 144, 175

Watson, B., Lashua, B. and Trevorrow, P. 4, 149–161
Weed, M. 2, 27–44
weight 106; loss 121, 122, 123
welfare state 116
well-being 69, 125, 165; measuring 193
wellness 95, 102
Westerbeek, H., *et al.* 4, 131–148
what works 150, 153–154
What Works Wellbeing Centre 193
whiteness 118
women 9, 97, 98, 115–127
working: collectives 53; conditions 56; practices 183
World Health Organisation (WHO) 8, 213; Commission on the social determinants of health 9, *17*; Global Action Programme (mhGAP) 63; *Investing in Mental Health: Evidence for Action* report (2013) 63; *Mental Health Action Plan 2013–2020* (2013) 63
World Health Report (2001) 63
Wright, P.M., Ressler, J.D. and Richards, K.A.R. 3, 213–215

young people 11, 45, 62, 66, 78, 138, 142, 206

Zambia 190